P L A B
SIMPLIFIED

STRIDOR
DYSPONEA
TRISMUS

P L A B
SIMPLIFIED

Wasim Shaikh MBBS
Manipal Academy of Higher Education

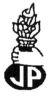

JAYPEE BROTHERS
MEDICAL PUBLISHERS (P) LTD
New Delhi

Published by
Jitendar P Vij
Jaypee Brothers Medical Publishers (P) Ltd
EMCA House, 23/23B Ansari Road, Daryaganj
New Delhi 110 002, India
Phones: 23272143, 23272703, 23282021, 23245672, 23245683
Fax: 011-23276490
e-mail: jpmedpub@del2.vsnl.net.in
Visit our website: http://www.jpbros.20m.com

Branches

- 202 Batavia Chambers, 8 Kumara Kruppa Road
  Kumara Park East, **Bangalore** 560 001, Phones: 2285971, 2382956
  Tele Fax : 2281761
  e-mail: jaypeebc@bgl.vsnl.net.in

- 282 IIIrd Floor, Khaleel Shirazi Estate, Fountain Plaza
  Pantheon Road, **Chennai** 600 008, Phone: 28262665 Fax: 28262331
  e-mail: jpmedpub@md3.vsnl.net.in

- 4-2-1067/1-3, Ist Floor, Balaji Building, Ramkote Cross Road,
  Hyderabad 500 095, Phones: 55610020, 24758498 Fax: 24758499
  e-mail: jpmedpub@rediffmail.com

- 1A Indian Mirror Street, Wellington Square
  Kolkata 700 013, Phone: 22451926 Fax: 22456075
  e-mail: jpbcal@cal.vsnl.net.in

- 106 Amit Industrial Estate, 61 Dr SS Rao Road
  Near MGM Hospital, Parel, **Mumbai** 400 012
  Phones: 24124863, 24104532 Fax: 24160828
  e-mail: jpmedpub@bom7.vsnl.net.in

PLAB Simplified

This book has been published in good faith that the material provided by author is original. Every effort is made to ensure accuracy of material, but the publisher, printer and author will not be held responsible for any inadvertent error(s). In case of any dispute, all legal matters to be settled under Delhi jurisdiction only.

First Edition : **2004**

ISBN 81-8061-193-0

Typeset at JPBMP typesetting unit
Printed at Gopsons Papers Ltd, A-14, Sector 60, Noida 201 301, India

This book is dedicated

to my dad...

Late Mr. Mustafa Shaikh

Preface

By the time I had cleared my PLAB part one, I found myself amidst this newfound revolution…wherein one and all around me aspired to pursue their post-graduate career in the United Kingdom. The rationale for this transformation were multiple… be it the complexity in obtaining a visa after clearing USMLE, or the sweeping changes in the admission patterns and fee configuration of colleges in India. For many, it was just that they recognised late, the fact that opportunities did exist outside India, opportunities, which in the long run could be more lucrative, in terms of glamour and riches.

Whatever the reasons might be, I noticed that anyone who decided on embarking to UK found him/herself in a position, where he/she did not know where to take the first step. If they did know how to begin, they would inevitably find some impediment in their path that they would find hard to overcome.

This book is a sincere effort to guide any plabber vis-à-vis how, when and where to take that first step; and to be of continuing assistance to them until the time they get their first job as a senior house officer. The purpose of this book is to SIMPLIFY the process involved. Moreover, I have also supplemented sections, which would be exceptionally useful for the revision of IELTS and PLAB exams.

I hope that this book will find its place in the hands of anyone and everyone who is planning to venture into this land of opportunities.

Wasim Shaikh

Acknowledgements

I am grateful to my buddies; Dr.Asha.N and Dr.Swathi Rao, for helping me with the sections on Revision for PLAB part one and the Mock exams. More importantly, they supported me all the way and made it possible to make each and every of the 324 pages of this book as enlightening yet as simple as possible.

I convey my thankfulness to the plabbers of Kasturba Medical College, Mangalore…their uncertainties provided me with the inspiration to come up with this book for PLAB.

Last but not the least…my mother, Mrs. Zaibunnisa M Shaikh. I don't have any words to state her goodness. All I can say is…

'Mom…I am here, because you were there!'

Table of Contents

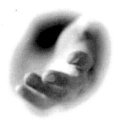

Introduction

WHY UK?

The United Kingdom welcomes doctors and dentists from overseas who wish to pursue postgraduate training in medicine or dentistry and who may choose to seek employment there. The tradition of training in the UK is time-honoured and has made a major donation to the health services of both developed and developing countries.

Each year several thousand doctors and dentists move to the UK to pursue their training. Doctors from less developed countries set off to the United Kingdom for training, supposedly because training is shoddier or non-existent in their own countries. However, many go there for a superior life and to live in a Western democracy, to enjoy the luxuries, the benefits and some drawbacks.

Professionally though, most of them would want to choose the speciality in which they are trained in, and to do well in them. The rest, freshly graduated, would want to start their training, initially by taking up a less competitive post and then progressing to their preferred field. However, overseas doctors often find themselves in a dilemma; they have to choose between struggling to stay on in the speciality of their choice or working in a related or very dissimilar speciality. This is not an easy decision, but if doctors have a pragmatic idea about their odds of career progression before they go there, then they are less likely to be disappointed.

In other words, if it's a life in Britain that you want, you may have to choose a specialty in which you have a realistic chance of progressing. If it is training in a particular specialty that you want, you might have to return home after you get the essential training in it.

Though higher training has become more structured bottlenecks exist. The widespread publicity about staff shortages in the NHS might also be sending conflicting signals to overseas doctors.

One of the big pluses of training in the UK is that the system recognises that to maintain a constant inflow of trainees in a programme that is quite prolonged requires a reasonable pay structure which allows for a comfortable and independent lifestyle. A good flow of trainees is essential to maintain a level of competitiveness, which in turn will provide towards establishing a high standard of healthcare services. A large stress factor related to financial dependency is, therefore, largely eradicated compared with trainees at a similar level in less developed countries like India.

To summarise, training in the UK is fairly "by the book", with structured, accountable training being the key factors. It is by no means easy, and not everybody makes it to the consultant grades. Competition is very stiff and a lax attitude can easily throw somebody into a medium grade non-progressive post.

WHEN TO GO?

Whether it is better to go over immediately after graduation in another country or later is not clear. As Part 1 of the Professional Linguistic Assessment Board (PLAB) examination is now held in many other countries, increasingly younger doctors are willing to go to the United Kingdom to sit Part 2, which can only be taken in Britain.

Advantages in Going Immediately after Graduation

1. Professionally, you are not too far down a particular career path and so are in a better position to choose a specialty that offers the best chance of progress at that time.
2. Socially, you are more likely to be free of the responsibilities that come with age and so are more ready to accept, for example, an academic position that may be good for your career but often brings a poorer salary.

Advantages of Going after Postgraduate Training Back Home

Better CV's and the advantage of prior experience in a medical speciality would significantly increase the probability of getting a job in your chosen field.

It actually is of little use consulting anyone regarding this matter, as you would get differing advices. One person would say, 'I think it is best for you to leave after your graduation, because you have a variety of options to choose from.' The very next moment someone else would say 'Hey, there is a variety of options, agreed. But remember, whatever post you apply for, there would be at least a hundred other applicants who would have had a postgraduate experience in that field.'

Therefore, what is recommended is, if you are ready to take a risk in order to make a big leap in your career; and if you feel that in spite of your inexperience, you deserve a job by virtue of your talents and achievements, try to take the flight as soon as you can!

One important point has to be mentioned here. February and August are the "beginning of the semesters" as you would call them, because the majority of the posts as Senior House Officer (SHO) begin from these two months. (See the Table 1 in the next page). Job adverts for these are placed in the BMJ and other journals, about four months before the jobs commence, i.e., in October and April. So it is recommended that you plan your journey in such a way that you have cleared the PLAB Part two and have your curriculum vitae (CV) ready by the beginning of these months.

WHICH SPECIALITY?

If you are going to the UK after postgraduation, there are not many choices other than your field of specialisation. A fresh graduate, however, has a plethora of subjects and fields to choose from. Some of them are relatively easy to get in (psychiatry and the non-clinical subjects), most are tough.

It is always better to target a couple of fields so that you can concentrate on ways to enhancing your prospects to get into that field. For example, targeting a job in accident and emergency would mean you could try to attend a Trauma course and probably pass the MRCS Part 1; these would significantly increase your chances in getting a job.

You can see from the table that certain specialities like Medicine and Paediatrics have a good deal more number of jobs than others. However, this does not imply that they are the easier ones to get in. Medicine and Paediatrics are amongst the most competitive fields at present, there could be more than 200 applicants for each job in these specialities. On the other hand, posts such as Psychiatry and Anaesthesia often have a very few job applicants (less than 10) and you have a realistic chance.

Summary of total number of jobs available throughout the UK in various specialities between 7 September 2003 and 5 December 2003. (See Table 1).

MEDICAL TRAINING IN THE UK

Postgraduate medical training in the UK involves

Table 1: Summary of total number of jobs available throughout the UK in various specialities between 7 September 2003 and 5 December 2003

Date	TOT	NEW	ME	SU	OR	OB	OP	PED	AE	AN	PS
7 - Sep	2028	1014	28	12	5	20	10	36	27	20	15
15 - Sep	2273	862	32	17	12	30	15	42	38	20	11
21 - Sep	2458	902	32	27	12	28	22	57	50	22	10
30 - Sep	2625	989	43	31	11	35	21	70	46	21	17
6 - Oct	2699	951	42	40	9	53	25	75	47	28	17
11 - Oct	2626	931	49	48	9	55	42	92	62	30	22
19 - Oct	2000	953	62	44	10	59	52	75	55	34	20
25 - Oct	2647	941	73	51	15	55	53	74	50	29	24
1 - Nov	2647	865	73	37	12	58	67	68	50	30	14
8 - Nov	1818	842	75	39	15	53	59	57	44	37	13
15 - Nov	1800	855	66	49	13	26	39	50	29	33	12
22 - Nov	1780	897	69	47	10	31	39	47	33	26	13
29 - Nov	1824	875	76	41	10	34	36	50	26	29	11
5 - Dec	2332	772	5	36	10	29	38	42	26	27	11

ME—Medicine	SU—Surgery	OR—Orthopedics
OB—OBG	OP—Ophthalmology	PD—Paediatrics
AE—Accident and emergency	AN—Anaesthesia	PS—Psychiatry

paid employment, service to patients, gaining clinical experience under supervision, while also studying and receiving tuition. Entry to a training programme is by successful appointment to a job, and not by enrollment on a course. In the hospital specialities this training is in three parts:

1. Pre-registration House Officer (PRHO) year.
2. Basic specialist training (BST) or general professional training (GPT) in the senior house officer (SHO) grade. This follows completion of pre-registration requirements, and lasts for two or three years, during which time the doctor takes the professional examinations of the relevant Royal College, which constitute the entry requirements for higher training.
3. Higher specialist training (HST) in the specialist registrar (SpR) grade. The old grades of registrar and senior registrar are obsolete. The full programme lasts for 4 to 6 years depending on specialty, consists of a structured rotation to give balanced experience, and leads to a Certificate of Completion of Specialist Training (CCST). Part of the programme may be advertised as a Locum appointment for training (LAT). Such a Locum period may

count towards specialist training, but only in the event of subsequent appointment to a definitive SpR post.

Not all SpR posts lead to a CCST. Fixed term training appointments (FTTA) are available to overseas doctors for a finite period of upto 2 years. This allows specific training in the speciality, but cannot lead to a CCST. A series of LAT posts cannot lead to a CCST. There are also Locum appointments for service (LAS), which do not count as training posts at all, even though some training may be available. These are only short-term posts.

The training for general practice (family medicine or primary care medicine) is a three-year vocational training scheme (GPVTS), with one year as a GP registrar in a training practice and two years in a variety of approved hospital posts (SHO). Funding for this scheme does not normally extend to overseas doctors, and Permit Free Training does not cover work in General Practice.

Appointment to all training posts is selective, following advertisement, application and competitive interview. Possession of the entry requirements and the desire to train in the speciality, however strong, are not sufficient to secure a training post. Doctors should realize that they might be unable to obtain a post in their chosen specialty even after numerous applications, especially in the more popular specialities.

In order to do any sort of clinical training a doctor must register with the General Medical Council (GMC), must satisfy the employing authority's regulations on health and other matters, and must have valid exemption from work permit regulations (Permit-free training).

Teaching will usually be a mixture of informal instruction in the workplace, clinical meetings and grand rounds, and sessions organized by speciality tutors to meet the needs of doctors in training. It is important that you make every effort to attend these educational sessions provided for you in the hospital, some of which will be in protected time, free of clinical commitments. All training posts have an entitlement to Study Leave with pay and expenses for attending relevant courses away from the workplace, subject to the approval of consultants and tutors.

Medical research is carried out in parallel with training and service provision. Some doctors in training undertake pure research posts for one to three years, usually working for a higher degree in a University appointment or on a research grant. If there is no clinical work at all involved then an overseas doctor doing research can have student status and need not have the GMC registration. If there is any clinical component to the work then all the GMC and work permit regulations apply.

APPLYING FOR A JOB

You will have to apply for posts in open competition. Jobs are advertised every Wednesday midnight by specialty in the Classified Section of the British Medical Journal, the latest copy of which should be available in any medical library. It can also be accessed online via:www.bmjcareers.com. All recognised posts will state in their ad: The Postgraduate Dean confirms that this placement and/or programme has the required educational and dean's approval.

For some posts you will need to request an application form and job description, others will ask you to send a CV. Check that the post is suitable for your needs. You may telephone the doctor who is currently in the post if you are not sure about this.

Remember to send in the application form and your curriculum vitae (CV) before the closing date. First class post in the UK has a guaranteed next day delivery but costs more (28 p for 60 gm) whereas a second-class post reaches within 3 days (20 p for 60 gm). If you have missed the closing date, then telephone to see if your application can still be accepted.

You may be short-listed and invited for interview. Do not be too disappointed if you are not, most jobs receive far more applicants than can be interviewed.

If you are invited for interview, try to give yourself time to look around and make enquiries beforehand. If you have to travel a long way, the hospital may provide overnight accommodation. Remember to apply for travel expenses.

In the interview you need to present yourself as well as possible to the panel, but remember that these are the British doctors. They will appreciate clear, direct, honest answers. They may seem rather unimpressed by what you have done overseas and by who you have worked for. They will be more impressed by what you know, how you think and what plans you have made.

You will usually be told at the end of the interview if you have been successful. If you are offered a post, then you may well be asked to give a firm commitment immediately. If you accept the post, then you must not withdraw at a later date, so be sure that you want the job. If you have doubts, then say so and ask for time or more information.

If you are unsuccessful, then it is perfectly reasonable to ask to see one of the interviewing consultants to ask why you were not successful and for advice on what you can do differently to improve your prospects of obtaining a post in the future. Try to make sure that you get specific advice rather than generalisations.

Tips in Getting a Job

*   *Keep an open mind about specializing*—Don't have unrealistic expectations about which specialty to work in. It may be easier, for example, to get ahead in anaesthesia or psychiatry than in surgery. Most overseas doctors struggle because their chosen field is competitive, and they may not realise this until they have started applying for jobs. Also, remember to choose a specialty that is under-represented in your own country.
*   *Do a clinical attachment*—Doing clinical attachments and even a UK degree (such as an MSc or Diploma) related to the profession and field of your interest may help your job prospects dramatically.
*   *Try to get your first job in a remote district general hospital*—These jobs may be relatively less competitive as such hospitals are usually extremely busy and opportunities for social activities may be limited. You are, however, likely to emerge as a better doctor with all that "hands on" experience with unselected emergencies. Also, concentrate on six-month jobs rather than on rotations, which can be reserved for later.
*   *Be prepared to move*—Be prepared to move anywhere in the United Kingdom where you think the best job is available, regardless of where your friends are working. You are here for the best training, and relocation is one of the sacrifices you should be prepared to make.
*   *Enhance your CV*—Your CV should always show that you are making steady progress in your career. Do not accept another six-month SHO post just because it is in the same hospital or area. You have only four years to prove that you are suitable for entry at the specialist registrar (SpR) grade. Stagnating at one level is not looked on favourably, and you should seek jobs that show commitment to your chosen specialty, or alternatively work as a more senior SHO or in Locum training posts while you look for that coveted training number.
*   *Attend interview skills courses*—Often overseas doctors are short-listed but do not get through the interview. Attending courses on interview skills or having mock interviews may help you overcome this problem.
*   *Attend House Officer induction courses*—These courses which can be taken up after passing your PLAB Part 2 in the UK give you an insight into the medical training, the process of application, CV building and so on.
*   *Do audits and presentations, and get published*—For various reasons many overseas doctors will not have opportunities in their own country to do audits and presentations or publish articles. However, it is an important component in the short-listing process in Britain. So the sooner you can do this, the better. Academic success seems to impress everyone. A huge emphasis is given to the philosophy of evidence based medicine and clinical governance in the UK today.
*   *Do something more*—Everyone who applies for a job will have passed the PLAB (Professional Linguistic Assessment Board) examination and also have other higher qualifications. However, to be short-listed and get the job, do something more than others, for example, computer and management courses. This may make you stand out from the crowd.

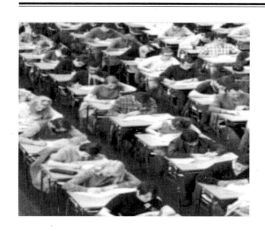

Section *One*

The IELTS Test

1 IELTS—Basics

> ◆ *This chapter is for the person who has little, if any idea about the IELTS. Described here is basic format of the examination, the scores and what they mean.*

The IELTS is the short form for the International English Language Testing System. Overseas doctors should begin the process of becoming eligible for limited registration by taking the IELTS in or near their home countries. The IELTS exam is a pre-requisite for admission to the PLAB test. The IELTS test can be taken in over 250 centres in more than 100 countries worldwide.

The IELTS tests the complete range of English language skills, which will commonly be encountered by students when studying or training in the medium of English.

The IELTS is jointly managed by the University of Cambridge Local Examinations Syndicate (ULCES), the British Council and IDP Education Australia. These three bodies are responsible for conducting the same IELTS examination throughout the world. Notions that each body conducts a different examinations, and that one is set at a higher difficulty level than the other, are false.

The IELTS examination gives you the option of taking up one of two modules—the Academic module or the General Training module. However, remember, the General Medical Council (GMC) will only accept the Academic Module of the IELTS examination. The emphasis of the general training module is on basic survival skills in a broad social and educational context.

MINIMUM ACCEPTABLE SCORES FOR IELTS

Speaking	:	7.0
Listening	:	6.0
Academic reading	:	6.0
Academic writing	:	6.0
Overall score	:	7.0

There are no exceptions to the above except for those doctors who are on the ODTS scheme or are accepted for exemption from the PLAB test. They are required to score 7.0 or above in each band of the IELTS test.

VALIDITY OF IELTS SCORE

The IELTS test results are valid for upto two years from the date, which appears on the IELTS certificate.

FORMAT OF THE TEST

The test consists of four parts, which are always held in the following order…

1. *Listening*	40 minutes
2. *Academic reading*	60 minutes
3. *Academic writing*	60 minutes
4. *Speaking*	15 minutes

Therefore, the total test time is approximately 2 hours 45 minutes.

TEST RESULTS

The IELTS examination is usually held on Saturdays and Sundays. You can expect the results on the third Monday, i.e., 15 to 16 days after the examination. Calling the British Council offices is generally of little use, as the results are *not* given over the telephone.

The test centre will communicate the results of the test directly to the General Medical Council if you had asked them to do so in your IELTS application form (See page 15).

At times, you will need the results of your IELTS examination earlier than two weeks, like when the last date for application for PLAB is approaching. You can then ask for the "Express Marking Service". A fee of INR 1000 is charged for this special service and the results are normally released on three working days after the test date. You can send the fee for the Express Marking Service along with your IELTS application or when you arrive at your test centre.

Candidates receive scores for each module of the test as well as an overall score. The scores are scaled from band 1 to 9.

Overall band scores as well as Listening and Reading band scores are reported in half bands; Writing and Speaking band scores are reported in whole bands.

A valid test report form bears a centre stamp, a validation stamp and the IELTS administrator's signature.

REPEATING THE IELTS TEST

Candidates should note that the IELTS test cannot be repeated within three months at any centre.

INTERPRETATION OF BANDS

Each band corresponds to a descriptive statement giving a summary of the proficiency in English of a candidate classified at that level. Overall band scores can be reported in either full or half bands.

The nine bands and their descriptive statements are as follows:

9—Expert User

Has operational command of the language: appropriate, accurate and fluent with complete understanding.

8—Very Good User

Has operational command of the language with only occasional unsystematic inaccuracies and inappropriacies. Misunderstandings may occur in unfamiliar situations. Handles complex detailed argumentation well.

7—Good User

Has operational command of the language, though with occasional inaccuracies, inappropriacies and misunderstandings in some situations. Generally handles complex language well and understands detailed reasoning.

6—Competent User

Has generally effective command of the language despite some inaccuracies, inappropriacies and misunderstandings. Can use and understand fairly complex language, particularly in familiar situations.

5—Modest User

Has partial command of the language, coping with overall meaning in most situations. Should be able to handle basic communication in own field.

4—Limited User

Basic competence is limited to familiar situations. Has frequent problems in understanding. Is not able to use complex language.

3—Extremely Limited User

Conveys and understands only general meaning in very familiar situations. Frequent breakdown in communications occur.

2—Intermittent User

No real communication is possible except for the most basic information using isolated words or short formulae in familiar situations and to meet immediate needs. Has great difficulty in understanding spoken and written English.

1—Non-User

Essentially has no ability to use the language beyond possibly a few isolated words.

0—Did Not Attempt the Test

No assessable information provided.

2 *Applying for the IELTS Exam*

> ◆ *If you go through the IELTS application form you will understand why I have included this chapter. Details regarding the application process, completing the form, addresses of the British council offices and the recommended reading for the IELTS are included.*

Candidates must remember a few important points before they begin the process of application for the IELTS exam.

- You cannot apply for the IELTS exam if you do not have a valid passport.
- You cannot repeat the IELTS exam within three months at any centre.

Having considered the above mentioned points, the process of application for the IELTS exam is as follows:

1. Log on to the website of the British council at www.britishcouncil.org/india and under the appropriate zone, search for the centres where you would like to give the exam. Note down at least three choices of centres and dates convenient to you. Under the 'How to register' section you can download a copy of the application form. Also, download the IELTS handbook.

2. Call up the British council office of the appropriate zone (see next page) and enquire about the availability of seats for the selected dates in the order of your priority.
   (*Note:* You can also get information on the centres and dates over the phone, but you would really be testing their patience by discussing the probabilities. It would be better to check the dates online in order to give yourself sufficient time to decide.)

3. Fill in the application form (Information on how to fill in the application form given later) and send it to the appropriate British council office. Enclose the following:
   a. Demand draft for the appropriate amount in favour of 'British Council-British Deputy High Commission'
   b. 1 Passport copy
   c. 4 passport size photographs.
   (*Note:* the fees for the IELTS exam has been revised to INR 5250/- and the fees for express marking is INR 1000/-).

4. Within two weeks you will receive a letter from the British council office confirming the dates, and two weeks before the exam, you will be sent the details of the venue and time of the exam.

5. Plan your journey (Booking tickets/Accommodation) taking into consideration your first priority date. Do this as soon as you get your first confirmation letter, or if your exam is within the next three weeks, even before you get the confirmation letter.

6. When you are going for the exam, make sure you carry the following with yourself:
   a. IELTS admission form
   b. Passport
   c. Additional photographs
   d. Stationery.

List of Centres for IELTS in India and their Contact Offices

NORTH ZONE
Delhi
Lucknow
Bhopal
Jalandhar
Chandigarh
Kanpur

British Council Division
British High Commission
17 Kasturba Gandhi Marg,
New Delhi 110 001
Tel +91 (11) 2-371 1401
Fax +91 (11) 2-371 0717
E-mail: delhi.enquiry@in.britishcouncil.org

SOUTH ZONE
Chennai
Bangalore
Trivandrum
Hyderabad

British Deputy High Commission
British Council Division,
737 Anna Salai,
Chennai 600 002
Tel +91 (44) 852 5002/ Fax +91 (44) 852 3234
Email:firstname.surname@in.britishcouncil.org

WEST ZONE
Mumbai
Pune
Ahmedabad

British Deputy High Commission
British Council Division,
Mittal Tower, C Wing, 1st Floor
Nariman Point,
Mumbai 400 021.
Tel +91 (22) 282 3530 /Fax +91 (22) 285 2024
Email:mumbai.enquiry@in.britishcouncil.org

EAST ZONE
Kolkata

British Deputy High Commission
British Council Division, L & T Chambers (First Floor),
16 Camac Street,
Kolkata 700017.
Tel +91 (33) 282 5370/ Fax +91 (33) 282 4804
E-mail: kolkata.enquiry@in.britishcouncil.org

FILLING IN THE APPLICATION FORM

The serial numbers mentioned below are as in the application form for the IELTS exam.

1. *Preferred date of test:* Fill in the date along with the centre name in order of priority.
2. *Family name:* You must have a family name, if you do not have one fill in the names apart from your first name here.
3. *Title:* Do not circle 'Dr' unless it says so in your passport.
4. *Other names:* Must be as in your passport.

5-11. As appropriate.

12. *Nationality:* For Indians – 089.
13. *First language:* Refer to IELTS handbook.
14. *Occupation:* Sector – 08/ Level – 07.
15. *Reason for…:* 04.
16. *Country…:* Circle United Kingdom and Ireland.
17. *Which module…:* Academic Module.
18. *Which IELTS…:* Pen and paper.

19-22. As appropriate.

23. *Where would….:* Mention the address of GMC. General Medical Council, 178, Great Portland Street, London, UK; band requirement—7.0.

RECOMMENDED READING FOR IELTS

Most of the books mentioned below will be available at your local book-seller. If not, log on to www.amazon.co.uk and place an order. The books will reach any international destination within ten days.

1. Insight into IELTS Cassette: The Cambridge IELTS course

Insight into IELTS cassette offers comprehensive preparation for the IELTS examination. It develops skills, language and familiarity with the test format for each paper progressively: exam-type exercises are a regular feature of the course, and it finishes with a complete practice test. It explores the exam thoroughly, paper by paper, and its flexible structure allows teachers or students working alone to pinpoint exactly aspects of the exam they most need to study.

2. Cambridge Practice Tests for IELTS 1 Cassette set

Cambridge Practice Tests for IELTS 1 contains four complete practice tests for the Academic module of the International English Language Testing System examination, plus extra reading and writing papers for the General Training module students. The cassettes contain listening material carefully chosen to reflect the reality of the exam in terms of timing, format and the types of speaker and accent used.

3. Check Your Vocabulary for the IELTS Examination: A Workbook for Users

Non-native speakers of English will find this instructional workbook a helpful source for improving and expanding their English language vocabulary in preparation for the IELTS examination. Over 60 activities are provided, including word games, puzzles, and quizzes that are specifically designed to target problem areas common to non-native speakers.

4. The IELTS Tutor

This video and book or CD-ROM and book have been designed to teach the skills they need to succeed in the IELTS test. It contains upto-date information that students need and very good strategies to use when doing the test.

5. 101 Helpful Hints for the IELTS Examination

- 2 Practice listening skill tests
- 4 Graded practice reading tests
- 4 Practice writing academic tests
- 2 Sets of speaking test questions.

6. British Council Preparatory Material for IELTS

Contains 1 sample test.

7. Books by Insearch UTS

The following products have been developed by Insearch UTS. The products are all adapted and geared towards the new IELTS speaking test.

- The New Prepare for IELTS: Academic Modules.
  5 complete practice tests for listening, reading, writing and speaking for the new IELTS test.
- The New Prepare for IELTS: General Training Modules.
  5 complete practice tests for listening, reading, writing and speaking for the new IELTS test.
  Website-www.uts.edu.au/international/ielts

Also, check out some IELTS books available at the following websites:

- www.nceltr.mq.edu.au/publications/books/ieltstra.htm
- www.conestogac.on.ca/ielts/ieltsprep.html
- www.oup.com.au/content/general.asp

8. Websites

1. www.ielts-test.com
2. www.ielts.org/index

9. Courses

a. IELTS Preparation Courses by British Council, Delhi

These specially, designed courses are run over

the four days just before each exam. However, seats are limited and admission will be on the first-come first-served basis. All you have to do is turn up at 0900 hrs on the first day of the course. You'll be asked to sit a placement test so that they can assess your English level and advise you on your eligibility. The course runs for the four days from 1400 to 1900 hrs.

Location: The British Council, Delhi

Duration: 20-hour 4-day intensive course—INR 5,300 or
32-hour 8-week course—INR 7,500

b. ielts secrets.com

The IELTS Secrets is only available as an instantly downloadable e-book from their site. It doesn't require any special software.

Cost: $ 19.95.

c. www.edict.com.hk/vlc/ielts/listening/tests/dlg1-test.htm

A completely free listening test with audio!

d. www.international.holmesglen.vic.edu.au/ IELTS01.htm

A whole load of free tests and tips.

e. www.onestopenglish.com

Useful site with free material.

f. ieltsonline.com

The official IELTS sample test, corrections and individual comments about each test module, an online practice speaking test, six essay corrections and suggestions for further study to improve your score.

Cost: $ 280!!!

g. www.englishworld.org/ielts/exam/listen.htm

3 *The Listening Component*

Almost everybody who has attempted the IELTS would agree with the statement that the listening component is the comparatively easy part of the entire exam.

The IELTS listening test takes approximately 30 minutes. The listening material is recorded on a cassette tape, which you will hear only once.

There are four sections in the listening test presented in order of increasing difficulty. The first two sections are on topics of general interest such as a report of a lost bag or an introduction to a public facility. Section one will be in the form of a dialogue, section two will be a monologue.

Sections three and four will have an education or training focus. There will be a lecture and a discussion between two and four people.

As you listen, you should write your answers on the question booklet. At the end of the recorded material you will be given ten minutes to copy your answers onto the answersheet.

It is very important that you take a number of timed practice listening tests before the actual exam day to become familiar with the style of questions asked, the speed of the speech and to develop the skill of recording your answers as you listen.

QUESTIONS

The following are the types of questions, which one would usually come across in the listening section:

1. Selecting Topics
2. Summary Completion
3. Multiple Choice
4. Form Completion
5. Sentence Completion
6. Short Answer Questions.

1. Sample Question One: Selecting Topics

You will be provided with a number of topics, three of which summaries parts of the listening text. The others are not discussed in the listening text. Your task is to decide which three topics are discussed.

2. Sample Question Two: Summary Completion

The input for this type of question will be a summary of all or part of the listening text. The summary will contain a number of gaps. All of the information in the summary will be contained in the listening text although the words used may be different. Your task is to complete the summary using not more than three words for each gap.

3. Sample Question Three: Multiple Choice

In this type of question you will be given a 'stem', which may be an incomplete sentence or a question. The stem will be followed by three or four options—one will be correct (the answer) and three may seem possible but are in fact incorrect in some way (the distracters).

4. Sample Question Four: Form Completion

You will be provided with an incomplete form, which covers information from the listening text. Your task is to complete the gaps in three words or fewer. The information in the form will be presented in the same order as the information you hear. In other words, you will hear the answer to question one before the answer to question two.

5. Sample Question Five: Sentence Completion

You will be provided with a number of incomplete statements, which you need to complete using information from the listening text. Generally you must complete the statement in three words or fewer, but confirm this with the instructions.

The questions will be presented in the same order as the answers in the listening text.

6. Sample Question Six: Short Answer Questions

You will be provided with a number of questions, which you have to answer. Generally your answers must be in three words or fewer, but confirm this with the instructions.

TIPS FOR THE LISTENING COMPONENT

Tip 1

As in any part of the exam, there are no lost marks for wrong answers. So, if you don't know—guess!

Tip 2

All the parts of the paper are heard only once—so don't do lots of textbook listening where they hear twice. It can be useful, however, to occasionally play the IELTS exam listening through again while they read the tape script.

Tip 3

Although the question papers will be collected in, only the answersheets will be marked. Students can therefore write anything they like on the question sheet. In fact, making a few notes as they listen will give students a chance to guess any answers they have missed during the time given to transfer answers to the answersheet.

Tip 4

Grammar, spelling and punctuation (e.g., capital letters) must also be correct for all answers.

Tip 5

There are things that students must get right to get the points which do not have anything to do with listening comprehension (e.g., getting grammar right, see Tip 4). These things can therefore be practiced in the classroom without even using a tape.

Tip 6

Of course, the best practice for the listening paper is to listen to as much English as possible. Students should try to listen to radio as well as watch TV, as they can't rely on visual prompts in the exam. If they want to watch movies, etc., then anything in an academic setting should include relevant vocabulary, e.g., *Educating Rita* or *The Dead Poet's Society*.

4 *The Reading Component*

> ◆ *I believe this chapter in itself will be a thorough preparation for the reading component of the IELTS. Details regarding the variety of questions, tips on how you can master them and finally a Sample reading test would do you a world of good!*

The IELTS reading test takes one hour. In this time you are required to read three texts of between 500 and 900 words each. The texts and questions increase in difficulty. There will be around 40 questions to answer and record on the answer sheet within the 60 minutes.

Most students come out of the reading test feeling that there was not enough time to complete the exam paper. For this reason, it is very important that you take a number of timed practice reading tests before the actual exam day to develop the skills of skimming and scanning and other time-saving strategies.

Common types of questions in the reading test:
1. Summary completion
2. Matching headings to paragraphs
3. Identifying the writer's views
4. Multiple choice
5. Selecting factors
6. Table completion
7. Matching causes and effects
8. Sentence completion
9. Short answer questions.

1. Summary Completion Questions—How to Approach

Step 1
Read the instructions carefully. In some questions, you may have been given the option of using each word more than once. Remember though that every IELTS test is different. So make sure that you read the instructions carefully even if you have practiced the type of question before.

Step 2
Skim through the summary to get an idea of the topic.

Step 3
Decide which section of the text does the summary cover. In some cases, the summary may cover the whole text.

Step 4
Read through the summary, referring to the list of words each time you reach a gap. Select one or more possible words from the list to fill each gap. Reject any words that do not fit grammatically, even if the meaning seems correct. Confirm your choice by referring to the relevant sections of the text.

Step 5
Quickly read your completed summary to check that it makes sense.

2. Matching Headings to Paragraphs— How to Approach

Step 1

Read the instructions carefully. Note that the heading you choose should sum up the main idea of the paragraph. Also note, which paragraphs you, need to look at, as you are often not required to do them all.

Step 2

Familiarize yourself with the list of paragraph headings by skimming through them quickly.

Step 3

Read the first paragraph for which you have to find a heading. Remember that you are reading to find out the main idea of the paragraph. Concentrate on the main idea or focus of the paragraph and try not to be distracted by details or by unfamiliar vocabulary.

Step 4

Choose the heading from the list, which best sums up the main point of the paragraph you have just read. If you cannot choose between two headings, go on to the next paragraph—you can come back to that question later. However, don't forget to make a choice before the end of the test because if you leave a blank or you have marked two answers on your answer sheet, you will be graded as incorrect for that question.

3. Identifying the Writer's Views— How to Approach

Step 1

Read the instructions carefully. Note that you are asked to identify the writer's opinion, which may not necessarily be the same as the facts. Note also the difference between the three categories you have to use, particularly.

No The statement contradicts the writer.

Not Given The writer does not give an opinion on this point.

Yes—The statement is in agreement with the writer.

Step 2

Skim through all of the statements to get an idea of the topics you will be searching for in your reading of the text.

Step 3

Read the first statement again more carefully. Note the main point or opinion given in the statement.

Step 4

Skim the text for the section, which refers to that idea. If you come across information relating to other statements, put a mark beside the section so that you can find it quickly again later.

Step 5

Once you have found the appropriate section of the text, read more carefully. Decide if the statement agrees with the view of the author or disagrees with the author or *Not Given*.

4. Multiple Choice Questions— How to Approach

Step 1

Read the instructions carefully.

Step 2

Skim all the questions briefly to get an idea of the topics for which you will be searching when reading the text.

Step 3

Read the first question again more carefully. Decide what you will need to read to answer the question. Is the question asking you for a particular detail that you need to find in the text? Alternatively, is the question asking you for an answer, which requires a global understanding of the whole text?

Step 4

Once you have decided the best strategy for dealing with the question (as above), you will need to proceed to read the text in the appropriate manner.

5. Questions Involving Selecting Factors—How to Approach

Step 1

Read the instructions carefully. Note that only three of the factors are correct.

Step 2

Read through the list of factors.

Step 3

Scan the text and find the sections or paragraphs, which discuss poor communication.

Step 4

Read those sections carefully and select the appropriate factors.

6. Table Completion Tasks— How to Approach

Step 1

Read the instructions carefully. Note that in the sample task you may use your own words if you wish, based on the information in the reading text. In other cases, you will be instructed to use the words from the reading text only. Note also that here you may write only three words or fewer.

Step 2

Look at the table and especially any headings. Decide which is the most useful way to read the table. Glance at the other information given in the table to get an idea of what information you will be searching for when you read.

Step 3

Look at the first row under the headings. Decide

what key ideas you will need to search for as you skim the reading text. Decide also what information you will need to complete the first gap.

Step 4

Skim the text for the appropriate paragraph or section.

Step 5

Read that section more carefully and decide on the best word or words to fill the gap. Remember that you will need to use the appropriate form of any verbs.

7. Matching Causes and Effects— How to Approach

Step 1

Read the instructions carefully.

Step 2

Look at the table and decide which list you should work from. In most cases, it would be most efficient to work from the shorter list (usually the causes).

Step 3

Read the first cause.

Step 4

Briefly familiarize yourself with the effects list. Which effects seem possible at this stage?

Step 5

Skim the reading text to find the section, which discusses the first cause.

Step 6

Read that section of the reading text carefully to find the effect.

Step 7

When you have found the effect in the reading

passage, refer back to the effects list and select the one which best paraphrases the information in the reading text. If none of the effects listed seem to match, then keep reading the text, as it is not unusual for causes to have more than one effect.

8. Sentence Completion Questions— How to Approach

Step 1

Read the instructions carefully. Note that in the sample task you must only use words from the reading passage, and that you may use no more than three words to complete each sentence.

Step 2

Briefly read all the incomplete sentences to get an idea of what information you will have to find in the text.

Step 3

Read the first sentence more carefully. Decide what information you will need. In this case, you will look for a section discussing inquiries about improving safety procedures.

Step 4

Once you have found the relevant section of the reading text, look back at the incomplete sentence and decide what specific information you need to complete it. In this case, you need to find what was initiated.

Step 5

Read that part of the text more carefully to find the answer. Remember that the correct answer you find in the text should fit the incomplete sentence grammatically. If not, you may need to look for another answer.

In some IELTS tests, the instructions will not say 'using words taken from the text', in which case you can use your own words or change the form of the words in the reading text.

9. Short Answer Questions— How to Approach

Step 1

Read the instructions carefully. Note that in the sample task you may use your own words but you may not use more than three words for each answer.

Step 2

Briefly read all of the questions to get an idea of what information you will have to find in the text.

Step 3

Read the first question more carefully. Decide what information you will skim for.

Step 4

Once you have found the relevant section of the reading text, look back at the question and decide what specific information you need to answer the question.

Step 5

Read that part of the text more carefully to find the answer.

Step 6

Your answer does not need to be a complete sentence but it does need to make sense grammatically.

SAMPLE READING TEST

Reading Passage 1

Personal Time Management
Since, the early work of Halberg (1960), the existence of human "circadian rhythms" has been well-known to biologists and psychologists. Circadian rhythms dictate that there are certain times of the day when we are at our best both physically and psychologically. At its simplest, the majority of us feel more alive and creative in

the mornings, while come the evenings we are fit only for collapsing with a good book or in front of the television. Others of us note that in the morning we take a great deal of time to get going physically and mentally, but by the evening are full of energy and bright ideas, while a very few of us feel most alert and vigorous in the late afternoon.

Irrespective of our personal rhythms, most of us have a productive period between 10 am and noon, when the stomach, pancreas, spleen and heart all appear to be in their most active phases. Conversely, the majority of us experience a low period in the hour or two after lunch (a time when people in some societies sensibly take a rest), as most of our energy is devoted to the process of digestion. The simple rules here are: don't waste too much prime time having a coffee break around 11 am when you should be doing some of your best work, and don't make the after-lunch period even less productive by overloading your digestion. A short coffee or tea break is, in fact, best taken on arrival at the office, when it helps us start the day in a positive mood, rather than mid-morning when it interrupts the flow of our activities. Lunch is best taken early, when we are just beginning to feel hungry, and we are likely to eat less than if we leave it until later. An early lunch also means that we can get back into our productive stride earlier in the afternoon.

Changes in one's attitude can also enhance personal time management. For example, the notion of pro-action is eminently preferable to reaction. To pro-act means to anticipate events and be in a position to take appropriate action as soon as the right moment arrives.

To react, on the other hand, means to have little anticipation and do something only when events force you to do so. Pro-actors tend to be the people who are always one step ahead of other people, who always seem to be in the right place at the

right time, and who are always better informed than anyone else. Many of us like an easy life, and so we tend to be reactors This means that we aren't alert to the challenges and opportunities coming our way, with the consequence that challenges bother us or opportunities pass us by before we're even properly aware they're upon us. We can train ourselves in pro-action by regularly taking the time to sit down and appraise the likely immediate future, just as we sit down and review the immediate past.

Psychologists recognise that we differ in the way in which we characteristically attribute responsibility for the various things that happen to us in life. One of the ways in which we do this is known as locus of control (Weiner, 1979), which refers to assigning responsibility. At its simplest, some individuals have a predominantly external locus of control, attributing responsibility to outside causes (for example, the faults of others or the help given by them), while with other individuals the locus of control is predominantly internal, in which responsibility is attributed to oneself (for example, one's own abilities or lack of them, hard work, etc.).

However, the picture usually isn't as simple as this. Many people's locus of control is more likely to be specific to a particular situation, for example internal in certain areas, such as their social lives, and external in others, such as their working lives. On the other hand, to take another example, they may attribute certain kinds of results to themselves, such as their successes, and certain kinds of results to other people, such as their failures. Obviously, the best kind of locus of control is one that is realistic and able to attribute every effect to its appropriate cause, and this is particularly important when it comes to time management. Certainly, there are occasions when other people are more responsible for our time loss than we are, but for most of us, and for most of the time, the blame must fall fairly and squarely upon ourselves.

QUESTIONS

Choose ONE phrase (A-J) from the list in the box below to complete each key point below. Write the appropriate letters (A-J) in boxes 1-6 on your answer sheet.

The information in the completed sentences should be an accurate summary of points made by the writer.

NB There are more phrases (A-J) than sentences, so you will not use them all. You may use any phrase more than once.

Questions 1-6

Time Management—Key Points

Example Our patterns of circadian rhythms... G
1. A proactive person...
2. A reactive person...
3. Analysing circadian rhythms...
4. The idea that the best time to work is in the morning...
5. The notion of feeling alert in the late afternoon...
6. Productivity appears to be enhanced...

List of Phrases

A. ...agrees with the circadian rhythms of most people.
B. ...makes us feel alive and creative.
C. ...conforms to the circadian rhythms of a minority of people.
D. ...if our energy is in a low phase.
E. ...is more able to take advantage of events when they happen.
F. ...enables one to gauge physical potential at particular times throughout the day.
G. ...can affect us physically and mentally.
H. ...when several specific internal organs are active.
I. ...takes a more passive attitude toward events.
J. ...when we eat lunch early.

Questions 7-13

Complete the sentences below with words taken from Reading Passage 1, "Personal Time Management".

Use NO MORE THAN THREE WORDS for each answer. Write your answers in *boxes 7-13* on your answer sheet.

Example Most people are less productive.....

Answer : After lunch

1. Our .... influence our physical and mental performance.
2. We are more likely to be productive in the afternoon if we have................
3. A person who reacts tends not to see .... when they are approaching.
4. Assessing the .... aids us in becoming proactive.
5. A person with a mainly internal locus of control would likely direct blame toward ....
6. A person with a mainly external locus of control would likely direct failure toward ....
7. A person with a healthy and balanced locus of control would attribute a result, whether negative or positive, to ....

Reading Passage 2

You are advised to spend about 20 minutes on Questions 14-25, which are based on Reading Passage 2, "The Muang Faai Irrigation System of Northern Thailand".

Questions 14-19

Reading Passage 2 has 7 sections.

Choose the most suitable heading for each section from the list of headings (A-L) below.

Write the appropriate letter (A-L) in boxes 14-19 on your answersheet.

Note: There are more headings than sections, so you will not use all of them.

List of Headings

A. Rituals and beliefs
B. Topography of Northern Thailand
C. The forests of Northern Thailand
D. Preserving the system
E. Agricultural practices
F. Village life
G. Water distribution principles
H. Maintaining natural balances
I. Structure of the irrigation system
J. User's rights
K. User's obligations
L. Community control

Example Section 5 A

    14. Section 1
    15. Section 2
    16. Section 3
    17. Section 4
    18. Section 6
    19. Section 7

The Muang Faai Irrigation System of Northern Thailand

Section 1

Northern Thailand consists mainly of long mountain chains interspersed with valley bottoms where streams and rice fields dominate the landscape. Most of the remaining forests of the North are found at higher altitudes. The forests ensure regular seasonal rainfall for the whole area and at the same time moderate runoff, so that there is water throughout the year.

Section 2

The lowland communities have developed an agricultural system adapted to, and partially determining, the distinctive ecosystems of their areas. Practicing wet-rice agriculture in the valley-bottoms, the lowlanders also raise pigs, ducks and chickens and cultivate vegetable gardens in their villages further up the slopes. Rice, beans, corn and native vegetables are planted in hill fields above the villages, and wild vegetables and herbal medicines are gathered and wild game hunted in the forests higher up the hillsides. The forests also serve as grazing grounds for cows and buffaloes, and are a source of wood for household utensils, cooking fuel, construction and farming tools. Fish are to be found in the streams and in the irrigation system and wet-rice fields, providing both food and pest control.

Section 3

In its essentials, a muang faai system consists of a small reservoir which feeds an intricate, branching network of small channels carrying water in carefully calibrated quantities through clusters of rice terraces in valley bottoms. The system taps into a stream above the highest rice field and, when there is sufficient water, discharges back into the same stream at a point below the bottom field. The water in the reservoir at the top, which is diverted into a main channel (Iam muang) and from there into the different fields, is slowed or held back not by an impervious dam, but by a series of barriers constructed of bunches of bamboo or saplings which allow silt, soil and sand to pass through.

Section 4

Water from the Iam muang is measured out among the farmers according to the extent of their rice fields and the amount of water available from the main channel. Also considered are the height of the fields, their distance from the main channel and their soil type. The size and depth of side-channels are then adjusted so that only the allocated amount of water flows into each farmer's field.

Section 5

Rituals and beliefs connected with the muang faai reflect the villagers' submission to, respect for, and friendship with nature, rather than an attempt to master it. In mountains, forests, watersheds and water, villagers see things of great value and power. This power has a favourable aspect, and one that benefits humans. But at the same time, if certain boundaries are overstepped and nature is damaged, the spirits will punish humans. Therefore, when it is necessary to use nature for the necessities of life, villagers take care to inform the spirits what they intend to do, simultaneously begging pardon for their actions.

Section 6

Keeping a muang faai system going demands cooperation and collective management, sometimes within a single village, sometimes across three or four different subdistricts including many villages. The rules or common agreements arrived at during the yearly meeting amount to a social contract. They govern how water is to be distributed, how flow is to be controlled according to seasonal schedules, how barriers are to be maintained and channels dredged, how conflicts over water use are to be settled, and how the forest around the reservoir is to be preserved as a guarantee of a steady water supply and a source of materials to repair the system.

Section 7

The fundamental principle of water rights under muang faai is that everyone in the system must get enough to survive; while many patterns of distribution are possible, none can violate this basic tenet. On the whole, the system also rests on the assumption that local water is a common property. No one can take control of it by force, and it must be used in accord with the communal agreements. Although there are inequalities in landholding, no one has the right to an excessive amount of fertile land. The way in which many muang faai systems expand tends to reinforce further the claims of community security over those of individual entrepreneurship. In the

gradual process of opening up new land and digging connecting channels, each local household often ends up with scattered holdings over the whole irrigation areas. Unlike modern irrigation systems, under which the most powerful people generally end up closest to the sources of water, this arrangement encourages everyone to take care that no part of the system is unduly favoured or neglected.

Questions 20-23

The chart below illustrates the agricultural system of the lowland communities.

Select words from Reading Passage 2 to fill the spaces in the chart. Use *up to three words* for each space. Write your answers in boxes 20-23 on your answer sheet.

Area	Activity
Example Forests	*Answer* grazing cows, buffaloes
Forests	- gathering ..... (20) ...., hunting wild animals
Hill fields	- cultivating .... (21) ....
Villages	- raising ..... (22) .... cultivating vegetables
Valley bottom	- growing................................... (23) ....

Question 24

From the list below, select the three main structures, which constitute the muang faai irrigation system. Write the *three* appropriate letters, in any order, in box 24 on your answer sheet.

A. channels
B. saplings
C. dam
D. barriers
E. reservoir
F. water

Question 25

From the list below, select two criteria for allocating water to farmers. Write *two* appropriate letters, in any order, in box 25 on your answersheet.

> A. field characteristics
> B. social status
> C. location of field
> D. height of barriers
> E. fees paid
> F. water available

READING PASSAGE 3

You are advised to spend about 20 minutes on Questions 26-39, which are based on Reading Passage 3 below.

The Origins of Indo-European Languages

The traditional view of the spread of the Indo-European languages holds that an U language, ancestor to all the others, was spoken by nomadic horsemen who lived in what is now western Russia north of the Black Sea near the beginning of the Bronze Age. As these mounted warriors roamed over greater and greater expanses, they conquered the indigenous peoples and imposed their own proto-Indo-European language, which in the course of succeeding centuries evolved in local areas into the European languages we know today. In recent years, however, many scholars, particularly archaeologists, have become dissatisfied with the traditional explanation.

The starting point of the problem of the origins of Indo-European is not archaeological but linguistic. When linguists look at the languages of Europe, they quickly perceive that these languages are related. The connections can be seen in vocabulary, grammar and phonology (rules for pronunciation), to illustrate the numbers from one to ten in several Indo-European languages. Such a comparison makes it clear that there are significant similarities among many European languages and also Sanskrit, the language of the earliest literary texts of India, but that languages such as Chinese or Japanese are not members of the same family (see Figure 1).

The Romance languages, such as French, Italian and Spanish are languages that developed from Latin. These languages served as the first model for answering the question. Even to someone with no knowledge of Latin, the profound similarities among Romance languages would have made it natural to suggest that they were derived from a common ancestor. On the assumption that the shared characteristic of these languages came from the common progenitor (whereas the divergences arose later as the languages diverged), it would have been possible to reconstruct many of the characteristics of the original protolanguage.

In much the same way, it became clear that the branches of the Indo-European family could be studied and a hypothetical family tree constructed, reading back to a common ancestor: proto-Indo-European.

This is the tree approach. The basic process represented by the tree model is one of divergence: when languages become isolated from one other, they differ increasingly, and dialects gradually differentiate until they become separate languages.

Divergence is by no means the only possible tendency in language evolution. Johannes Schmidt, introduced a "wave" model in which linguistic changes spread like waves, leading ultimately to convergence; that is, growing similarity among languages that were initially quite different.

Today, however, most linguists think primarily in terms of linguistic family trees. It is necessary to construct some explicit models of how language change might occur according to a process-based view. There are four main classes of models.

The first is the process of initial colonisation,

ENGLISH	OLD GERMAN	LATIN	GREEK	SANSKRIT	JAPANESE
ONE	AINS		THRIJA	FIDWOR	FIMF
TWO	TWAI	DUO	DUO	DVA	FUTATSU
THREE	THRIJA	TRES	TREIS	TRYAS	MITTSU
FOUR	FIDWOR	QUATTOUR	TTTARES	CATVARAS	YOTTSU
FIVE	FIMF	QUINQUE	PENTE	PANCA	ITSUTSU
SIX	SAIHS	SEX	HEKS	SAT	MUTTSU
SEVEN	SIBUM	SEPTEM	HEPTA	SAPTA	NANATSU
EIGHT	AHTAU	OCTO	OKTO	ASTA	YATTSU
NINE	NIUN	NOVEM	ENNEA	NAVA	KOKONOTSU
TEN	TAIHUM	DECEM	DEKA	DASA	TO

Fig.1: Words for numbers from one to ten show the relations among Indo-European languages and the anomalous character of Japanese, which is not part of that family. Such similarities stimulated interest in the origins of Indo-European languages.

by which an uninhabited territory becomes populated; its language naturally becomes that of the colonisers. The second are the processes of divergence, such as the linguistic divergence arising from separation or isolation mentioned above in relation to early models of the Indo-European languages. The third group of models is based on processes of linguistic convergence. The wave model, formulated by Schmidt in the 1870's, is an example, but convergence methods have not generally found favor among linguists.

Now, the slow and rather static operation of these processes is complicated by another factor: linguistic replacement. That factor provides the basis for a fourth class of models. In many areas of the world, the languages initially spoken by the indigenous people have come to be replaced, fully or partially, by languages spoken by people coming from outside. Were it not for this large complicating factor, the world's linguistic history could be faithfully described by the initial distribution of *Homo sapiens,* followed by the gradual, long-term workings of divergence and convergence. So linguistic replacement also has a key role to play in explaining the origins of the Indo-European languages.

Questions 26-32

Below is a summary of part of Reading Passage 3, "The Origins of Indo-European Languages".

Read the summary and then select the best word or phrase from the box below to fill each gap according to the information in the Reading Passage.

Write the corresponding letters (A-L) in boxes 26-32 on your answer sheet.

Note: There are more words and phrases than you will need to fill the gaps. You may use a word or phrase more than once if you wish.

Summary—Models of Language Change

Example There are four main models of language .... (Ex) .....

Answer: K

The first is the process of initial colonisation where an uninhabited territory becomes populated: the language spoken will therefore be that of the .....(26)..... Processes of .....(27)..... occur where different dialects, and then languages, develop from a common .....(28)..... Many of the original characteristic of this common ancestor can be reconstructed from what we know of the present separate .....(29).....

Processes of linguistic .....(30)..... occur when languages, which were initially different, become more similar through contact. The wave model, formulated by Schmidt in the 1870s, is an example. The final model is that of linguistic

.....(31)..... In this model, a new language replaces the language spoken by the .....(32).....

A colonisers	G languages
B invader	H waves
C proto-language	I replacement
D indigenous people	J convergence
E linguists	K development
F model	L divergence

Questions 33-36

Several aspects of language development discussed in Reading Passage 3 are listed below.

Match each aspect with the appropriate model from the box below, according to the information in the Reading Passage. Write the appropriate letter (A, B, C, or D) in boxes 33-36 on your answersheet.

Aspects of Language Development

Example Population of territory
Answer: A
  33. "wave" model
  34. Romance languages
  35. Proto-Indo-European
  36. European languages

Models

A Colonisation	C Convergence
B Divergence	D Replacement

Questions 37-39

Answer the following questions using *not more than three words*, according to the information in the Reading Passage 3. Write your answers in boxes 37-39 on your answer sheet.

37. What are three ways in which the languages of Europe are related?
38. On what basis does the author decide that Chinese and Japanese are not related to European languages?
39. According to the tree model, what was the original proto-language for English?

PRACTICE SAMPLE READING TEST ANSWERS

Reading Passage 1: Personal Time Management
  1. E
  2. I
  3. F
  4. A
  5. C
  6. H
  7. circadian rhythms.
  8. (an) early lunch
  9. opportunities // challenges // challenges and opportunities
  10. (likely) immediate future // immediate past
  11. himself // herself
  12. others // other people // outside causes // faults of others
  13. (its) appropriate cause(s)

Reading Passage: 2 The Muang Faai Irrigation System;
  14. B
  15. E
  16. I
  17. G
  18. L
  19. J
  20. Two correct out of: vegetables, herbal medicines, herbs, wood.
  21. Two correct out of: rice, beans, corn, (native) vegetables.
  22. Two correct out of: pigs, ducks, chickens.
  23. (wet) rice / (fish).
  24. E, A, D [any order].
  25. Two correct out of: F, A, C [any order].

Reading Passage 3: The Origins of Indo-European Languages
  26. A
  27. L
  28. C
  29. G
  30. J
  31. I
  32. D
  33. C
  34. B
  35. D
  36. B
  37. Vocabulary, grammar, phonology [all three must be correct]
  38. Comparison of words/vocabulary/numbers/features // compare (the) words
  39. Proto-Indo-European

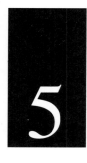 **5** *The Writing Component*

> ◆ Here, I will be taking you back to your school days to give you a little coaching on English grammar. Again, a few tips on how to get a better score and a Sample writing test with answers is included.

The IELTS writing test takes one hour. In this time you are required to complete two tasks.

Task One

It is a report based on some graphic information provided on the question paper. With a few exceptions, the graphic information will come in one of five forms—a line graph, bar graph, pie chart, table or diagram illustrating a process. You are required to describe the information or the process in a report of 150 words. This task should be completed in 20 minutes. It is important that you are familiar with the language appropriate to report writing generally and to each of the five types of report.

Task Two

It is an essay based on a topic given on the question paper. You should write at least 250 words in 40 minutes. It is important that you keep within the advised time limits as Task Two carries more weight in your final band score than Task One. Remember that illegible handwriting will reduce your final score.

Writing Tasks

1. Single Line Graphs
2. Double Line Graphs
3. Bar Charts
4. Tables
5. Pie Charts.

STRATEGIES FOR IMPROVING YOUR SCORE

We shall discuss this under the following headings:
1. Selecting Information
2. Report Structure
3. Grammar and Vocabulary
4. Expressing
5. Comparing and Contrasting
6. Describing Parts of the Chart.

1. Selecting Information

It is important that you describe the whole graph fully. However, this does not mean that you should note every detail. In most cases, there will be too much information for you to mention each figure. You will therefore need to summarise the graph by dividing it into its main parts. This is what we mean by describing the trends.

> The number of cases of X disease started at 50 in 1965 and then went up gradually to 100 in 1965 and continued up to 200 in 1970 and then went up more sharply to 380 in 1975.

While this way of describing the information may be accurate, it does not meaningfully sum up the information in the graph.

2. Report Structure

Your report should be structured simply with an

introduction, body and conclusion. Tenses should be used appropriately.

Introduction

Use two standard opening sentences to introduce your report. These opening sentences should make up the first paragraph. Sentence one should define what the graph is about; that is, the date, location, what is being described in the graph, etc. For example:

> The graph shows the number of cases of X disease in Scotland between the years 1960 and 1995 ...

Notice the tense used. Even though it describes information from the past, the graph shows the information in the present time. Notice that the sample opening sentence does not simply copy the words used on the graphic material. Copied sentences will not be assessed by the examiner and so you waste your time including them.

Describing the Overall Trend

Sentence two (and possibly three) might sum up the overall trend. For example:

> It can be clearly seen that X disease increased rapidly to 500 cases around the 1980s and then dropped to zero before 1999, while Y disease fell consistently from a high point of nearly 600 cases in 1960 to less than 100 cases in 1995.

Notice the tense used. Here we are talking about the occurrence of the disease in the past.

Describing the Graph in Detail

Line graphs generally present information in chronological order and so the most logical order for you to write up the information would, most probably, be from the earliest to the latest. Bar graphs, pie charts are organised in different ways and so you need to decide on the organisation of each one.

Concluding Sentences

Your report may end with one or two sentences which summarise your report to draw a relevant conclusion.

3. Grammar and Vocabulary

Avoiding repetition

For example, the candidate who writes the following:

> The number of cases of X disease started at 50 in 1965 and then went up to 200 in 1970 and then went up to 500 in 1980.

will lose marks for being repetitive. You should therefore, practice writing reports using a wide variety of terms to describe the different movements in the graphs and different structures to vary your writing.

Describing Trends

There are three basic trends:

Expressing Movement: Nouns and Verbs
The following is a list of terms that could be used to describe various trends:

Trends	Verbs	Nouns
↗	Rose (to)	A rise
	Increased (to)	An increase
	Went up (to)	Growth
	Climbed (to)	An upward trend
	Boomed	A boom
↘	Fell (to)	A decrease
	Declined (to)	A decline
	Decreased (to)	A fall
	Dipped (to)	A drop
	Dropped (to)	A slump
	Went down (to)	(a dramatic fall)
	Slumped (to)	A reduction
	Reduced (to)	
	Leveled out	Maintained the same level
←→	Did not change	A leveling out
	Remained stable	No change
	Remained steady	
	Stayed constant	
↑↓↑↓	Fluctuated (around)	A fluctuation
	Peaked (at)	Reached a peak (of)
	Plateaued (at)	Reached at plateau (at)
	Stood at	

Describing the Movement
Adjectives and Adverbs

Sometimes we need to give more information about a trend as follows:

> There has been a *slight* increase in the value of the dollar (degree of change).
>
> Unemployment fell *rapidly* last year (the speed of change).

Remember that we modify a noun with an adjective (a **slight** increase) and a verb with an adverb (to increase **slightly**).

Describing the degree of change

Adjectives	Adverbs
Dramatic	dramatically
sharp	sharply
huge	hugely
enormous	enormously
steep	steeply
substantial	substantially
considerable	considerably
significant	significantly
marked	markedly
moderate	moderately
slight	slightly

Describing the speed of change

Adjectives	Adverbs
rapid	rapidly
quick	quickly
swift	swiftly
sudden	suddenly
steady	steadily
gradual	gradually
slow	slowly

4. Expressing Approximation

We use words to express approximation when the point we are trying to describe is between milestones on the graph.

just under	just over
well under	well over
roughly	nearly
approximately about	around

5. Comparing and Contrasting

One Syllable

Adjectives with one syllable form their comparatives and superlatives like this:

cheap	cheaper	cheapest
large	larger	largest
bright	brighter	brightest

Exceptions

good	better	best
bad	worse	worst

Two Syllables

Some adjectives with two syllables form their comparatives and superlatives like this:

pretty	prettier	prettiest
happy	happier	happiest

But many form their comparatives and superlatives like this:

striking	more striking	most striking

Although some can form their comparatives and superlatives like this:

common	more common	most common
clever more	clever/cleverer	most cleverest

Three or More Syllables

All adjectives with three or more syllables form their comparatives and superlatives like this:

attractive	more attractive	most attractive
profitable	more profitable	most profitable
expensive	more expensive	most expensive

6. Describing Parts of the Chart

Starting with the adjective

The highest	percentage of	women	• are employed in X category
The greatest	proportion of	cars sold	• are red
The lowest	number of	holiday makers	• come from Spain
The most	most		
A significant			
The smallest			
The largest			
• Red is the	most	popular prevalent	• car colour
• Professional is the	second/third most	common	• employment category
• Spain is the	least		• holiday destination

↑
Starting with the noun

EXAMPLE QUESTION FOR WRITING

The graph, for example, shows the pass marks for different nationalities of students over the last five years. Write a report for a university lecturer describing the information shown below.

Tip 1

The data that the students must describe is given in a graphic form (e.g., a graph or bar chart) or as a table of figures.

Tip 2

They have to write 150 words in 20 minutes, in well-organised paragraphs, with a conclusion—so time is of the essence! All class work should be closely timed, be it brainstorming, discussion or actual writing.

Tip 3

Tenses they are likely to need to know for this part are the contrast between present perfect for unfinished actions and the simple past, the use of present continuous to describe things in the process of happening, and future with will for predictions.

Tip 4

The other language they are likely to need is that of trends. A great source for this is Business English teaching books.

Tip 5

The thing students most often forget, and the obvious way to start the piece of writing is to describe what the graph actually represents—'This graph shows.../the axes represent...'.

Tip 6

The obvious way to liven up classes practicing this point is to speak about the graphs before writing about them. It is possible to play games like pair work information gap activities and Bingo to add a bit more fun.

Tip 7

The other way to add interest for the students is to use data that means something to them personally. For example, graphs from local government or newspapers, or having them give presentations on something that interests them.

SAMPLE WRITING TASK 1 SINGLE LINE GRAPH

Task Description

You will be given a graph with a single line. Your

task is to write a 150-word report to describe the information given in the graph. You are not asked to give your opinion.

You should spend around twenty minutes on the task. Task one is not worth as many marks as task two and so you should make sure that you keep within the recommended twenty minute time frame.

Sample Task

You should spend about 20 minutes on this task. Write a report for a university lecturer describing the information in the graph below. You should write at least 150 words.

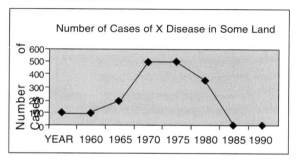

Guidelines for a Good Answer

Does the report have a suitable structure?
- Does it have an introduction, body and conclusion?
- Does it include connective words to make the writing cohesive within sentences and paragraphs?

Does the report use suitable grammar and vocabulary?
- Does it include a variety of sentence structures?
- Does it include a range of appropriate vocabulary?

Does the report meet the requirements of the task?
- Does it meet the word limit requirements?
- Does it describe the whole graph adequately?
- Does it focus on the important trends presented in the graphic information?

SAMPLE ANSWER

The graph shows the number of cases of X disease in Someland between the years 1960 and 1995. As an overall trend, it is clear that the number of cases of the disease increased fairly rapidly until the mid-seventies, remained constant for around a decade at 500 cases before dropping to zero in the late 80s.

In 1960, the number of cases stood at approximately 100. That number rose steadily to 200 by 1969 and then more sharply to 500 in 1977. At this point the number of cases remained stable until 1984 before plummeting to zero by 1988. From 1988 to 1995 Someland was free of the disease.

In conclusion, the graph shows that the disease was increasingly prevalent until the 1980s when it was eradicated from Someland.

SAMPLE WRITING TASK 2

The style of essay required for Task 2 of the IELTS writing test is standard to academic courses. There are several published textbooks available to assist you to improve your writing skills for this part of the test.

Structure and cohesion should be evident at the essay level, within and between paragraphs and within and between sentences. Structure and cohesion have a very important effect on the readability and clarity of your essay as a whole.

The structure of your essay should show a clear development from introduction, through your points and on to the conclusion. Your essay needs to have an introduction, body and conclusion.

Structure and cohesion should also be apparent within and between paragraphs. Each paragraph will typically contain a topic sentence, which states the main point of your paragraph. The topic sentence is usually the first one. This will be followed by the evidence, which supports the point of the paragraph. The final sentence will typically lead into the point of the following paragraph.

Write an essay expressing your views on the following topic:

Technology can bring many benefits, but it can also cause social and environmental problems. In relation to new technology, the primary duty of Governments should be to focus on potential problems, rather than benefits.

SAMPLE ANSWER

It is true that new technologies can create serious social and environmental problems. The question is whether governments should focus on these problems when they are formulating policies relating to new technology.

Some people would argue that governments have an important watchdog role to play and that they should attempt to establish whether a proposed technology is likely to have any harmful effects. This is seen as an aspect of government looking after the public interest and showing concern for the welfare of its citizens. These people would invest government with the power to veto the introduction of certain technologies.

The problem with this approach, however, is that it is very difficult to know in advance what the full effects of any new technology will be. The history of science and technology has many fascinating examples of unexpected developments. Sometimes a technological advance in one area can lead to a surprising breakthrough in another, seemingly unrelated area. For example, technology, which originated from the US space program has been further developed and applied in many other areas of life. And one certainly cannot depend on government bureaucracies to make accurate assessments about these matters. Another problem is that, where one government might decide to ban the use of a new technology, another country may well go ahead with its introduction. In an increasingly competitive global economy the first country may severely disadvantage itself by such an action.

New technology is essential for a country's economic development. The best approach is to positively encourage the development of new technologies and to focus on their benefits. Any problems that may arise can be dealt with after implementation (279 words).

6 *The Speaking Component*

The IELTS speaking test takes between 11 and 14 minutes and is in the form of an oral interview between the candidate and an examiner. During the interview you will need to answer questions asked by the interviewer, speak at length on a topic selected by the interviewer and give and justify your opinions on a range of issues related to that topic.

The Interview has Three Main Parts

- Some general questions about yourself, your life and your interests.
- A short talk on a particular topic.
- A discussion of issues linked to the talk in Part 2.

It is important that you relax and speak as confidently as you can. Candidates who are not able to participate fully in the conversation may not achieve their potential band score. This may be because they haven't been able to demonstrate the level of language they are capable of producing.

How the Speaking Component is Assessed

The aim of the test is to assess your ability to communicate effectively. The interviewer considers this ability in four different ways:

- *Fluency and Coherence*

This measures your ability to speak without too many pauses and hesitations. It is also to do with how easily and clearly your ideas can be understood.

- *Lexical Resource*

This refers to your use of words and the range and accuracy of the vocabulary you choose to use. Not only how you select words but also how well you use them will be considered.

- *Grammatical Range and Accuracy*

The variety of grammar you use and how correctly you use it are both judged by the interviewer. So, the range of tenses as well as the appropriate use of them is important in all parts of the speaking test.

- *Pronunciation*

Here it is not only individual words but also the whole sentences, which are considered. The interviewer will be considering how easily he can understand what you are saying.

GENERAL TIPS

Tip 1

Part of the reason they start the speaking test with

'giving personal information' is to put students at their ease, so the examiner gets a chance to see what students are capable of during the test. Therefore, students should just relax and answer the questions as naturally as possible.

Tip 2

Students should not just provide one-word answers, but it is not necessary to stretch one question out to the whole 4 or 5 minutes either. Extended speaking is tested in Part 2 of the speaking paper. In other words, the answer to 'Do you have any brothers or sisters?' is not 'Yes', but it is not 'My eldest sister is 5 foot 2 inches tall and her birthday is 7 weeks after mine....' either. Again, be natural.

Tip 3

Students should remember that the different parts of the speaking test do not have separate marks, so it isn't the end of the world if they start slowly just as long as they have showed what they can do by the end of the test.

Tip 4

The examiner has had a long hard day, and is human too—so be interesting!

Tip 5

A good warmer, and practice for providing interesting extended answers to the questions, is getting students to ask their partners exactly the same question over and over again. Each time they answer the question, students should give a different response. For example:

A: 'Where are you from?'
B: 'Seaford.'
A: 'Where are you from?'
B: 'A small town on the south coast of England.'
A: 'Where are you from?'
B: 'A really boring place to grow up, etc.'

Tip 6

Another good practice activity for this is to have play the 'Don't answer yes or no' game. Basically, one student sits in front of the class and answers all the questions the other students ask them. If they say 'Yes' or 'No' at any time, they are out, and another student takes their place. The winning student is the one who stays there the longest.

Tip 7

A simpler warmer is just getting students to question each other in detail about a different one of the possible topics (e.g., 'your education') at the beginning of each lesson.

Tip 8

Getting students to concentrate on communicatively important things, such as keeping eye contact and not fidgeting, can help some students by taking their attention off the actual language they are using.

Tip 9

A range of times and tenses may come up in this part, and it is a good opportunity for students to show they can talk about the past, present and future as the topics are less demanding than in the other parts of the speaking exam.

THE INTERVIEW: PART 1

Task Description

Part 1 of the interview starts with an introduction in which the interviewer asks you basic questions about yourself and asks to see your identification. The interviewer will then go on to ask you further questions about yourself, your family/ hometown, your job or studies and a range of similar topic areas that are familiar to you. This section of the test lasts 4 to 5 minutes and in it you may need to give longer answers to questions to ensure you display your best ability.

What is Being Tested is Your Ability to:

- Provide full answers to all questions.
- Give longer responses to some questions.
- Give information by describing and explaining.

Sample Questions

The interviewer will ask for general information about topics such as the following:

- Your country of origin
- Your hometown
- How long you have lived there
- What you do: Work or study
- Your interests and future plans.

It is not possible to predict what topics may be discussed at this point in the interview; however, some familiar topics related to you or your country could include:

- Family and family relationships
- Modern and traditional lifestyles
- Traditional or modern buildings
- Tourism and tourist sites
- Celebrations and cultural activities
- Schooling and the education system
- City and country living.

The introductory section of the test will go something like this:

1. The interviewer greets the candidate and introduces him or herself.
2. The interviewer asks the candidate to state his or her name clearly for the cassette and confirms the candidate's country of origin.
3. The interviewer then asks to see the candidate's identification.

The remainder of part 1 of the test will follow this format:

1. The interviewer will ask the candidate set questions about his hometown or his occupation.
2. The interviewer will then ask set questions about a familiar topic of general interest.

3. He could ask three to five questions which will extend or develop this topic.
4. The interviewer may ask the candidate about more than one topic.

Typical questions for this stage of the test might be:

What is your name?
What country do you come from?
Describe your hometown to me.
Where do you live?
Tell me about your family members.
What are you studying?
What do you dislike most about your studies?
Do you like eating in restaurants? Why?
What type of transport do you use most? Why?
Where would you like to go on holidays? Why?
Tell me who you would most like to go on vacation with.

Strategies for Approaching the Task

- Carefully consider what you know about each of the topics above. Try to think of all the questions that someone who was trying to get to know you might ask, and make sure that you have all the vocabulary you need to discuss the topics in depth. Check and practice the pronunciation of any new vocabulary. Practice extending your answers to questions.
- You will perform better in the IELTS interview if your speech is fluent.

THE INTERVIEW: PART 2

Task Description

Part 2 is the long turn. The examiner will give you a card with prompts relating to a particular topic. These prompts are to help you prepare a short talk of 1 to 2 minutes. You will be given a minute to organise your thoughts and you can make some notes. The examiner will ask one or two follow-up questions to finish this part of the test. Part 2 will take three to four minutes, including the one-minute preparation for your talk.

What is Being Tested is Your Ability to
- Talk at length on a topic.
- Develop your ideas into a talk.
- Use grammar correctly and speak clearly.

Sample Topic
The examiner tells you your topic and gives you a card like this:

Long Turn Card
Describe a person from your youth who had a great influence on you:
You should say:
• Where you met him/her.
• What relationship this person was to you.
• What was special about him/her.
In addition, explain how his person influenced you so much.

Strategies for Approaching the Task
- Before the test, you need to practice talking about topics for one or two minutes, making notes appropriate to the topic beforehand, to help you. Record yourself and then play back the recording, listening to how clearly you are pronouncing and how well you select vocabulary.
- It is very important that you use examples from your own life. These you can speak about more easily than stories you have made up or read somewhere else. Try to relax and enjoy the experience of telling the interviewer as much interesting information about yourself as you can.
- You are likely to be more fluent if you have already thought about the topic and have some ideas to express.
- Before the test, prepare the language you will need in order to discuss topics like these. This doesn't mean memorising or rehearsing a speech because you can never be sure.
- You should also be prepared to use the past, present and present perfect tenses to describe your current situation. For example, 'I have

been studying English for two years since I moved to the city'.

THE INTERVIEW: PART 3
Task Description
After asking one or two follow-up questions the interviewer will lead you into an extended conversation discussing issues related to the Part 2 topic you spoke on. The interviewer will enlarge on things which were discussed in the second part of the test, possibly starting by asking you to describe something, then asking you to attempt something a little more difficult like comparing, evaluating or speculating; the questions will become a little more difficult as Part 3 proceeds.

Finally, the interviewer will conclude the Speaking test by simply saying something like:

"Thank you, that is the end of the Speaking test."

What is Being Tested is Your Ability to
- Give in-depth answers to questions about the topic.
- Use the language of description, comparison and speculation.
- Explain and justify your opinions, assumptions, predictions, reasons, etc.

Sample Questions
It is not possible to predict what questions will come up at this point in the test except that you can be sure that the topic will be related to your long turn topic. Some questions will arise naturally from the discussion and the information you are giving as this section progresses.

For example, consider the following sample topic:

Describe a piece of music that has had a big effect on you.

Possible related topics may be:
- *Music in society*
- *Cultural aspects of music*
- *Commercialization of music*

Thus, the interviewer may start the discussion on the first related topic (*Music in society*) by asking you to describe how music is important to everyday life in your country. After you have talked about this, the interviewer may ask you to compare the importance of music now with how it was when your grandparents were young; and then may even go on to ask what you think will be the effects of music on future societies.

Strategies for Approaching the Task

- Expose yourself to everyday topics as often discussed in newspapers or on radio and TV programmes. Make it your habit to read newspaper and magazine articles, particularly those that discuss issues and contain arguments and opinions. Also, listen to radio discussions like talk-back and watch interviews on current affairs programmes on the television.
- Not only does this give you some excellent listening practice, but also it will build your background knowledge for the issues that may come up in both the Speaking and the Writing tests.
- Choose an issue. Record all the vocabulary you will need to discuss that issue—note words raised in the news article or programmes (TV, radio, newspapers). Try to do one of these everyday. When you consider an issue, decide what would be your position on the issue, especially the steps you will need to take to reach your desired position and how you would overcome any possible problems in discussing it.
- Be prepared to use descriptive and comparative language, for example, in respect to the *Music in society* example given earlier: "In my country, traditional music plays a more important role in society than it seems to here, in Australia. It is played at important events like festivals and official ceremonies, as well as at special occasions such as weddings and funerals."

- Practice using conditional sentences to discuss, for instance, hypothetical issues from a broad or world view; for example: "If the world economy becomes more global, all nations will lose their cultural independence." *or*

  "If the leaders of the world were to spend more money on the poor, many of the problems of global conflict would be resolved."
- Be ready to use a good range of tenses and a variety of grammar, for instance, to speculate on what may be possible in the future. For example:

Interviewer: What future role do you see for music in society?

Candidate: Well, I'd (or I've) always hoped that all the peoples of the world could benefit by sharing their common experience of music. *or*

Candidate: If different cultures could see the common features of music in other countries, they may be less fearful of each other and understand one another's cultures better.

Be prepared to speculate about the future:

> *I hope that …*
> *It's possible that…*
> *I can see that …*
> *If possible, I'd like to see …*
> *We should plan to …*
> *It might be that …*
> *We can assume that …*
> *Probably, …*

SAMPLE TOPICS

- Your home
- The school you went to
- The role of sport today
- Public transport in your city
- A favourite object
- Your hobbies
- How would you improve the education system in your country?
- The importance of leisure activities in our lives

today—a culture comparison between your country and England
- The media as an invasion of privacy
- What you do in your spare time
- The future of communication systems
- Environmental problems of the third millennium
- Travel nowadays compared with travel in my grandparents' days
- A book you have read
- How you got here today
- Public transport versus private transport
- Your best friend
- The importance of friends.

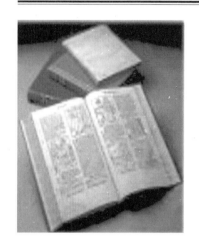

Section *Two*

PLAB Part 1—The EMQ's

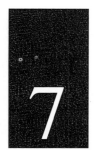

7 Introduction to the PLAB Part 1 Exam

> ◆ So, everybody knows that the Part 1 exam consists of 200 EMQ's! You will find in this chapter, however, the details concerning the format of the exam, the eligibility requirements, the syllabus, and guidelines on how to approach the exam.

ELIGIBILITY

Before a candidate enters the Examination, he or she must have obtained:

a. A primary medical qualification acceptable for limited registration.

b. The following scores in the IELTS test 1 (academic module), obtained a maximum of two years before the date on which the candidate takes the Examination:

1. A minimum overall band score of 7.0.
2. A minimum band score of 7.0 in the speaking section.
3. A minimum band score of 6.0 in each of the following sections: listening, academic reading and academic writing.

STANDARD OF THE EXAMINATION

A pass in the PLAB test will demonstrate that the successful candidate has the ability to practice safely as a senior house officer (SHO) in a first appointment in a UK hospital. This is the standard laid down by the General Medical Council for the PLAB test.

FORMAT OF THE EXAMINATION

Part 1 of the test consists of an Extended Matching Question (EMQ) Examination, referred to throughout this annex as the Examination. The Examination paper will contain 200 questions divided into a number of themes. It will last three hours.

Four groups of skills will be tested in approximately equal proportions:

Diagnosis

Given the important facts about a patient (such as age, sex, nature of presenting symptoms, duration of symptoms) you are asked to select the most likely diagnosis from a range of possibilities.

Investigations

This may refer to the selection or the interpretation of diagnostic tests. Given the important facts about a patient, you will be asked to select the investigation, which is most likely to provide the key to the diagnosis. Alternatively, you may be given the findings of investigations and asked to relate these to a patient's condition or to choose the most appropriate next course of action.

Management

Given the important facts about a patient's condition, you will be asked to choose from a range of possibilities the most suitable course of treatment. In the case of medical treatments, you will be asked to choose the correct drug therapy and will be expected to know about side effects.

The Context of Clinical Practice

This may include:

1. *Explanation of disease process:* The natural history of the untreated disease.
2. *Legal ethical:* You are expected to know the major legal and ethical principles set out in the General Medical Council publication *Good Medical Practice.*
3. *Practice of evidence-based medicine:* Questions on diagnosis, investigations and management may draw upon recent evidence published in peer-reviewed journals. In addition, there may be questions on the principles and practice of evidence-based medicine.
4. *Understanding of epidemiology:* You may be tested on the principles of epidemiology, and on the prevalence of important diseases in the UK.
5. *Health promotion:* The prevention of disease through health promotion and knowledge of risk factors.
6. *Awareness of multicultural society:* You may be tested on your appreciation of the impact on the practice of medicine of the health beliefs and cultural values of the major cultural groups represented in the UK population.
7. *Application of scientific understanding to medicine:* You may be tested on the scientific disciplines, which underpin medicine. Examples include anatomy, genetics and pathology.

CONTENT

The *content* to be tested is, for the most part, defined in terms of patient presentations. Where appropriate, the presentation may be either acute or chronic. Questions in the Examination will begin with a title, which specifies both the skill and the content, for example, the management of varicose veins.

You will be expected to know about conditions that are common or important in the United Kingdom for all the systems outlined below. Examples of the cases that may be asked about are given under each heading and may appear under more than one heading.

Accident and Emergency Medicine (to include trauma and burns)

Examples: Abdominal injuries, abdominal pain, back pain, bites and stings, breathlessness/ wheeze, bruising and purpura, burns, chest pain, collapse, coma, convulsions, diabetes, epilepsy, eye problems, fractures, dislocations, head injury, loss of consciousness, non-accidental injury, sprains and strains, testicular pain.

Blood (to include coagulation defects)

Examples: Anaemia's, bruising and purpura.

Cardiovascular System (to include heart and blood vessels and blood pressure)

Examples: Aortic aneurysm, chest pain, deep vein thrombosis (DVT), diagnosis and management of hypertension, heart failure, ischaemic limbs, myocardial infarction, myocardial ischaemia, stroke, varicose veins.

Dermatology, Allergy, Immunology and Infectious Diseases

Examples: Allergy, fever and rashes, influenza/ pneumonia, meningitis, skin cancers.

ENT and Eyes

Examples: Earache, hearing problems, hoarseness, difficulty in swallowing, glaucoma, 'red eyes', sudden visual loss.

Gastrointestinal Tract, Liver and Biliary System, and Nutrition

Examples: Abdominal pain, constipation,

diarrhoea, difficulty in swallowing, digestive disorders, gastrointestinal bleeding, jaundice, rectal bleeding/pain, vomiting, weight problems.

Metabolism, Endocrinology and Diabetes

Examples: Diabetes mellitus, thyroid disorders, weight problems.

Nervous System (both medical and surgical)

Examples: Coma, convulsions, dementia, epilepsy, eye problems, headache, loss of consciousness, vertigo.

Orthopaedics and Rheumatology

Examples: Back pain, fractures, dislocations, joint pain/swelling, sprains and strains.

Psychiatry (to include substance abuse)

Examples: Alcohol abuse, anxiety, assessing suicidal risk, dementia, depression, drug abuse, overdoses and self harm, panic attacks, post-natal problems.

Renal System (to include urinary tract and genitourinary medicine)

Examples: Haematuria, renal and ureteric calculi, renal failure, sexual health, testicular pain, urinary infections.

Reproductive System (to include obstetrics, gynaecology and breast)

Examples: Abortion/sterilization, breast lump, contraception, infertility, menstrual disorders, menopausal symptoms, normal pregnancy, post-natal problems, pregnancy complications, vaginal disorders; scrotal swelling, testicular pain, torsion of the testes.

Respiratory System

Examples: Asthma, breathlessness/wheeze, cough, haemoptysis, hoarseness, influenza/pneumonia.

Disorders of Childhood (to include non-accidental injury and child sexual abuse; fetal medicine; growth and development)

Examples: Abdominal pain, asthma, child development, childhood illnesses, earache, epilepsy, eye problems, fever and rashes, joint pain/swelling, loss of consciousness, meningitis, non-accidental injury, testicular pain, urinary disorders.

Disorders of the Elderly (to include palliative care)

Examples: Breathlessness, chest pain, constipation, dementia, depression, diabetes, diarrhoea, digestive disorders, headache, hearing problems, influenza/pneumonia, jaundice, joint pain/swelling, loss of consciousness, pain relief, terminal care, trauma, urinary disorders, vaginal disorders, varicose veins, vertigo, vomiting.

Peri-operative Management

Examples: Pain relief, shock, pre-operative assessment, post-operative management.

Please remember that this is just a list of examples. Other similar conditions may occur.

HOW TO APPROACH THE EXAMINATION

- The Examination paper will contain 200 questions in the extended matching format, divided into a number of themes.
- Each theme has a heading which tells you what the questions are about, in terms both of the clinical problem area, for example, chronic joint pain and the skill required, for example, diagnosis.
- Within each theme, there are several numbered items, usually between three and six. These are the questions—the problems you have to solve.

- Begin by reading carefully the instruction, which precedes the numbered items. The instruction is very similar throughout the paper and typically, reads *'For each patient described below, choose the SINGLE most discriminating investigation from the above list of options. Each option may be used once, more than once or not at all.*

- Consider each of the numbered items and decide what you think the answer is. You should then look for that answer in the list of options (each of which is identified by a letter of the alphabet). If you cannot find the answer you have thought of, you should look for the option, which, in your opinion, is the best answer to the problem posed.

- For each numbered item, you must choose ONE, and only one, of the options. You may feel that there are several possible answers to an item, but you must choose the one most likely from the option list. *If you enter more than one answer on the answersheet, you will gain no mark* for the question even though you may have given the right answer along with one or more wrong ones.

- In each theme there are more options than items, so not all the options will be used as answers. This is why the instruction says that some options may not be used at all.

- A given option may provide the answer to more than one item. For example, there might be two items, which contain descriptions of patients, and the most likely diagnosis could be the same in both instances. In this case, the option would be used more than once.

- You will be awarded one mark for each item answered correctly. Marks are not deducted for incorrect answers nor for failure to answer. The total score on the paper is the number of correct answers given. You should, therefore, attempt all items.

- Names of drugs are those contained in the most

recent edition of the British National Formulary.

- Some questions relate to current best practice. They should be answered in relation to published evidence and not according to your local arrangements. If necessary, you should take steps to familiarise yourself with the range of equipment routinely available in teaching hospitals.

- You will have two marksheets on the day—a purple one for questions 1 to 100 and a pink one for questions 101 to 200. Instructions on how to complete the marksheet are at the top of the first sheet.

ARRIVAL AT THE EXAMINATION

You must make your own arrangements for travel and accommodation. It is important that you ensure that, having been allocated a place in the Examination, you are not prevented from attending by factors such as your ability to obtain leave from employment, or the availability of transport, or visa or other immigration formalities.

DURATION OF THE EXAMINATION

The invigilator's instructions will take about 30 minutes. The Examination will last three hours and collecting the Examination materials will take a further fifteen minutes. You will be required to be at the Examination centre for a *minimum* of three and three-quarter hours. The letter offering you a place will tell you the time you should arrive at the Examination. If you arrive after the first half an hour of the Examination has passed, you will not be allowed to enter the Examination hall. You will not be permitted to leave the Examination hall in the first half hour or in the last half hour of the Examination.

PROOF OF IDENTITY

You must take proof of your identity to the Examination together with the letter from the General Medical Council or British Council offering you a place in the Examination. These will be checked at the Examination. The following are acceptable forms of identification. To be accepted, the identification document *must* bear your photograph.

- Your passport
- Your UK Immigration and Nationality Department identification document
- Your Home Office travel document
- Your UK driving license.

If the name on your identification document is different from that on the letter from the General Medical Council or British Council offering you a place in the examination, you *must* provide original evidence that you are the person named in that letter. The following will suffice as evidence:

- Your marriage certificate.
- A declaration from the awarding body which granted you your IELTS certificate or your primary medical qualification, stating that both names relate to you.

CONDUCT DURING THE EXAMINATION

You will be provided with all the materials you need during the Examination. You may not use or refer to any other materials. You should not write down details of questions to take out of the examination hall.

MARKING THE EXAMINATION

The Examination will be marked in the UK by computer.

Standard setting For the first sitting of the Examination, the Professional and Linguistic Assessments Board (PLAB) determined the standard required to pass in accordance with a recognized method of standard setting. This standard is maintained by test equating. This means that the standard for each examination will be the same, but the pass mark may vary, reflecting the difficulty of the questions set in the Examination.

NOTIFICATION OF RESULTS

At the end of the Examination, you will be told the date on which your results will be available. For Examinations held in the UK, results will be put in the post on that date. Results cannot be collected from the General Medical Council's offices. For Examinations held in all other countries, **you can collect your results on that date from the British Council office in the city where you took the Examination. Results not collected will be put in the post the following day.**

IF YOU PASS

If you pass the Examination you will be sent an application form and information pack for Part 2 of the test—the OSCE—together with your results. You can only take Part 2 of the test in the UK.

IF YOU FAIL

If you fail the Examination you may re-apply. The GMC will send you another application form with the letter informing you of your results.

FEEDBACK ON YOUR PERFORMANCE

Your results will include information about your position in relation to the pass mark and the performance of the other candidates.

8 Applying for the PLAB Part 1 Exam

> ◆ Includes help with completing the application form and details about the cancellation procedure and charges.

COMPLETING THE APPLICATION FORM

The following notes are intended to help you complete your application form.

Name

You should use the name you gave to the General Medical Council when you made your first enquiry.

If this name differs from:

- The name on your IELTS certificate;
- The name on the proof of identity you intend to use at the Examination;
- The name shown on your diploma or other evidence of qualification,

You will be required to provide *original* documentary evidence that the names on the different documents refer to you. IELTS result.

You must insert the date you took the IELTS test and the scores you obtained. If this is your first application in the country in which you wish to sit the Examination, you must enclose your original IELTS certificate. For subsequent attempts in that country, you need not enclose a certificate as the office will have kept a record from your first application.

Date on which you would Like to Take the Examination

Please choose your preferred centres and dates from the list. An up-to-date list can also be found at the GMC website: *www.gmc-uk.org*

Enclosures

Fees: The fee of £145 must be paid in advance in sterling. Personal callers to the General Medical Council's office in London may pay fees in cash. Otherwise, fees paid in the United Kingdom must be in the form of a cheque, money order or postal order payable to 'General Medical Council'. Fees sent from other countries, or paid in other countries, must be by sterling bank draft or money order. These must be made payable to 'General Medical Council'. Please remember, where appropriate, to take bank charges into account when paying the fee.

IELTS Certificate

If this is your first application in the country in which you wish to take the Examination, please enclose your IELTS certificate.

Do not enclose evidence of your primary qualification at this stage. This will be checked by the General Medical Council when you apply for limited registration.

Declaration

Please check the form carefully to ensure that the information is correct, and sign and date it. Then return it with the appropriate enclosures to the address at the end of the form.

Notification of a Place

Once your form has been processed, you will be sent a letter offering you a place in the Examination and a map showing you where the Examination centre is located. If there are no places available, they will write to you about other Examination dates.

Cancellation by a Candidate

If you want to cancel your place, please give the office, which offered you the place, as much notice as possible. You must return the letter offering you an Examination place. If you cancel early, the office may be able to offer your place to another candidate waiting to take the Examination. You may not pass the letter offering you a place to anyone else.

If you cancel your place, you will be charged a fee. This will normally be deducted from the fee you paid to enter the Examination. The amount charged depends on the amount of notice you give.

Cancellation Charges

The current cancellation charges are as follows:

UK Centres

Period of notice	*Cancellation charge*
Four months or more	£70
Between 21 days and four months	£100
Less than 21 days	£145

Overseas Centres

Period of notice	*Cancellation charge*
Before closing date	£20
After closing date	No refund

9 Review of Preparation Material for Part 1

> ◆ An arsenal of books is available for practicing the EMQ. You need not have all of them, but to select the best ones amongst the lot, we provide here, the compiled details of all available books. The books have been graded with respect to their content, accuracy of answers, presentation and cost.

EXTENDED MATCHING QUESTION (EMQ) BOOKS

1. PLAB—1000 Extended Matching Questions

Author	:	Una F. Coales
Publisher	:	Royal Society of Medicine Press
Edition	:	2000
Pages	:	282
EMQ's	:	1000
Price	:	£ 18.50 + postage
Order	:	www.amazon.co.uk
Content	:	✷ ✷ ✷
Presentation	:	✷ ✷ ✷ ✷ ✷
Accuracy	:	✷ ✷ ✷ ✷ ✷
Cost	:	✷

Though this book burns a hole in your pocket, it is still worth buying when you consider its excellence in terms of accuracy and presentation. The themes, although not divided into subjects encompass almost the entire gamut of themes. Simple but dependable information is provided for most of the answers.

2. PLAB Digest

Author	:	Atish Pratap Mathur
Publisher	:	Paras Medical Publishers
Edition	:	2002
Pages	:	740
EMQ's	:	3000
Price	:	INR 275
Order	:	Any Medical Bookshop
Content	:	✷ ✷ ✷ ✷ ✷
Presentation	:	✷ ✷ ✷
Accuracy	:	✷ ✷
Cost	:	✷ ✷ ✷ ✷

Exhaustive book wherein the themes have been well divided into various subjects. But there are quite a number of questions with ridiculous answers. Overall, a book that, if you have the corrected answers, will make you confident of doing well in the exam.

3. PLAB Plus

Author	:	Madhu Babu Paladugu
Publisher	:	Kalam Books
Edition	:	2002
Pages	:	740
EMQ's	:	1500
Price	:	INR 225
Order	:	Any Medical Bookshop
Content	:	✷ ✷ ✷ ✷
Presentation	:	✷ ✷ ✷ ✷
Accuracy	:	✷ ✷ ✷ ✷
Cost	:	✷ ✷ ✷ ✷

The themes and questions are essentially the same as those in PLAB Digest (though they are less in number), but the difference is that the answers are accompanied by detailed explanations and there are not many mistakes as in PLAB Digest. There is also a section on the themes and questions of a few past papers, and a table of useful laboratory values.

4. First Aid for PLAB

Author	:	Tyagi/Vidyarthi
Publisher	:	Jaypee/ Blackwell
Edition	:	2003
Pages	:	740
EMQ's	:	1000
Price	:	INR 690/ £ 27.99
Order	:	Any Medical Bookshop/amazon

Content	:	✱ ✱ ✱ ✱
Presentation	:	✱ ✱ ✱
Accuracy	:	✱ ✱
Cost	:	✱ ✱ ✱

A pretty good book to practice mocks after you have done with all the other books. It gives a thorough explanation of all the answers together with a note on the 'confusas' for each question. You may find some explanations unexplainable and irrelevant.

There is also a section on the so-called high-yield topics, such as drugs in pregnancy, medical ethics and fitness to drive, which are pretty useful.

5. Pastest Series

Author	:	J.Treml, Peter Krocker
Publisher	:	Pastest
Edition	:	2002
Pages	:	100
EMQ's	:	200 each
Price	:	£ 8 each + postage
Order	:	www.amazon.co.uk/ www.pastest.co.uk

Content	:	✱ ✱
Presentation	:	✱ ✱ ✱ ✱
Accuracy	:	✱ ✱ ✱ ✱ ✱
Cost	:	✱ ✱

This series of three books are essentially three mock tests with some very good explanations for the answers. A good book to buy if you don't mind spending the money.

6. EMQ's for PLAB

Author	:	Matthews
Publisher	:	India Book House Limited/ Science
Edition	:	2000
Pages	:	220
EMQ's	:	500
Price	:	INR 170/ £ 10 + postage
Order	:	Any Medical Bookshop

Content	:	✱ ✱
Presentation	:	✱ ✱ ✱
Accuracy	:	✱ ✱ ✱
Cost	:	✱ ✱ ✱ ✱

This book will only be an adjunct to your other EMQ books. You can read it when you are tired of reading the other bulky books. One-line explanations for a few answers are not particularly impressive. This book is quite difficult to procure in India.

7. EMQ's for PLAB

Author	:	Henry Mokbel
Publisher	:	Petroc Press
Edition	:	1999
EMQ's	:	600
Price	:	£ 10 + postage
Order	:	www.amazon.com

Content	:	✱ ✱ ✱
Presentation	:	✱ ✱ ✱
Accuracy	:	✱ ✱ ✱
Cost	:	✱ ✱ ✱

I would recommend this book when you have mastered the other books like PLAB Digest and

PLAB Plus. It contains themes, which you would not have encountered before, and some of them are very difficult. Again, this is a book which is hard to find in India.

8. Fischtest PLAB Journal

Edition	:	2000
Pages	:	740
EMQ's	:	750
Price	:	£ 35
Order	:	www.fischtest.co.uk
Content	:	✶ ✶ ✶
Presentation	:	✶ ✶ ✶
Accuracy	:	✶ ✶ ✶
Cost	:	✶ ✶

By far, the costliest of all the books for PLAB, this book is actually designed to accompany the Fischtest Part—1 course. Otherwise, having just 750 **EMQ's**, it is not worth the **price**.

9. Recent Manual of PLAB

Author	:	Nitin Maheshwari
Publisher	:	Jaypee Brothers/ Blackwell
Edition	:	2002
Pages	:	600
EMQ's	:	1500
Price	:	INR 230/ £ 11 + postage
Order	:	Any Medical Bookshop, www.amazon.co.uk
Content	:	✶ ✶ ✶ ✶
Presentation	:	✶ ✶ ✶
Accuracy	:	✶ ✶ ✶
Cost	:	✶ ✶ ✶ ✶

This book too will provide you with some different supplementary **EMQ's** packed in very little space. It also provides you an insight into the PLAB exam and contains some useful information on PLAB Part 2 as well. All in all, a good buy!

10. Plab Made Easy

Author	:	Parveen Babu

Publisher	:	Jaypee Brothers/ Blackwell
Edition	:	2001
Pages	:	400
EMQ's	:	1000
Price	:	INR 180/ £ 11 + postage
Order	:	Any Medical Bookshop/ www.amazon.co.uk
Content	:	✶ ✶ ✶
Presentation	:	✶ ✶ ✶
Accuracy	:	✶ ✶ ✶
Cost	:	✶ ✶ ✶ ✶

If you have this book, you don't need to buy the Fischtest journal. Almost all the questions from the journal are incorporated here with some additional EMQ's.

11. RXPG EMQ Digest for PLAB Part 1

Author	:	Himanshu Tyagi/Vidyarthi
Publisher	:	Paras Medical Publishers
Edition	:	2003
Pages	:	740
EMQ's	:	2500
Price	:	INR 266
Order	:	Any Medical Bookshop
Content	:	✶ ✶ ✶ ✶
Presentation	:	✶ ✶ ✶ ✶
Accuracy	:	✶ ✶ ✶ ✶
Cost	:	✶ ✶ ✶ ✶

A very recently published book, it is based on the sequence of chapters in the Oxford handbooks and for almost all questions, the relevant page in Oxford is mentioned.

12. MCQ's for the PLAB

Author	:	Kavita Dutta
Publisher	:	Butterworth Heinmann
Edition	:	1998
Price	:	INR 212
Order	:	Any Medical Bookshop

13. Handbook of PLAB

Author	:	Kunal Goyal
Publisher	:	Jaypee/ Blackwell

Edition	:	2001
EMQ's	:	3000
Price	:	INR 248/ £ 10 + postage
Order	:	Any Medical Bookshop, www.amazon.co.uk

14. 4000 EMQ's for PLAB
Author	:	U.N.Panda
Publisher	:	All India Traveller BK Seller AITBS
Edition	:	2000
Price	:	Rs. 135
Order	:	Any Medical Bookshop

15. PLAB Basics
Author	:	Ranjeetha Bakashi
Publisher	:	Paras Medical Publisher
Edition	:	2003
Price	:	INR 405
Order	:	Any Medical Bookshop

16. Extended Matching Questions for the PLAB—Medicbyte Series
Author	:	Asrar Rashid
Publisher	:	Medicbyte series
Edition	:	2002
Price	:	£ 32 each + postage
Order	:	www.amazon.co.uk

17. The Complete PLAB EMQ's
Author	:	Afzal Mir
Publisher	:	Churchill Livingstone
Edition	:	2004
EMQ's	:	1000
Price	:	£ 20 + postage
Order	:	www.amazon.co.uk

18. Passing PLAB Part 1: A Self Assessment Workbook
Author	:	Peter Kabunga
Publisher	:	Radcliffe Medical Press
Edition	:	2003
EMQ's	:	1250

Price	:	£ 25 + postage
Order	:	www.amazon.co.uk

OTHER RECOMMENDED READING FOR PART 1
1. Oxford Handbook of Clinical Medicine
2. Oxford Handbook of Clinical Specialities
3. Oxford Handbook of Acute Medicine
4. Clinical Medicine—Kumar and Clark
5. ECG made easy—John Hampton
6. Lecture notes in Orthopedics
7. Lecture notes in Emergency Medicine
8. Lecture notes in Surgery
9. Lecture notes in Ophthalmology
10. Lecture notes in Obstetrics and Gynaecology
11. Lecture notes in Psychiatry.

RECOMMENDED WEBSITES FOR PART 1
1. www.mcqs.com.

   This website provides more than 1000 **EMQ's** with detailed explanations. Though some of the questions are not anything close to what would be asked in the exam, this site is worth $ 38. The forums on this site have been very popular and going through these you can find:
   - A number of EMQ's
   - Past papers with conflicting answers
   - Views of others regarding the exam
   - Information about UK
   - Second-hand books for sale in your country
   - Review of books and courses
   - A little of nonsense!

2. www.onexamination.com

   Contains more than 1000 'difficult' EMQ's with very satisfying explanations. Costs about £ 35.

3. www.7plus7.com.

   Contains one free + seven paid mocks without explanation.

4. www.rxpg.com.

   Contains forums which could prove useful for discussion.

10 *Courses for PLAB Part 1*

> ◆ There are not many courses available for preparation for the part one exam, at least not as many as for the OSCE. I have highlighted here the important aspects of the more popular courses in India as well as in UK.

1. MEDICBYTE PLAB 1 HOME STUDY COURSE

About the Course

The course is online and is supplemented by Medicbyte PLAB specimen papers.

You will meet tutors online who are fully registered UK doctors.

If you invest in the home study course, you get all three PLAB part one books with CDROM and the online PLAB course tutor sessions. EXTRA questions will be sent to you to discuss with the tutor to ensure you are on the right learning tract. The total investment you will need to make is £300 (ex vat). On payment the question papers are sent to you and dates are arranged for the online tutoring.

What the Course Covers

* Specimen papers that cover important concepts.
* Technique is emphasised.
* The PLAB 1 examination is emulated so that you are ready for the examination.
* The course will be over four weeks.
  For further information
  Email: courses@medicbyte.com

2. MEDICBYTE PLAB-1 COURSE AT HYDERABAD

Medicbyte also conducts one-week courses at its laboratory in India. The normal course duration is two weeks, but for outstation doctors they allow extra hours for Centre access, so that they complete the course in one week.

Excellent hostel accommodation with good food can be arranged very reasonably, at a location convenient to you for Centre access.

Contact them at www.medicbyte.com
Tel: 91-40-682 5867 / 91-40-682 5868
Mobile: 98491 63751

3. PLAB-1 COURSE BY VISHWA MEDICALS

The PLAB Part I Intensive Revision Course is conducted in India. Those who have attended the course in the past have found the course helpful. Above all, the results of the past course candidates have been very encouraging. These courses are conducted in Mumbai, Bangalore and Delhi and last for four days.

TEACHING AIDS INCLUDE

* Past exam question revision
* Group Discussions
* CD-ROM's
* Videocassettes
* Mock exam
* Online discussions with UK faculty.

The course fee is INR 6000/- (including accommodation)—*All the candidates are eligible for a free stay and an access to the library for five days before the exams only in Mumbai.*

For further information look up:
www.vishwamedical.com

4. PLABMASTER WORKSHOP IN INDIA

During this workshop, there would be an elaborate discussion on the important topics in Medicine, Surgery, Obs/Gyn. etc., repeatedly stressed upon in PLAB.

Dr. Mahadeo Bhide who has been coaching students for PLAB in the U.K. for past five years would be here to guide you and explain the nuances of the exam. Your queries on job opportunities in the U.K., prospects after the PLAB, lodging and boarding in the U.K. etc., will also be answered.

For further information contact:
Y.B.E.S., 4, "Neelkamal", Near "Daya Kshama Shanti", Bhaskar Colony, S.V. Road, Naupada, Thane (W) - 400 602.

Website: www.plabmaster.com

5. MEDVARSITY PLAB 1 COURSE AT HYDERABAD

This is a 15-day course, which costs Rs.7000/-.

The EMQs and Clinical situation discussions.

- Over 1000 EMQs as tests and discussion.
- All subjects covered for Part-1.
- Daily Mock Test based on PLAB master / Past test series pattern.
- Clinical cases based discussion.
- Technique of answering EMQs.
- Counselling by doctors who have worked in the UK.

For further details, please contact:
www.medvarsity.com

PLAB PART 1 COURSES IN UK

1. The PLAB Course

Outline of Programme, Fees, and Prices

1. Revision day   £45, one full day before your exam
2. Weekend course   £145, Saturday, Sunday, and a Revision day.
3. One-week course £295, Monday through Friday, plus Revision day, plus Guarantee
4. Past papers   £30 for three of my past papers
5. Individual assessment   £45, one full day by appointment

Contact: info@plab.co.uk
7 Arundel Place, Islington
London N1 1LS
Tel : +44 (0) 207 607 3165
+44 (0) 207 700 0969

2. PLABMASTER Course

Costs of the Course: £335+17.5% VAT (i.e. UK Gov.Tax) = £394

If you pay upfront, you pay only £335 (you save £59, we pay the VAT)

If you wish to pay part payment *only if you have all the documents:* Reg.= £100chq. payable to **"PLABMASTER"**

a. Photocopy of the admit card.
b. Photocopy of the first 4 pages of the passport.
c. Photocopy of the Degree certificate.
d. 2 passport size photos.
e. You sign contract in the UK and pay remaining amount = £319 when you pass.

Contact: 1st Floor, 2A Burges Road, EastHam, London E6 2BH

3. Pastest PLAB Part 1 Course

Course material includes EMQs with answers and

teaching notes, an EMQ examination, tips on examination technique, detailed lecture notes for each subject and a recommended reading list.

You will receive a MOCK EMQ Examination prior to the start of the course to give you maximum practice before you arrive.

Cost: £ 630 for 5 days course.

Contact: PasTest, Egerton Court, Parkgate Estate, Knutsford, WA16 8DX

4. The Fischtest Course

This is an intensive EMQ-based weekend course covering all the subject areas candidates are expected to know.

Subject Areas

- General Medicine
- Obstetrics and Gynaecology
- Paediatrics and Child Health
- Psychiatry
- Pharmacology
- Surgery
- Ethics of Medicine
- Emergency Medicine.

In Addition

All course participants are given a:
- Pre-course practice EMQ exam;
- Technique and tactics session;
- Practice questions to take home.

Course Fee

Either:

£300.00 (includes tuition, course File, lunch and refreshments) full payment before the course; or:

£100 (includes tuition, course File, sandwich lunch and refreshments) part payment before the course, then £400 payable within the first month of employment as Doctors within the UK (total cost £500).

Contact:

Fischtest Ltd
7 Miller House
Westgreen Road
London
N15 3DR
United Kingdom
Tel: 0870 429 4739

5.   North Central London College PLAB Course

Contact:

67, Elliot Road
Hendon,
London NW4 3 EB
Tel: 0208 457 3962/ 0796 105 3077

11 Revision Aid for PLAB Part 1

◆ *During my preparation for the Part 1, I always felt the need for a book, which could convey to me 'THE' investigation of choice, 'THE' definitive investigation and/or management for a particular condition. In this chapter, I have tried to provide you with the same. Where there is just one investigation/management mentioned, it is 'THE' definitive investigation/management for that condition. If more than one is mentioned, the one mentioned before is 'THE' first investigation/management.*

RESPIRATORY SYSTEM

Disease	Clinical Features	Investigation	Management
Bronchiectasis	Cough with copious purulent sputum, haemoptysis.	CXR Def: CT chest	Postural Drainage, antibiotics, bronchodilators
Pneumonia	Fever, rigours, malaise, cough, Rusty sputum, chest pain	CXR Sputum for M & C	Oxygen antibiotics IV fluids
Lung abscess	Swinging fever, cough, foul smelling purulent sputum, pain	CXR Bronchoscopy for specimens	Antibiotics for 4-6 weeks, postural drainage
Pleural effusion	Fever, breathlessness, chest pain on insp, O/E—Abs BS ↑ Hemithorax, ↓ movements,	CXR Def: Pleural Aspiration	Underlying condition, pleural drainage
Empyema	Like lung abscess with high fever	CXR, Def: Aspiration	Cefuroxime + Metronidazole, drainage
Pneumothorax	Sudden breathlessness, chest pain, O/E—Abs BS, Hyper-resonant, ↑ hemithorax	CXR after needle thoracocentesis	Needle thoracocentesis, underwater drainage
Acute bronchitis	Cough initially unproductive, chest tightness, dyspnoea, O/E—Wheeze/ Creps	Neutrophil Leucocytosis	Respond spontaneously or Amoxicillin 250 mg TID
Chronic bronchitis	Morning productive cough, wheeze, dyspnoea, smoker, O/E –rhonchi/creps	Def: Lung function tests, ABG	Bronchodilators, steroids if FEV1 >15% improvement
Emphysema	Exertional dyspnoea, wheeze, smoker, O/E—barrel chest, rhonchi/creps	CXR Def: Lung function	Bronchodilators, steroids as above, surgery
Obstructive sleep apnea	Snoring, daytime sleepiness, restless sleep	24 hour Oximetry polysomnographic studies—Def	CPAP

Contd...

Contd...

Disease	Clinical Features	Investigation	Management
Cystic fibrosis	Recurrent RTI, clubbing, polyps, breathlessness, pancreatic, GI and skeletal	Sweat chloride test Def: Blood DNA analysis	Antibiotics, human DNase Gene therapy
Bronchial asthma	Nocturnal cough, wheezing and episodic dyspnoea, family history, O/E—rhonchi	Bronchodilator/ steroid trial, PEFR, histamine provocation trial	See later
Acute severe asthma	RR> 25/min, tachycardia >110, PEFR< 50 % normal, silent chest, cyanosis	Def: PEFR	Nebulised dilators, Hydrocortisone Prednisolone
Tuberculosis	Low grade fever, night sweats, cough O/E—varied	CXR, Def: Sputum for M and C	Rifampicin, Ethambutol, INH, Pyrazinamide
Sarcoidosis	Dull chest pain, fever, malaise, dyspnoea, skin, eye and bone inv	Serum ACE Def: Transbronchial biopsy	Spontaneous recovery or Prednisolone
Wegener's granulamatosis	Rhinorrhoea, haemoptysis and kidney involvement	Transbronchial biopsy, ANCA positive, Anti-GBM antibodies	Cyclophosphamide, Prednisolone
Churg-Strauss syndrome	Rhinitis, asthma, eosinophilia and systemic vasculitis	ANCA positive	Prednisolone
Allergic bronchop'nary aspergillosis	Episodes of wheeze, cough and fever, firm plugs	CXR Sputum— Mycelia High IgE	Prednisolone and itraconazole
Tropical pulmonary eosinophilia	Cough, wheeze, fever, lassitude, weight loss	CXR—hazy mottling, High Eosinophil	DEC
Goodpasture's syndrome	Haemoptysis, URTI, glomerulonephritis, anaemia	CXR Anti-GBM antibodies	Prednisolone, plasmapheresis
Cryptogenic fibrosing alveolitis	Breathlessness, cyanosis, O/E– clubbing, insp creps Acute– Hamman Rich syn	CT scan Def: Biopsy	Prednisolone, Azathioprine, Cyclophosphamide
Extrinsic allergic alveolitis	Cough, fever and malaise after exposure. O/E—Tachypnoea, wheeze, creps, cyanosis	Lung function tests, bronchoalveolar lavage	Prednisolone
Pneumoconiosis	Dry cough, black sputum, breathlessness	CXR Lung function tests	Symptomatic
Bronchogenic carcinoma	Cough, breathlessness, chest pain, haemoptysis, malaise, clubbing, consolidation EP manifestations	CT scan Def : Fibreoptic bronchoscopy	Small cell—chemotherapy, non-small cell-surgery

NEPHROLOGY

Disease	Clinical Features	Investigation	Management
Nephrotic syndrome	Facial puffiness, leg oedema, frothy urine.	24-hr urinary protein, serum albumin	Sodium restrictions, thiazides, treat the cause.
Nephritic syndrome	Post-streptococcal infection, hypertension, oedema, oliguria, haematuria, uremia	Anti-streptrolysin titre, renal biopsy	Salt/fluid restriction, frusemide, penicillin
Haemolytic uremic syndrome	Following viral infection, pallor, bleeding and renal failure, affects children	CBC Schistocytes on blood film	Heparin, platelet aggregation inhibitors, fresh frozen plasma
TTP	Young adults, fever, anaemia fluctuating CNS signs, thrombosytopenia, ARF	CBC	Fresh frozen plasma, platelet infusion, steroids
Cholesterol emboli	In arteriopathy–eosinophilia, livido reticularis, GI bleeding, purpura, myalgia	Cholesterol clefts seen in renal biopsies	Statins
Pyelonephritis	Fever, rigours, vomiting, loin pain and tenderness	MSU for microscopy– casts, USG abdomen	Cefuroxime
Cystitis	Frequency, dysuria, urgency, strangury, suprapubic pain	MSU	Trimethoprim
Prostatitis	Flu-like symptoms, low back ache, few urinary symptoms, swollen and tender prostate	MSU	Ciprofloxacin
Renal TB	Fever, night sweats, frequency dysuria and haematuria, epididymal discomfort	Sterile pyuria IVU	ATT
Acute interstitial nephritis	Fever, arthralgia, skin rashes, renal failure	Eosinophilia, renal biopsy	Withdraw offending drugs, steroids
Renal artery stenosis	Hypertension, renal failure	Spiral CT, MRI Definitive: renal arteriography	Transluminal angioplasty and stent insertion
Renal vein thrombosis	Loin pain, haematuria, proteinuria, renal enlargement, renal failure	Doppler USG, renal angiogram	Warfarin, Streptokinase to lyse acute thrombosis
Ureteric calculi	Loin pain radiating to groin, nausea, vomiting, restlessness	KUB, USG, IVU if haematuria	<5 mm – expectant < 2 cm–lithotripsy Diclofenac, antibiotics
Retroperitoneal fibrosis	Backache, hypertension, palpable kidney, oedema	USG	Retrograde stent placement, steroids
ARF	Features of cause, anorexia, nausea, vomiting, pruritis, drowsiness, fits, coma	Blood urea and creatinine	Manage hyperkalemia and pulmonary oedema (dialysis), cause
Bladder calculi	Pain on micturition, strangury, infection	KUB, USG	Endoscopic lithotripsy or open surgery
CRF	Nocturia, itching, parasthesia, anaemia, hypertension	Blood urea and creatinine, USG	Control complications, renal replacement

Contd...

Contd...

Disease	Clinical Features	Investigation	Management
Polycystic kidney	Hypertension, loin pain, haematuria, SAH, uremia	USG, CT	Surgery, control BP
Medullary sponge kidney	Renal colic, haematuria, skeletal abnormalities	IVU	Manage renal failure
RCC	Haematuria, loin pain and mass in flank	IVU	Nephrectomy
Wilms' tumour	< 3 years, abdominal mass, hematuria	IVU	Nephrectomy, radiotherapy, chemo
BPH	Frequency, urgency, hesitancy, terminal dribbling	USG	TURP
Ca Prostate	As BPH + haematuria + wt.loss	USG, biopsy PSA	Surgery
Ca Bladder	Painless hematuria, wt.loss, symptoms of obstruction	Urine for cytology, IVU	Local cystodiathermy and/or resection
Ca Testis	Swelling–painless or painful, lymph nodes, metastasis	CT	Chemo/ surgery/radio for seminomas

ENDOCRINOLOGY

Disease	Clinical Features	Investigation	Management
Hypogonadism–male	Impotence, poor libido, loss of secondary sexual hair	Testosterone, LH, FSH, pituitary MRI	Androgens, LH/FSH
Hypogonadism–female	Amenorrhoea/oligomenorrhoea, loss of libido, loss of pubic hair	FSH, LH, oestrogen and prolactin	Treat the cause
Hyperprolactinaemia	Galactorrhoea, subfertility oligo/amenorrhoea, decreased libido, headache, vision defect	MRI pituitary, prolactin	Bromocriptine, transphenoidal surgery
PCOS	Oligo/Amenorrhoea, hirsuitism, obesity, diabetes	Increased LH/FSH, ovarian USG	Clomiphine, steroids, oestrogens
Acromegaly	Change in appearance, large tongue, spade-like hands and feet, interdental separation	GTT	Transphenoidal surgery, octreotide
Hyperthyroidism	Weight loss, diarrhoea, goitre, tremor, tachycardia, heat intolerance, exophthalmos	T3 and TSH	Antithyroid drugs, radioiodine surgery
Hypothyroidism	Weight gain, decreased appetite, peaches and cream complexion, bradycardia, cold intolerance, menstrual disturbances	T4 and TSH	Throxine
Hashimoto's thyroiditis	Goitre, firm and rubbery	Thyroid microsomal Ab	Thyroxine
Thyroid CA	Goitre, hoarseness of voice, weight loss, secondaries	FNAC	Surgery

Contd...

Contd...

Disease	Clinical Features	Investigation	Management
De Quervain's thyroiditis	Fever, malaise, pain, tachycardia, thyroid tenderness	ESR, thyroid scan	Aspirin, prednisolone
Addison's disease	Weakness, weight loss, hypoglycaemia, pigmentation, postural hypotension, vitiligo	Synacthen or short ACTH stimulation test	Prednisolone and fludrcortisone
Cushing's syndrome	Weight gain, amenorrhoea, acne, hypertension, striae, buffalo hump, moon face	48 hr low-dose dexamethasone suppression test	Surgery, metyrapone
Cong. adrenal hyperplasia	Fused labia, enlarged clitoris, collapse, hypotension, hirsuite	ACTH	Glucorticoid, Mineralocorticoid
Diabetes insipidus	Polyuria, nocturia, polydipsia	Water deprivation test	Desmopressin
SIADH	Confusion, nausea, irritability, coma, no oedema	Low plasma osmolality, plasma sodium	Fluid restriction, Demethylchlor–tetracycline
Conn's syndrome	Hypokalemia, hypertension, muscle weakness and nocturia	Plasma aldosterone, rennin	Surgery, Spirinolactone
Pheochromo-cytoma	Panic attacks, palpitation, tremour, constipation, diarrhoea hypertension, sweating	Urinary VMA	β-blockade preceded by α-blockade

RHEUMATOLOGY

Disease	Clinical Features	Investigation	Management
Rheumatoid arthritis	Involves small joints of hands (PIP) symmetrically, early morning stiffness, tender joints with swelling, characteristic deformities and EA features	RA factor X-ray	NSAID's, DMARD's such as gold, sulphasalazine, methotrexate
Osteoarthritis	Involves large joints and DIP joints, joint pain, worse in evening, joint gelling and instability, crepitus	X-ray	Paracetamol, NSAID's, joint replacement
Ankylosing spondylitis	Teenagers, pain in buttock and lower back, fixed flexion deformity of hip, uveitis.	X-ray –bamboo spine, syndesmophytes HLA studies– B27	NSAID's
Psoriatic arthritis	DIP involved, onycholysis, sausage finger, cutaneous lesion	X-ray – pencil in cup appearance	NSAID's, steroid injections
Reactive arthritis	Preceding diarrhoea, burning micturition, acute asymmetrical	Stool culture	NSAID's and steroids
Reiter's–arthritis, urethritis and conjunctivitis	Lower limb arthritis, Achilles tendonitis, circinate balanitis, keratoderma blenorrhagica, conjunctivitis.		

Contd...

Contd...

Disease	Clinical Features	Investigation	Management
Gout	Acute onset of severe monoarticular pain– MTP joint, history of diuretic use or alcohol	Joint fluid—needle shaped positively birefringent	Ibuprofen Colchicine Allopurinol
Pseudogout	History of chronic inflammation or disease–presentation usually with U/L knee pain	Joint fluid–Rhomboidal –ve/ weakly birefringent	NSAID's Colchicine
SLE	Butterfly rash, Raynaud's, small joint arthritis, anaemia, glomerulonephritis	Anti-Ds DNA	Steroids, immunosuppressive drugs
Antiphospho-lipid syndrome	Arterial, venous thrombosis, abortions, livedo reticularis	Anti-cardiolipin antibodies	Aspirin, warfarin
Systemic sclerosis–limited, also known as CREST	Calcinosis, Raynaud's, oesophageal involvement, sclerdactyly, telangectasia, beak nose, microstomia	Anti-centromere antibodies	Steroids, immunosuppressive drugs
Systemic sclerosis–diffuse	Features similar to CREST but skin changes appearing before Raynaud's	Anti-topoisomerase antibodies	Steroids, immuno-suppressive drugs
Polymyositis	Proximal muscle weakness, fever, malaise, weight loss	Electromyography, CPK	Steroids, immuno-suppressive drugs
Dermatomyositis	Purple heliotrope rash, Collodion patch	Electromyography, CPK	Steroids, immuno-suppressive drugs
Primary Sjögren's syndrome	Keratoconjunctivitis sicca, dry mouth, skin, vagina, no associated autoimmune disease	Schirmer tear test	Artificial tears and salivary replacement
Polymyalgia rheumatica	> 50 yrs, pain and stiffness of shoulders, hip, neck	ESR	Steroids
Giant cell arteritis	Headache, scalp tenderness, jaw claudication	ESR, temporal artery biopsy	Steroids
Takayasu's arteritis	Pulseless disease- Absent peripheral pulses, hypertension, ↓ vision, syncope –young females	Biopsy	Steroids
PAN	Abdominal pain, GI h'ge, hypertension, MI, subcutaneous nodules	Aortography, ESR	Prednisolone
Kawasaki's disease	< 5 yrs, fever, conjunctival conges-tion, red palms and soles cervical lymphadenopathy	Clinical	IV Gamma globulin
Behcet's disease	Triad of genital ulcers, eye and skin lesions	Pathergy test	Immunosuppressive agents, Steroids
HSP	Purpura on buttocks, extensor surfaces, nephritis, abdominal pain	Renal biopsy	Steroids

Contd...

Contd...

Disease	Clinical Features	Investigation	Management
Hypertrophic pulmonary osteoarthropathy	Pain, swelling in wrists and ankles, last stage of clubbing, associated with Ca bronchus	X-ray	Treat cause
Osteoporosis	Pathological fractures in post-menopausal women	Bone scan	HRT, Bisphosphonates
Rickets/ Osteomalacia	Muscle or bone pain, proximal myopathy	Biochemical and radiological	Vitamin D
Paget's disease	Pain and enlargement of skull, clavicle femur, sabre tibia, nerve deafness, pathological fractures	Alkaline phosphatase	Calcitonin, Di sodium Etidronate
Hypercalcemia	Bones, stones, groans and psychic moans, polyuria. polydipsia, hypertension	Investigate cause	Rehydration, Bisphosphonates
Hypocalcemia	Tetany, depression, carpo pedal spasm, Trousseau's and Chvostek's signs	Investigate cause	Calcium supplements
Osteomyelitis	Painful, warm and tender affected part	MRI	Antibiotics, Immobilisation
Osteopetrosis	Brittle bones, anaemia, deafness, thrombocytopenia, optic atrophy	Acid phosphatase	No treatment

DERMATOLOGY

Disease	Clinical Features	Investigation	Management
Impetigo	Weeping exudative areas, honey coloured crusts	Skin swab	Antibiotics- Flucloxacillin
Cellulitis	Hot tender confluent erythema of skin	Streptococcal titres	Penicillin, Erythromycin
Boils	Deep seated painful red swellings	Clinical	Antibiotics, Antiseptics, I & D
Hidradenitis Suppurativa	Painful discharging chronic inflammation of axilla, groin	Clinical	Antibiotics, oral retinoids
Herpes Zoster	Prodrome of tingling followed by painful, tender blistering rash in dermatomal fashion	Clinical	Analgesia, Acyclovir
Viral Warts	Papular lesions with coarse surface	Clinical	Cryo, Cautery, Keratolytics
Molluscum contagiosum	Small multiple translucent umbili-cated papules	Clinical	No treatment
Tinea	Itchy asymmetrical scaly patches with central clearing	KOH mount	Miconazole, Clotrimazole
Pityrosporum	Hypo or hyper pigmented scaly macules	Skin scrapings or Wood's light	Selinium sulphide
Scabies	Itchy red papules in Circle of Hebra, Burrows	KOH mount	Malathion, Permethrin

Contd...

Contd...

Disease	Clinical Features	Investigation	Management
Eczema	Itchy erythematous scaly patches in flexures	Clinical, RAST	Topical steroids, emollients, antibiotics, antihistaminics
Psoriasis	Pinkish silvery plaques on extensor surfaces, nail changes	Clinical	PUVA, Tar, Calcipotriol, Topical steroids
Pityriasis rosea	Herald parch, Oval pink macules with scaly collar	Clinical	No treatment
Lichen planus	Purple polygonal pruritic papules, Wickham's striae	Clinical	Topical steroids
Pemphigus vulgaris	Mucosal involvement, flaccid blisters, Nikolsky's sign, Intercellular Ig G deposition	Skin biopsy	Oral steroids, Immunosuppressants
Bullous pemphigoid	Large tense blisters, itchy, Ig G deposition in basement membrane	Skin biopsy	Prednisolone, Azathioprine

OPHTHALMOLOGY

Disease	Clinical Features	Investigation	Management
Chalazion	Residual swelling of Hordeolum internum, point inwards, opens on to conjunctiva	Clinical	Incision and curretage, fusidic acid
Blepharitis	Burning itchy red eyelid margins, scales	Clinical	Saline bathing, fusidic acid
Dendritic ulcers	Photophobia, epiphora	1% fluorescein drop stains the lesion	Aciclovir ointment
Keratocon-junctivitis sicca	Dry eye	Schirmer's test	Artificial tears
Orbital cellulitis	Fever, eyelid swelling, proptosis, immobility of eye	Clinical	Cefuroxime IV
Carotico-cavernous fistula	Engorged blood vessels, edema of lids and conjunctiva		Carotid ligation or spontaneous resolution
Acute glaucoma	Uniocular Pain, nausea, haloes around lights, ↓ vision, circumcorneal redness, ovoid fixed dilated pupil	Clinical + IOP measurement	Pilocarpine + Acetozolamide
Acute iritis	Photophobia, blurred vision, lacrimation, ciliary congestion, small irregular pupil	Slit-lamp, Talbot's test	Steroids with cyclopentolate
Ulcerative keratitis	Pain, photophobia, blurred vision	Fluorescein drops in bright light, diagnostic smear	Antibiotics

Contd...

Contd...

Disease	Clinical Features	Investigation	Management
Episcleritis	Inflammatory nodule, sclera may look blue under the engorged vessels, which can be moved over the area	Clinical	Steroid drops
Scleritis	Oedema of conjunctiva, thinning of sclera, vessels cannot be moved	Clinical	Steroid drops
Conjunctivitis	Itch, burn and lacrimation, red conjunctiva, vision, pupil, cornea N	Conjunctival swab	Antibiotics
Subconjuncti-val H'ge	Red eye	Clinical	No treatment
CRAO	Sudden loss of vision, RAPD	Fundoscopy–pale with cherry red spot	Globe pressure
CRVO	Sudden loss of vision	Fundoscopy– stormy sunset, Fluorescein angiography	No treatment
Vitreous H'ge	Visual loss	Absent red reflex, Fundus cannot be seen	Treat cause, spontaneous resolution
Amaurosis fugax	Temporary loss of vision, curtain descending down	Clinical	Treat cause
Optic neuritis	Uniocular ↓ acuity, pain on eye movements, red desaturation	RAPD, swollen optic disc	Treat cause
Senile macular degeneration	Loss of acuity, reduced central vision	Normal disc with pigment, exudate and H'ge at macula	No treatment
Chronic glaucoma	Visual loss	Cupping, scotomas, pale disc	β-blockers, Trabeculectomy
Cataract	Blurred vision, Dazzling, monocular diplopia	Clinical, slit-lamp	ECCE
Retinal detachment	Floaters, flashes field loss, falling acuity	Ophthalmoscopy–grey opalescent retina ballooning forward	Scleral buckling, Cryo, laser coagulation
Retinitis pigmentosa	Night blindness in adolescents	Ophthalmoscopy– black pigments in fundus	No treatment
Retinoblastoma	< 3 yrs, Leukocoria, squint, absent red reflex	MRI	Enucleation
Toxoplasma	Features of uveitis	Punched out pigmented chorioretinal scars	Pyrimethamine

Contd...

Contd...

Disease	Clinical Features	Investigation	Management
Diabetic retinopathy	Features of diabetes with reduced vision	Ophthalmoscopy– dot and blot h'ges, cotton wool spots, vitreous h'ge, hard exudates	Glucose control
Hypertensive retinopathy	Features of hypertension	Hard exudates, macular edema, h'ge and papilloedema	Aspirin
CMV retinitis	Asymptomatic, sudden visual loss	Pizza pie fundus, flame h'ges	No treatment
Trachoma	Lacrimation, erythema, follicles, corneal ulceration	Depending on the site involved	Tetracycline + sulfadimethoxine
Xerophthalmia	Night blindness, loss of corneal lustre, dry conjunctiva, Bitot's spots	Clinical	Vitamin A
Foreign bodies	Chemosis, subconjunctival h'ge, abnormalities with iris, pupil retina or lens	Metal–Orbital X-ray; high velocity FB–USG	Removal

NEUROLOGY

Disease	Clinical Features	Investigation	Management
Bell's palsy	Unilateral facial weakness, loss of taste in anterior 2/3 rd of tongue	Clinical	Steroids, cosmetic surgery
Subarachnoid h'ge	Thunderclap headache, coma, vomiting, neck stiffness	CT, LP	Bed-rest, supportive
Subdural h'ge	Fluctuating headache, drowsiness, confusion, unequal pupils	CT– concavo-convex	Evacuation via burr holes
Extradural h'ge	Drowsiness, lucid interval, progressive hemiparesis, stupor, coning, Hutchison's pupil	CT–biconvex	Burr holes
Intracerebral h'ge	Sudden focal deficit, headache, coma	CT	Supportive
Parkinson's disease	Tremour, rigidity, bradykinesia, shuffling gait	Clinical	L-dopa, carbidopa
Huntington's chorea	Progressive chorea and dementia in middle age, + family history	Clinical	Phenothiazines
Gilles de la Tourette	4-6 yrs, Motor and phonic tics, obscene verbal gestures	Clinical	Haloperidol
Multiple sclerosis	Relapsing and remitting optic neuritis, weakness, spasticity, altered sensation, autonomic dysfunction Uhthoff's sign, Lhermitte's sign	MRI, CSF– oligoclonal bands	ACTH, steroids, immunosuppressors, β-interferons

Contd...

Contd...

Disease	Clinical Features	Investigation	Management
Encephalitis	Fever, headache, altered sensorium, seizures	CT, MRI	Acyclovir, anticonvulsants and supportive measures
Tabes dorsalis	Lightening pain, ataxia, stamping gait, Charcot's joints, AR pupil	TPHA	Benzylpenicillin
Benign intracranial hypertension	Obese females, headache, papilloedema, VI nerve palsy	Fundoscopy, CT	Thiazides, acetozolamide
Normal pressure hydrocephalus	Dementia, urinary incontinence, gait apraxia	CSF pressure studies are normal	No treatment
Syringomyelia	Pain in upper limbs, dissociated sensory loss, loss of reflexes, brain-stem signs, neuropathic joints of shoulder	MRI	Surgical decompression
Myasthenia gravis	Fatiguability of extraocular muscles, proximal limb muscles, muscles of speech	Clinical, Tensilon test	Thymectomy + oral anticholinesterases
Myasthenic syndrome/ Eaton-Lambert syndrome	Autonomic involvement, hyporeflexia, exercise ↑ muscle strength	Chest X-ray, associated with bronchial small cell Ca	Diaminopiridine

CARDIOVASCULAR SYSTEM

Disease	Clinical Features	Investigation	Management
Angina	Exertional retrosternal heavy tight or gripping sensation, radiating to jaw and arms. < 30 min. Relieved by rest and nitrates	ECG	Sublingual nitrate, Aspirin, β-blockers CABG, PTCA.
Myocardial infarction	Retrosternal gripping pain > 30 mins. Sweating, dyspnoea impending doom, hypotension, arrhythmias, 4th sound, JVP	ECG Cardiac Enzymes	IV Morphine, Aspirin, β-blocker, Streptokinase
Rheumatic fever	Children, migrating polyarthritis, murmurs, cardiomegaly, pericardial rub, nodules, fever, erythema marginatum, chorea	Prolonged P-R int, throat swab, ASO titre, ESR, CRP	Benzyl Penicillin, Aspirin. If carditis–Steroids.
Infective endocarditis	Malaise, clubbing, murmurs, splenomegaly, hematuria, Oslers nodes, roth spots, splinter hemorrhages.	Blood culture, Echocardiography	Antibiotics
Pericarditis	Pain worse on inspiration, lying flat, relief by sitting forward, friction rub.	ECG	NSAID, Prednisolone if recurrent or severe

Contd...

Contd...

Disease	Clinical Features	Investigation	Management
HOCM	Family history of sudden death, angina, palpitations, syncope, double apex, jerky carotids, ESM, PSM, 4th heart sound	Echocardiogram	β-blockers, Amiodarone, Pacing, Alcohol ablation
Dilated C'pathy	Features of heart failure, syncope and arrhythmias	Echocardiogram	Manage Heart failure and arrhythmias
Restrictive cardiomyopathy	Dyspnoea, fatigue and embolic symptoms, signs of constrictive pericarditis	Echocardiogram, Endomyocardial biopsy	– do –
Constrictive pericarditis	Features of RVF, Quiet heart sounds, diastolic knock, Kussmaul's sign, Friedreich's sign and pulsus paradoxus.	Echocardiography, cardiac catheterisation, MRI	Surgical excision
Pericardial effusion	Dyspnoea, JVP, Ewart's sign, soft heart sounds	Echocardiography	Pericardiocentesis
Cardiac tamponade	JVP with diastolic collapse, fall in BP, quiet heart sounds (Beck's triad), Signs of constrictive pericarditis	Echocardiography	Pericardiocentesis
Myocarditis	Fatigue, dyspnoea, chest pain, palpitations, Soft S1, S4 gallop	ECG, Serology	Treat the cause
Ruptured aortic aneurysm	Severe sharp tearing abdominal pain radiating to back, Shock, Expansile pulsations	Abdominal USG	Immediate surgery
Dissecting aortic aneurysm	Hypertensive, severe chest pain radiating to back and arms, shock, neurological signs	Transesophageal ECHO	Immediate surgery
Left heart failure	Dyspnoea, orthopnoea, PND, tachycardia, S3 gallop, crackles	Echocardiography	Digoxin, ACEI, vasodilators
Right heart failure	Dyspnoea, oedema, ascitis, JVP, S3, tachycardia	- do -	Diuretics, digoxin vasodilators,
Pulmonary oedema	Dyspnoea, orthopnoea, pink frothy sputum, crackles, gallop	CXR, ECHO	Oxygen, morphine, frusemide

HEPATOLOGY

Disease	Clinical Features	Investigation	Management
Hepatitis A	Malaise, anorexia, nausea and distaste for cigarettes. Then jaundice, hepatomegaly	Antibodies to HAV	Rest and dietary measures
Hepatitis B	Like HAV, and serum sickness like syndrome–rashes, polyarthritis.	HBs antigen + other markers	Symptomatic

Contd...

Contd...

Disease	Clinical Features	Investigation	Management
Hepatitis C	Flu-like illness with jaundice. Arthritis, glomerulonephritis, porphyrea cutanea tarda	HCV RNA	Interferon in acute case
Chronic hepatitis	Asymptomatic with mild slowly progressive jaundice	HbsAg + HBV DNA + IgM AntiHBc	Interferon if deranged LFT, Lamivudine
Autoimmune hepatitis	Fatigue, signs of chronic liver disease, hepatosplenomegaly, cutaneous striae, features of other auto-immune disease	Autoantibody	Prednisolone Azathioprine
Cirrhosis	Ascitis, oedema, haematemesis, pruritis, gynaecomastia, loss of hair, test. atrophy, jaundice, spider naevi, dupuytren's contracture, splenomegaly	USG Liver biopsy	Manage complications
Alcoholic liver	Jaundice, signs of chronic liver disease	GGT 5-nucleotidase	Thiamine IV
Budd-Chiari	Abdominal pain, nausea, vomiting, tender hepatomegaly, ascites	USG	Underlying cause, transplant
Amoebic liver abscess	Fever anorexia, weight loss, malaise, tender hepatomegaly, pleural effusion	Serology USG	Metronidazole + Diloxanide furate + Aspirate
Liver tumours	Weight loss, anorexia, fever, pain, ascites. Enlarged irregular tender liver	Liver biopsy	Surgical resection
Alpha-1 antitrypsin def	Cirrhosis and respiratory problems	Liver biopsy	Replacement, Transplantation
Wilson's disease	Children–Hepatic problems, KF ring Adults–tremour, dysarthria, dementia	Liver biopsy	Penicillamine Trientine HCl
Hemo-chromatosis	Bronze skin pigmentation, hepato-megaly, diabetes, hypogonadism, chondrocalcinosis heart failure, arrhythmias	Liver biopsy, MRI	Repeated Venesection Desferrioxamine
Primary biliary cirrhosis	Hepatomegaly following pruritis, jaundice, xanthelesma on eyelids and hands	AMA Liver biopsy	Cholestyramine Ursodeoxycolic Acid
Sclerosing cholangitis	Pruritis, jaundice, associated with IBD	ERCP, MRCP and biopsy	Liver transplantation
Hepatic encephalopathy	Personality change, hyper-reflexia, ↑ tone, fetor hepaticus, flapping tremour, constructional apraxia	Clinical, LFT	Lactulose, Neomycin, Rifaximin

Contd...

Contd...

Disease	Clinical Features	Investigation	Management
Portal hypertension	Hematemesis, malena, ascites, encepalopathy	Endoscopy	Sclerotherapy, Tamponade
Biliary colic	Severe constant pain crescendo type, radiate to right shoulder and scapula, nausea, vomiting	USG Scintiscan	Cholecystectomy
Cholecystitis	Severe localized right upper quadrant pain, tenderness, guarding and rigidity.	USG HIDA scan	Supportive + Cholecystectomy
Acute pancreatitis	Epigastric pain develops quickly reaching maximum within minutes, constant, relieved by leaning forwards, nausea and vomiting, may follow an alcoholic binge	Serum Amylase USG	Supportive
Chronic pancreatitis	Epigastric pain radiating to back, episodic, weight loss, steatorrhoea, diabetes	Spiral CT	NSAIDs, Opiate Enzyme suppl
Pancreatic tumour	Jaundice, abdominal pain radiating back, anorexia, weight loss, GB palpable, mass	USG CT	Surgery
Insulinoma	Fasting hypoglycaemia, diplopia, sweating, palpitation, confusion, LOC	FBS /Insulin levels	Surgery Diazoxide
Glucagonoma	Migratory necrolytic dermatitis, weight loss, diabetes, DVT, anaemia, hypoalbuminaemia	Serum glucagon	Surgery Octreotide

HEMATOLOGY

Disease	Clinical Features	Investigation	Management
Iron Defeciency Anaemia	Koilonychia, bald tongue, angular stomatitis, post-cricoid Web – Plummer-Vinson syndrome	Serum Ferritin	Iron
B12 defeciency anaemia	Angular stomatitis, glossitis, lemon yellow tinge, subacute combined degeneration	Serum Vitamin B_{12} and peripheral blood film	Hydroxycobalamin
Folate deficiency Anaemia	As above except for neurological manifestations	Red cell folate	Folate supplements with B_{12}
Aplastic Anaemia	Pallor, bleeding and infections	Pancytopenia Hypocellular marrow	Cause, Ig Cyclosporin BM transplant
Hereditary Spherocytosis	Jaundice, gallstones, leg ulcers, splenomegaly	Peripheral film, osmotic fragility	Splenectomy
Thalassemia	Failure to thrive, chipmunk facies, hepatosplenomegaly	Electrophoresis	Desferrioxamine Transfusions

Contd...

Contd...

Disease	Clinical Features	Investigation	Management
Sickle cell anaemia	Recurrent crisis–infarctive, sequestration, hemolytic, aplastic	Electrophoresis Blood Film	Supportive/Hydroxyurea
Warm AIH anaemia	Remitting and relapsing anaemia and jaundice, associated with lymphoma, CLL, SLE	Direct antiglobulin test	Steroids Immunosuppressive
Cold AIH anaemia	Acrocyanosis after exposure to cold. Associated with Glandular fever, lymphoma, Mycoplasma.	Direct antiglobulin test	Underlying cause
Paroxysmal nocturnal Haemoglobinuria	Recurrent thrombotic episodes, urine at night and in morning is dark	Ham's test	Supportive/Anticoagulate
Polycythaemia	Tiredness, depression, tinnitus, visual disturbance, Severe itching after hot bath, splenomegaly	Hemoglobin, PCV	Venesection, Hydroxyurea
Myelofibrosis	Lethargy, splenomegaly, abdominal pain, bleeding episodes	Bone marrow aspiration	Supportive
Myelodysplasia	Anaemia, infection and bleeding	$\uparrow$ cellularity Pancytopenia	Supportive
ITP	Easy bruising, purpura, epistaxis, menorrhagia	Platelet count	Steroids/Splenectomy
Haemophilia A	Family history, easy bruising, haemarthrosis and joint deformity	APTT	Factor VIII
von Willebrand's disease	As in Haemophilia and ITP	APTT + BT	Synthetic Vasopressin
Vitamin K deficiency	Bleeding manifestations	BT + APTT	Phytomenidione
DIC	Underlying infections, obstetric malignancies etc. Bleeding sites	FDP	Cause, Replacements
ALL	Younger age group. Features of pancytopenia. Lymphadenopathy	Blood Film	Chemotherapy
AML	Older age group pancytopenia. Hepatosplenomegaly	Blood Film	Chemotherapy
CML	Anaemia, sweating, blurred vision headache, hepatosplenomegaly	Ph Chromosome Blood Film	Alpha-interferons
CLL	Pancytopenia, lymphadenopathy and splenomegaly	Blood film	Chlorambucil
Hairy Cell	Similar to CLL	cyt. projections	2-CDA
Hodgkin's lymphoma	Picket fence fever, weight loss, night sweats, hepatosplenomegaly, contiguous lymphadenopathy. alcohol-induced nodal discomfort	Tissue biopsy– Reed Sternberg cells	MOPP regime

Contd...

Contd...

Disease	Clinical Features	Investigation	Management
Non-Hodgkin's lymphoma	Fever, weight loss, Noncontiguous lymphadenopathy, epitrochlear nodes involved	Tissue biopsy	CHOP regime
Multiple myeloma	Pancytopenia, bone destruction, Hyperviscosity, renal stones	Protein Electrophoresis	Chemotherapy
Waldenstroms macroglobuli-naemia	Multiple myeloma + lymphadenopathy	- do -	Chemotherapy Plasmapheresis
Varicose veins	Visible veins, cramps, tingling, ulcers, heaviness, restless leg, oedema, eczema	Doppler	Sclerotherapy, Stripping of veins
DVT	Calf tenderness, fever, pitting oedema, Homan's and Moses sign	Doppler	Heparin, compression bandage
Dissecting aortic aneurysm	Tearing chest pain with radiation to back, hemiplegia, unequal arm pulses	Transesophageal Echo	Hypotensives
Ruptured aortic aneurysm	Abdominal pain, collapse, expansile abdominal mass	Abdominal USG	Treat shock, surgery
Diverticulitis	Altered bowel habits, colicky left sided abdominal pain, GI h'ge, pyrexia	CT	Nill by mouth, IV fluids, antibiotics
TAO	Smoker, claudication pain in the calves, ulceration and other signs of ischaemia–absent pulse, cold leg, atrophic skin	Arteriography	Stop smoking, Aspirin, Vasodilators, Angioplasty, Bypass
Atherosclerosis	As above but involves larger vessels. Other vessel signs such as stroke, renal bruit, ischaemic heart disease	ABPI Doppler Arteriography	Balloon angioplasty, Aspirin, Grafts, Angioplasty
Embolism	Pain, pallor, parasthesia, pulselessness, paralysis	Arteriography	Immediate–Embolectomy, TPA
Volvulus of caecum	Abdominal pain, vomiting, constipation	Abdominal X-ray	Right hemicolectomy
Intestinal obstruction	Abdominal colic, vomiting, distension constipation, increased bowel sounds	AXR	Supportive, Definitive Mx is Surgery
Hypertrophic pyloric stenosis	Projectile vomiting after feeds, pyloric mass during a feed, VGP	Endoscopy– Bull's eye sign	Ramstedt's pyloromyotomy
Intussusception	5-12 months, episodic drawing up of legs with pain, red current jelly stools, vomiting, sausage-shaped mass	Barium enema– claw sign	USG with reduction by air enema

Contd...

Contd...

Disease	Clinical Features	Investigation	Management
Colorectal Ca	Symptoms of intestinal obstruction with or without diarrhoea + mass + bleeding PR + weight loss	Sigmoidoscopy followed by Ba enema, C'scopy	Surgery, Radiotherapy, Chemotherapy
Ca stomach	Abdominal pain, dyspepsia, vomiting, Haematemesis, weight loss, mass	Gastroscopy + Biopsy	Surgery
Branchial cyst	Swelling along the anterior border of SCM.	Clinical	Excision
Cystic hygroma	Brilliantly transilluminant swelling in anterior triangle	Clinical	Surgery or hypertonic saline sclerosant
Carotid body tumour	Soft pulsatile mass in anterior triangle. Moves only horizontally. No bruit	DSA	Extirpation
Laryngocele	Singers, lump in anterior triangle, painless, made worse by blowing.	Laryngoscopy	Excision by dual approach
Thyroglossal cyst	Fluctuant mass in the region of hyoid bone that moves on protruding tongue	USG, Thyroid scan	Excision. For fistula – SISTRUNK operation
Anal fissure	Painful defecation, bleeding PR (blood on paper), sentinal pile	Sigmoidoscopy after PR	Lignocaine, GTN ointment
Pilonidal sinus	Foul smelling discharge, painful bottom– Jeep bottom	Clinical	Excision ± primary closure
Rectal prolapse	Incontinence, mass protruding, mucus	Clinical	Thiersch's wiring, Surgery
Haemorrhoids	Large volume blood 'splash in the pan', constipation, mucus and pruritis	Clinical	Haemorrhoidectomy
Inguinal hernia	Lump pointing to the groin above the inguinal ligament, cough impulse +,	Clinical	Herniorrhaphy
Femoral hernia	Lump below and medial to the inguinal ligament and points to the leg.	Clinical	Surgical repair
Torsion testis	Sudden onset of pain in one testis, vomiting, nausea, relief on elevation	USG	Urgent surgical exploration
Epididymo orchitis	Fever, gradual onset testicular pain worse on elevation of testis, urethritis	Three glass test MSU	Antibiotics
Epididymal cyst	Swelling lying above and behind the testis	USG	Removal

Contd...

Contd...

Disease	Clinical Features	Investigation	Management
Hydrocoele	Enlargement of scrotum, fluctuation, transilluminance.	Clinical	Jabaolay's repair or Lord's plication
Achalasia	Dysphagia more to liquids initially, Regurgitation.	Barium swallow	Dilatation
GERD	Dysphagia more to solids, pain more on stooping and at night, regurgitation, heart burn, water brash	pH monitoring, Oesophagoscopy	Omeprazole, Surgery
Ca oesophagus	Dysphagia, weight loss, retrosternal chest pain, hoarseness, cough	Ba swallow and oesophagoscopy	Surgery and Radiotherapy
Hiatus Hernia	Dysphagia, Regurgitation, GERD	Barium Swallow	Surgical repair
Peptic Ulcer	Epigastric pain related to food, vomiting, anorexia.	Gastroscopy	*H. pylori* eradication Ranitidine, Omeprazole

OTORHINOLARYNGOLOGY

Disease	Clinical Features	Investigation	Management
Furunculosis	Tender tragus, pain worse on jaw movement	Clinical	Heat, analgesia, Icthammol and glycerine pack, flucloxacillin
Otitis externa	Pain and thick discharge, pain worse on movement of auricle	Clinical	Topical antibiotics
Otitis media	Pain, fever, sensation of pressure in the ear, hearing loss, drum is dull, bulged	Culture of discharge	Penicillin in adults, amoxycillin in children
Serous otitis media	Hearing loss, concave lustreless drum + radial vessels, -ve pneumatic otoscopy	Clinical, culture of middle ear fluid	If symptoms > 4mths, myringotomy, insertion of grommet
Mastoiditis	Pain, fever, ↓hearing, foul discharge, swelling behind the ear with downward displacement of pinna	Clinical	IV antibiotics, myringotomy, mastoidectomy
Otosclerosis	Females, bilateral, conductive deafness, hearing is better in background noice	Impedence audiometry	Stapedectomy
Presbyacusis	Senile change, loss of acuity for high frequency sounds	Audiometry	Hearing aids
Benign positional vertigo	Sudden onset rotational vertigo, provoked by head turning, common after head injury	Provocative test	Habituation, Epley head exercises
Vestibular neuronitis	Follows a viral febrile illness, sudden vertigo, vomiting exacerbated by head movement	Clinical	Cyclizine

Contd...

Contd...

Disease	Clinical Features	Investigation	Management
Meniere's disease	Repeated attacks of deafness, vertigo, tinnitus, vomiting	Audiometry	Cyclizine, Diuretic, Decompression
Foreign body in ear	Deafness, Pain, Foul smelling discharge	Clinical	Removal by suction
Acoustic neuroma	Progressive ipsilateral tinnitus, sensorineural deafness, cerebellar sign, ↑ICP signs	MRI	Surgery if possible
Acute sinusitis	Yellow green discharge, fever, pain worse on bending, sinus tenderness	Sinus X-ray	Antibiotics, Steam inhalation, analgesics
Tonsillitis	Sore throat, fever, dysphagia and neck lymph nodes.	Throat swab	Penicillin, Analgesia Tonsillectomy
Quinsy	Difficulty in swallowing + trismus, Tonsil obscured by soft palate	Clinical	Drainage
Croup	Stridor, barking cough following URTI	Clinical	Oxygen, epinephrine
Acute epiglottitis	Fever, cough, drooling of saliva, respiratory distress	Throat swab	Penicillin + Cefuroxime
Laryngomalacia	Present since birth, Stridor during sleep and excitement.	Clinical	Resolve by 2 years
Ca larynx	Progressive hoarseness, stridor, loss of weight, dysphagia, earache, hemoptysis	Laryngoscopy and biopsy	Radiotherapy, Total Laryngectomy
Pharyngeal pouch	Halitosis, regurgitation of food, neck lump	Barium swallow	Surgery
Naso-pharyngeal Ca	Epistaxis, diplopia, nasal obstruction, neck lump and conductive deafness, CN palsies	Post rhinoscopy and biopsy	Radiotherapy
Ramsay Hunt syndrome	Pain in ear precedes facial nerve palsy, vesicles in ear, vertigo, deafness	Clinical	Acyclovir, Steroids
Temperomandibular joint dysfunction	Relapsing orofacial pain, joint noises, restricted jaw function— worsened by stress, anxiety	Clinical	Education, NSAIDs, antidepressants, surgical arthrotomy
Aerotitis	Sensations of pressure, pain and deafness	Clinical, seen in divers and air travellers	Spontaneous resolution, prevent by decongestants, Valsalva manoeuvres

PSYCHIATRY

Disease	Clinical Features	Investigation	Management
Delirium	Toxic confusional state, abnormal perception and mood, Visual hallucinations	Clinical	Diazepam, Haloperidol if severe

Contd...

Contd...

Disease	Clinical Features	Investigation	Management
Alzheimer's Dementia	Consciousness not clouded, impaired memory, personality, judgement, apraxia, agnosia.	Clinical	Donepezil, Vitamin E, Seleigiline
Pick's Dementia	As Alzheimer's but loss of inhibitions, speaking to strangers	Clinical	As for Alzheimer's
Schizophrenia	Auditory hallucinations, Thought withdrawal/insertion/ broadcasting, Delusions, External control of emotions, Somatic passivity	Clinical	Phenothiazines...if two or more fail– Clozapine.
Depression	Low mood, early morning awakening, suicidal feelings, loss of libido, retarded	Clinical	Tricyclics , SSRI's Antidepressants,
Mania	Elevated mood, Flight of ideas, Restless, Grandiose delusions, Insomnia, Disinhibition	Clinical	Chlorpromazine, Haloperidol, Px Lithium for MDI
Dysthymia	Depression lasting for > 2 years	Clinical	Fluoxetine
Cyclothymia	Alternate episodes of depression and mania.	Clinical	Carbamazepine
Anxiety Neurosis	Dry mouth, Palpitations, Dyspnoea, Hyperventilation, Sleep disturbances	Clinical	Behavioural therapy, Benzodiazepines
OCD	Irresistable desire to repeat an act with varying degrees of depression, anxiety and depersonalization	Clinical	Behavioural therapy SSRI's Chlorpromazine
Conversion disorder	Symptoms and signs in the absence of pathology produced unconsciously	Clinical	Behavioural therapy Abreaction
Munchausen's syndrome	Symptoms relating to single system–with no pathology- laparotimophilia migrans, hemorrhagica histrionica, neurological diabolica, cardiopathia fantastica	Clinical	Cognitive therapy
Briquet's syndrome	More than 13 unexplained symptoms in various organs	Clinical	Cognitive therapy
Somatoform disorder	Patients who repeatedly present with physical symptoms and complaints, but negative findings on investigations	Clinical	Behavioural and relaxation therapy
Post-traumatic stress disorder	Delayed response to a stressful event, flashbacks	Clinical	Psychoanalytical therapy
Alcohol Dependence	Inability to keep limits, memory lapses, morning retching, withdrawal fits	Clinical	Diazepoxide Disulfuram

Contd...

Contd...

Disease	Clinical Features	Investigation	Management
Alcohol Withdrawal DeliriumTremens	Disorientation, agitation, tremours and visual hallucinations, Tachycardia, Pyrexia	Clinical	Diazepam Chlordiazepoxide
Fugue	Patient loses memory and wanders away from usual surroundings and deny all memory of wherabouts	Clinical	Counselling
Anorexia nervosa	BMI < 17.5, Amenorrhoea, wish to be thin, fear of fatness, lanugo, binging	LH and FSH	Cognitive and behavioural therapy
Bulimia	BMI > 17.5, Binge eating, self-induced vomiting, laxative and diuretic abuse	Clinical	As above
Paranoid	Oversensitive, suspicious, defensive, hyperalert with limited emotional response		
Schizoid	Shy, introvert, withdrawn, avoids close relationships		
Schizotypal	Superstitious, socially isolated, suspicious, limited interpersonal ability, odd speech		
Dissocial	Selfish, callous, promiscuous, impulsive, unable to learn from experience		
Histrionic	Dependent, immature, seductive, egocentric, vain and emotionally labile		
Narcissistic	Exhibitionist, grandiose, lacks interest in others, high self-esteem		
Anankastic	Obsessive compulsive – excessive doubt and caution, perfectionism		
Dependent	Passive, overaccepting, lacks confidence with poor self esteem		
Borderline	Impulsive, suicidal, aggressive behaviour, feelings of emptiness, drug abuse		
Avoidant	Fierce rejection, hyper-reaction to rejection and failure, poor social endeavour		

OBSTETRICS AND GYNAECOLOGY

Disease	Clinical Features	Investigation	Management
Uterine retroversion	Discomfort and retention of urine when pregnant	Clinical	Treat the cause Ventrosuspension
DUB	Heavy and irregular bleeding in the absence of any pathology	USG, HSG, FBC, TFT	NSAIDs, Anti-fibrinolytic, OCP
PMS	Tension, irritability, depression, bloating, breast tenderness, headache	Clinical	Progestogens, Bromocriptine
Menopause	Hot flushes, sweating, palpitations, fractures, dyspareunia	FSH and LH	HRT, Raloxifene
Abortion	Bleeding PV with or without clots, pain, history of amenorrhoea	USG	D and C
Ectopic Pregnancy	Amenorrhoea, bleeding PV following pain abdomen	β HCG, USG	Resuscitation and laparotomy
Trophoblastic disease	Morning sickness, pre-eclampsia, PV bleeding, abdominal pain, hyperthyroidism	USG–Snow storm appearance	Suction evacuation

Contd...

Contd...

Disease	Clinical Features	Investigation	Management
Cervical Ectropion	Pregnancy, OC pills, puberty, PV bleeding, Red ring around os	Cervical Smear	Cautery
Cervical CA	Post-coital bleeding, Pain, discharge, metrorrhagia, fixity of mass, friable,	Pap Smear, Colposcopic Biopsy	Surgery
PID	Abdominal pain, fever, menstrual disturbance, Uterine tenderness	USG, Endometrial swab for culture	Doxycycline, Metronidazole
Fibroids	Nulliparous, menorrhagia, infertility, pain, mass, urinary problems	USG	Progestogens, Myomectomy
Endometrial CA	Post-menopausal inter menstrual bleeding, weight loss	Uterine sampling	Radiotherapy, surgery
Ovarian CA	Family history, mass, urinary frequency, ascites, menstrual problem	USG	Surgery
Endometriosis	Cyclical pelvic pain, infertility, menorrhagia, uterosacral knobbing	Laparoscopy	See later
Prolapse	Mass per vaginum, stress incontinence, frequency, dysuria	Clinical	Pessary, surgery
Urge incontinence	Sudden uncontrollable desire to empty bladder, large amounts lost	Urodynamic studies	Oxybutinin Bladder drill
Stress incontinence	Incontinence during increased abdominal pressure, small amounts	Urodynamic studies	Exercises, surgical repair
Urethral syndrome	Frequency, dysuria, dyspareunia with negative MSU	MSU	Vaginal oestrogens, lubricants
Ovarian hyperstimulation	Due to GnRH use, lower abdominal pain, ascites, cystic ovarian mass	USG	Supportive with IV fluids
Placenta previa	Painless unprovoked vaginal bleeding, no tenderness, FHR norm	USG	Conservative. If severe deliver.
Abruptio Placentae	Shock out of proportion, Pain, tender, tense uterus, PIH, FHR ↑	USG	As above
PIH	Headache, epigastric pain, vomiting, visual disturbance, hyper-reflexia	Urine protein	Methyl-dopa Hydralazine
Multiple pregnancy	Aggravated normal symptoms, large for date, 2 FHR, multiple fetal parts, history of ART	USG	More frequent ante-natal visits, diet, rest
Hyperemesis gravidarum	Inability to keep food or fluids down, weight loss, dehydration	PCV, Urea, TFT, USG	IV fluids Metoclopramide
Polyhydramnios	Large for date, Breathlessness, palpitations, ↑ vomiting, oedema	USG	Indomethacin, Amniocentesis

Contd...

Contd...

Disease	Clinical Features	Investigation	Management
Uterine rupture	Pain, tenderness, vaginal bleeding, unexplained tachycardia, disappearance of presenting part	Clinical	Immediate laparotomy
Uterine inversion	Hemorrhage, shock, partial or completely revealed uterus	Clinical	Hydrostatic replacement
Amniotic fluid embolism	Dyspnoea, hypotension, may be preceded by seizures, DIC	Platelet studies	Oxygen supportive

PEDIATRICS

Disease	Clinical Features	Investigation	Management
Coeliac disease	Diarrhoea, anaemia, abdominal distension, other autoimmune diseases	Anti-endomysial Ab Anti-reticulin Ab Conf – Biopsy	Gluten free diet
Gastroenteritis	Diarrhoea, vomiting, dehydration	Stool culture	Oral Rehydration salts
UTI in infants	Septicaemia, collapse, FTT, PUO	MSU, MCU	Trimethoprim
PEM	Growth retardation, diarrhoea, apathy, skin hair depigmentation	Serum albumnin	Manage complications gradually ↑ diet
Hypothyroidism	Prolonged neonatal jaundice, excessive sleeping, inactivity, coarse hair, protruded tongue, hypotonia	Guthrei's test – Heel prick test for T3	Thyroxine
Hirschsprung's disease	Infrequent narrow stools, features of GI obstruction, PR–pellet-like faeces	Barium enema, biopsy	Excision of aganglionic segment
Cerebral palsy	Weakness, paralysis, learning disability, scissoring of gait, epilepsy	Clinical	Supportive rehabilitation
Homocystinuria	Paraplegia, fits, friable hair, emboli, cataracts	Urine analysis for cystine	Low methionine cystine suppl. diet
Phenylketonuria	Fair hair, fits, eczema, musty urine	Blood levels of phenyl alanine	Phenyl alanine low diet
Diaphragmatic hernia	Respiratory distress, bowel sounds in one hemithorax, cyanosis	CXR	Surgical repair
Undescended testis	Absent testis in one or both sides (cryptorchidism), palpaple along path of descent, prone for infection and malignancy	USG abdomen	Orchidopexy
Neonatal sepsis	Unusual crying, sleepiness, shock, apnoea, hypotonia, rashes, hyper/ hypothermia, bradycardia	Blood culture	Antibiotics

Contd...

Contd...

Disease	Clinical Features	Investigation	Management
RDS	Worsening tachypnoea hours after birth, grunting, intercostal recession	CXR	Surfactant
Necritising enterocolitis	Premature infant, blood and mucus PR, distension, tenderness, shock	Culture faeces, AXR	Metronidazole, penicillin, netilmicin
HDN	2-7 days post-partum, unexplained bruising and bleeding	PT, APTT, platelets	Phytomenidione IV
Non-accidental injury	Inconsistent history, late presentation to unknown doctor, odd mode of injury, parent not accompanied	Clinical	Inform social services.

ORTHOPAEDICS

Disease	Clinical Features	Investigation	Management
Supraspinatis tendonitis	Painful arc	Clinical	NSAIDs and active exercise
Frozen shoulder	Pain worse at night, reduced active and passive movements, ↓ abduction +/− ↓ external rotation	Clinical	NSAIDs and intra-articular steroids
Dupuytren's contracture	Flexion at the MCP joints of the ring and little finger	Clinical	Surgery
de Quervain's syndrome	Pain over the radial styloid process	Finklestein's sign (pain on forcible adduction and flexion of the thumb)	Hydrocortisone injection
Trigger finger	Full extension of the ring and middle fingers cannot be achieved, click may be felt in the flexor tendon	Clinical	Steroid injection into the region of the nodule
Volkmann's ischaemic contracture	Flexion deformity of the wrist and elbow, passive finger extension is painful, absent radial pulse	Clinical	Surgery
Lumbar disc prolapse	Lumbago, sciatica, pain on coughing, limited forward flexion and extension, weak reflexes	MRI	Bedrest, pain relief and surgery
Spondylolisthesis	Young adults, low back pain +/− sciatica	Plain X-ray	Wearing a corset, nerve release and spinal fusion
Lumbar spinal stenosis	Spinal claudication—pain worse on walking with aching and heaviness in one or both legs, pain on extension, −ve SLR	Myelography and MRI	NSAIDs, epidural steroid injection, corset, canal decompression
Perthes' disease	Male child, 5-10 years of age, pain in hip or knee, limp, all movements at hip are limited	X-ray	Bedrest

Contd...

Contd...

Disease	Clinical Features	Investigation	Management
Slipped upper femoral epiphysis	Males, 10-15 years of age, limp, spontaneous pain in the groin or knee, foot lies eternally rotated	Lateral X-ray	Surgery
CDH, DDH	Females 1-5 years of age	Ortolani's, Barlow's US,	Double nappy, von Rosen splint, closed
Club foot	Males, inversion, adduction of forefoot, plantar flexion		Foot manipulation and strapping, ORIF
Cruciate ligament injury	Drawers, Lachman, pivot shift tests, effusion or haemarthrosis	Clinical	Immobilization in plaster cylinder or surgery
Meniscal injury	McMurray's test, Apley's grinding test, joint line tenderness, mechanical locking	MRI, arthroscopy	Surgery
Osteoarthritis	Pain ↑ on exercise, crepitus, loose bodies, varus deformity	X-rays - ↓ joint space, subchondral sclerosis, cysts, osteophytes	Weight reduction, analgesics and physiotherapy
Prepatellar bursa	Housemaid's knee—swelling over the anterior inferior patella	Clinical	Aspiration, hydrocortisone injection, excision
Infrapatellar bursa	Vicar's knee—swelling over the anterior superior patella	Clinical	Aspiration, hydrocortisone injection, excision
Hammer toe	Extension at the MTP and DIP, hyperflexion at PIP	Clinical	Arthrodesis at PIP, tenotomy of extensor tendons
Claw toe	Extension at MTP, flexion at both PIP, DIP	Clinical	Girdlestone operation
Hallux valgus	Toe deviates laterally at MTP	Clinical	Keller's operation Mayo's operation
Morton's metatarsalgia	Pain between metatarsals	Clinical	Excision of neuroma
Giant cell tumour	Young adults, epiphysis, osteolytic progressive	X-ray – soap bubble appearance	Curettage
Ewing's sarcoma	Children, diaphysis, limb girdles	X-ray–large soft tissue mas, onion peel sign	Chemo, surgery, radiotherapy
Osteosarcoma	Adolescents, metaphysis	X-ray– sunray, Codman's triangle	Surgical resection and chemo
Chondrosarcoma	Middle age, slowly increasing mass	X-ray – cotton wool calcification	Surgical excision
Osteoid osteoma	Males, long bones, severe pain which is aspirin responsive	X-ray – cortical sclerosis	Local excision
Osteogenesis imperfecta	Blue sclera, brittle translucent bones	X-ray – trefoil pelvis, wormian bones	Prevent injury, correct deformity by osteotomy
Achondroplasia	Large head, normal trunk length, short limbs, fingers are all of the same length	X-rays – short bones with wide eiphysis	No treatment

Contd...

Contd...

Disease	Clinical Features	Investigation	Management
Mallet finger	Inability to extend the middle finger	Clinical	Splinting in extension
Ruptured Achilles tendon	Sudden ankle pain while running or jumping, cannot stand tip toe	Simmonds' test	Tendon repair
Ruptured long head of biceps	Discomfort after 'something has gone when lifting or pulling' ball in muscle on elbow flexion	Clinical	Repair not required
Carpal tunnel syndrome	Tingling pain in median nerve distribution, wasting of thenar eminence, ↓ palm sense	Phalen's test, nerve conduction studies	Wrist splint, steroid injection, treat cause
# Clavicle	Fall on outstretched hand or birth injury	X-ray	Broad sling
Anterior shoulder dislocation	Flat deltoid, deltoid paralysis, absent sensation on apatch below the shoulder	X-ray	Opioids, reduction by Kocher's, Hippocratic method
Posterior dislocation	Seizures or ECT	AP X-ray – light bulb appearance	Reduction
Supracondylar #	Child, fall on outstretched hand	X-ray	Broad sling, reduction
Pulled elbow	Child, pulled by the arms	X-ray	Elbow rotation
Colles' #	Dinner fork deformity—dorsal displacement of the distal fragment	X-ray	Reduction and plaster cast immobilisation
Smith's #	Garden spade deformity—volar displacement of distal fragment	X-ray	Reduction and plaster cast immobilisation
Bennett's #	# dislocation of carpometacarpal joint	X-ray	Reduction and plaster cast immobilisation
Scaphoid #	Pain, swelling on wrist movement, tenderness	X-ray –scaphoid view, bone scan	Immobilisation in glass holding pos
Intracapsular # of the hip	Minimal external rotation, no swelling, nonunion common	X-ray	Multiple screw fixation or Garden screws
Intertrochanteric	Fully externally rotated, marked local swelling, malunion common	X-ray	Dynamic hip screw
Femoral fracture	Shock, swelling, deformity, tenderness of thigh	X-ray	Intramedullary nail
Posterior hip dislocation	Dashboard injury, leg is flexed, adducted and shortened	X-ray	Reduction
Pott's #, Bimalleolar #	Pain, swelling, deformity of the ankle	X-ray	Above knee X-ray plaster or internal fixation
Dupuytren's trimalleolar #	Pain, swelling, deformity of the ankle	X-ray	Open reduction screw fixation
Cauda equina compression	Saddle anaesthesia, incontinence, paralysis	MRI	Bedrest, pain relief and surgery

MANAGEMENT OF EMERGENCY CONDITIONS

Emergencies	Management
Cardiorespiratory arrest	• Precordial thump • Basic life support • Defibrillator
Anaphylactic shock	• Secure airway, oxygen • IM adrenaline • Chlorpheniramine, hydrocortisone
Acute MI	• Oxygen • Aspirin, morphine • GTN, thrombolysis
Heart failure	• Sit the patient upright, oxygen • IV Diamorphine • Frusemide
Cardiogenic shock	• Oxygen, diamorphine • Dobutamine if PCWP > 15 mm Hg • Plasma expander if PCWP < 15 mm Hg
Acute severe asthma	• Sit patient up, oxygen • Nebulised salbutamol • IV hydrocortisone
Exacerbation of COPD	• Oxygen (24-28%) • Nebulised salbutamol, IV hydrocortisone, Amoxycillin
Tension pneumothorax	• 14-16 gauge needle with syringe partially filled with 0.9% saline in the 2nd intercostal space in the mid-clavicular line done before chest X-ray
Massive pulmonary embolism	• Oxygen • IV morphine • Heparin
Acute upper GI bleeding	• Rapid IV colloid • Urgent endoscopy +/– sclerotherapy
Status epilepticus	• Protect airway, oxygen • Diazepam • Phenytoin, phenobarbitone, if not controlled use thiopentone sodium
Raised ICP	• Elevate head of the bed to 30-40° • Hyperventilate • IV mannitol
Diabetic ketoacidosis	• 0.9% saline IVI • IV soluble insulin • Potassium replacement and sodium bicarbonate
HONK coma	• 0.9% saline IVI • Wait for an hour before giving insulin

Contd...

Contd...

Emergencies	Management
Hypoglycemic coma	• 50 ml of 50% dextrose IV fast
Thyrotoxic storm	• IVI 0.9% saline • Propranolol • High-dose digoxin • Carbimazole, IV hydrocortisone
Addisonian crisis	• Take blood for cortisol and ACTH • Hydrocortisone sodium succinate IV stat • IV plasma expansion • Monitor blood glucose
Phaeochromocytoma	• Phentolamine IV • Phenoxybenzamine oral • Propranolol
Acute renal failure	• Manage pulmonary oedema with diuretics and or dialysis • Manage hyperkalemia with calcium gluconate • Dialysis

CHROMOSOMAL SYNDROMES

Syndrome	Abnormality	Features
Down's syndrome	Trisomy 21	Flat face, Mongoloid eyes, epicanthic folds, simian crease, hypotonia, ↓IQ, endocardial cushion defect, short stubby fingers
Patau's syndrome	Trisomy 13	Low-set ears, cleft lip and palate, polydactyly, micro-ophthalmia, ↓ IQ
Edward's syndrome	Trisomy 18	Low-set ears, micrognathia, rocker bottom feet, mental retardation
Fragile X syndrome/Martin-Bell syndrome		Most common inherited cause of learning difficulty in males, macro-orchidism
Turner's syndrome	45X0	Primary amenorrhoea, short stature, webbed neck, cubitus valgus, coarctation of aorta, normal IQ
Klinefelter's syndrome	47 XXY	Eunuchoid, testicular atrophy, infertility, gynaecomastia, learning difficulties
Laurence-Moon-Biedl syndrome		Obesity, polydactyly, small genitals, retinitis pigmentosa, squint, cataract, azoospermia, renal anamolies, ↓IQ
Klippel-Feil syndrome		Fusion of cervical vertebrae, nystagmus, deafness, CNS signs
Lesch-Nyhan syndrome		Orange crystals in nappy, motor delay, ↓IQ, self-mutilation, choreoathetosis, fits

Contd...

Contd...

Syndrome	Abnormality	Features
Ehlers-Danlos syndrome		Soft, hyperelastic, poor healing, easy bruising skin, hypermobile joints, GI bleeds, perforation
Beckwith-Wiedemann syndrome		Large tongue and kidneys, hemihypertrophy, microcephaly, hypoglycemia, feeding difficulty, omphalocoele

POISONING

Poison	Clinical Features	Management
Benzodiazepine	CNS depression, drowsiness, ataxia, dysarthria, nystagmus, coma	Flumazenil
Tricyclic antidepressants	Drowsiness, convulsions, hypertonia, hyper-reflexia, fixed dilated pupils, urinary retention, HT, tachycardia	Gastric lavage, activated charcoal, sodium bicarbonate
Lithium	Vomiting, diarrhoea, coarse tremour, decreased consciousness, ataxia, increased muscle tone, hypokalemia	IV fluids and haemodialysis
Digoxin	↓cognition, yellow-green visual haloes, nausea, vomiting, cardiac arrhythmias	Digoxin specific antibody fragments
Neuroleptic malignant syndrome	Hyperthermia, rigidity, extra-pyramidal signs, autonomic dysfunction, mutism, confusion, coma	Dantrolene
Opiate poisoning	Pinpoint pupils, respiratory depression	Naloxone
β blockers	Severe bradycardia or hypotension	Atropine, glucagons
Cyanide	Dizziness, headache. Breathlessness, shock, no cyanosis, odour of bitter almonds	Oxygen, sodium nitrite and sodium thiosulphate, dicobalt edetate
Methanol	Headache, breathlessness, photophobia, papilloedema, optic atrophy, blindness	Gastric lavage, bicarbonate infusion, ethanol
Ethylene glycol (anti-freeze)	GI upset, neurological involvement, cardiorespiratory collapse, ARF	Gastric lavage, bicarbonate infusion, ethanol + IV calcium
CO	Pink skin, headache, vomiting, tachycardia, tachypnoea, fits, coma, cardiac arrest	100% hyperbaric oxygen, mannitol for cerebral oedema

Contd...

Poison	Clinical Features	Management
OP	Salivation, lacrimation, urination, diarrhoea, sweating, small pupils, bradycardia, respiratory distress, muscle fasciculation	Atropine and pralidoxime
Paraquat	Diarrhoea, vomiting, painful oral ulcers, alveolitis, renal failure	Activated charcoal
Ecstacy/Amphetamine	Nausea, muscle pain, blurred vision, confusion, hyperthermia, tachyarrhythmias,↑/↓ BP, ARF, hyperkalemi, hepatocellular and muscle necrosis	Gastric lavage, chlorpromazine, α and β blockade, dantrolene
Salicylate	Vomiting, dehydration, hyperventilation, tinnitus, vertigo, sweating, initial respiratory alkalosis followed by metabolic acidosis	Sodium bicarbonate, IV fluids, electrolyte supplements, alkaline diuresis
Paracetamol	Vomiting, RUQ pain, jaundice, encephalopathy	N-Acetyl cysteine
Lead poisoning	Nausea, vomiting, blue line on gums, abdominal colic, constipation, wrist drop, foot drop, lead encephalopathy	Calcium edetate, D-Penicillamine
Arsenic	Vomiting, abdominal pain, diarrhoea, rain drop pigmentation	Rehydration, Dimercaprol

INFECTIOUS DISEASES MANAGEMENT

Infection	Management
Staphylococcal infections	Flucloxacillin, fusidic acid
Scarlet fever	Phenoxymethyl penicillin
Diphtheria	Benzyl penicillin
Tetanus	Antitoxin, Penicillin
Botulism	Antitoxin
Gas gangrene	Penicillin, Antitoxin
Anthrax	Penicillin
Brucellosis	Doxycycline + Rifampicin
Pertusis	Erythromycin
Cholera	Supportive
Traveller's diarrhoea	Ciprofloxacin
Typhoid	Ciprofloxacin
Shigellosis	Ciprofloxacin
Plague	Streptomycin or tetracycline
Campylobacter	Erythromycin

Infection	Management
Actinomycosis	Penicillin
Tuberculosis	ATT
Leprosy	Rifampicin, Dapsone
Syphilis	Benzyl penicillin
Leptospirosis	Penicillin
Lyme disease	Doxycycline
Typhus	Tetracycline
Herpes Simplex	Acyclovir
CMV	Ganciclovir
Influenza	Ribivarin
Rabies	Supportive
Candidiasis	Ketoconazole
Leishmaniasis	Sodium stibogluconate
Toxoplasmosis	Pyrimethamine + sulphadiazine

Contd...   *Contd...*

Contd...

Infection	Management
Malaria	Chloroquine + Primaquine
Amoebiasis	Metronidazole
Giardiasis	Metronidazole
Filariasis	DEC
Hookworm	Albendazole
Roundworm	Levamisole
Pinworm	Albendazole
Tapeworm	Niclosamide

Contd...

Infection	Management
Chlamydiae	Doxycycline
Gonorrhoea	Penicillin
LGV	Tetracycline
H.Ducreyi	Azithromycin
Granuloma inguinale	Tetracycline
Trichomoniasis	Metronidazole
Bacterial vaginosis	Metronidazole
HIV	Anti-retroviral therapy

12 Explaining the Confusing Themes

> ◆ *One can never say, 'I am finally done with my preparation for PLAB 1'. That's because if you have prepared thoroughly, you will have scores of doubts traversing your brains.* 'Would the ideal contraceptive in this case be OC pills, or would it be a barrier method…it could be an IUCD…' *Don't panic my friend, help is at hand…Enjoy!*

1. DIFFERENTIAL DIAGNOSIS OF GENITAL ULCERS

Disease	Clinical Features	Diagnosis	Treatment
PRIMARY SYPHILIS	Chancre —painless ulcer, rubbery. Inguinal lymphadenopathy.	Dark field illumination	Procaine Penicillin
SECONDARY SYPHILIS	Snail track ulcers on mucosal surfaces. Symmetrical non-itchy maculopapular rash	Serology	Procaine Penicillin
HERPES SIMPLEX	Multiple painful shallow ulcers which may coalesce, tender inguinal lymphadenopathy	Isolation of virus	Lignocaine gel Acyclovir
LYMPHO-G VENEREUM (*Chlamydia trachomatis*)	Painless ulcerating papule on genitalia followed by regional lymphadenopathy. Nodes become compressed by inguinal ligament– Groove sign. Nodes–Buboes	Complement fixation	Doxycycline Erythromicin
CHANCROID (*H.ducreyi*)	Multiple shallow painful ulcers with irregular edges and localized l'pathy	Isolation in culture	Azithromycin Ciprofloxacin
GRANULOMA INGUINALE (*Klebsialla granulomatis*)	Also known as Donovanosis. Discrete papules which enlarge to form beefy red painful ulcers which heal by fibrosis. (*K.granulomatis* previously *C.granulomatis*)	Donovan bodies, PCR	Doxycycline Azithromycin

2. DIFFERENTIAL DIAGNOSIS OF VAGINAL DISCHARGE

Disease	Candidiasis	Bacterial Vaginosis	Trichomoniasis
Causative organism	Candida Albicans	*Gardenella vaginalis,* bacteroides, mobiluncus, mycoplasma hominis	Trichomonas vaginalis
Itching	++	−	+++

Contd...

Contd...

Disease	Candidiasis	Bacterial Vaginosis	Trichomoniasis
Smell	Yeasty	Fishy	Offensive
Colour	White	White/Yellow	Green/Yellow
Consistency	Curdy	Thin homogenous	Thin homogenous
pH	> 4.5	4.5-7	4.5-7
Microscopy	Fungal hyphae	Clue cells	Punctuate haemorrhage– Strawberry cervix
Management	Clotrimazole pessary	Metronidazole or Clindamycin cream	Metronidazole/ Clotrimazole pessary

3. INFECTIONS IN PREGNANCY

Features Disease	Clinical Features	Diagnosis	Management
Rubella	M–Macular rash, suboccipital lymph'pathy B– Cataract, cardiac lesions, deafness	IgM Ab	Vaccination
CMV	M–Fever, sore throat, lymphadenopathy C–Rubella, microcephaly, choroidoretinitis	Paired sera	Symptomatic
Toxoplasmosis	M–Glandular fever + Eosinophilia C–Micro/Hydrocephaly, cerebral calcification-epilepsy, chorioretinitis	Serology	Spiramycin + Sulfadiazine + Folinic acid
Syphilis	F–Snuffles, rash, hepatosplenomegaly, lymphadenopathy, anaemia	Serology	Procaine Penicillin
Listeria	M–Fever, myalgia, sore throat, vaginitis F–Fetal distress, pneumonia, convulsions, rash	Culture- CSF, blood, mecon	Ampicillin + Gentamicin

4. CHOICE OF CONTRACEPTION

Features method	Mechanism of action	Indications	Contra-indications	When to prescribe
Male condom	Barrier + Spermicidal	Multiple sexual partners, starting relationship, presence of STD	Latex allergy	As per indications
Female condom	Barrier + Spermicidal	Missed Pill, Post-child-birth, latex allergy, dyspareunia	None	As per indications
IUCD	Prevents implantation	Multipara who wants reversible contraception for 1-2 yrs, as a post-coital pill up to 5 days. Mirena = IUCD + levonorgestrol	Nullipara, PID, DUB, fibroids, suspected pregnancy, postpartum/ Abortal.	4 weeks' postpartum, or immediately after menses
COC	Prevents ovulation	Nullipara, stable relationship, mennorhagia, emergency contraception-Yuzpe method	Migraine with aura, liver disease, GTD, thrombo-embolic disease,	5th day of cycle, continue for 21 days

Contd...

Contd...

Features method	Mechanism of action	Indications	Contra-indications	When to prescribe
			DUB, >35 years, hyperlipidaemia	
POP	Renders cx mucus hostile to sperms	COC contraindicated, breastfeeding mother, Post-coital–Ho/Kwan	Arterial and venous diseases	If B/F–21st postpartum, else 1st cycle day
Depo-Provera	-do-	Major surgery, sickle cell disease, epileptics, After vasectomy, bowel disease, non-compliance with COC (shift workers)	-do-	Not B/F–5 days postpartum If B/F–6 weeks postpartum

5. EXAMINATION FINDINGS IN RESPIRATORY DISEASE

Condition	Mediastinal displacement	Percussion	Breath sounds	Added sounds	VR/VF
Consolidation	None	Dull	Bronchial	Crackles	↑
Collapse	Towards lesion	Dull	↓/Absent	None	↓/absent
Fibrosis	Towards lesion	Dull	Bronchial	Crackles	↑
Pleural effusion	Away from lesion	Stony dull	↓/Absent	None	↓
Pneumothorax	- do -	Hyper-resonant	↓/Absent	None	↓
Asthma	None	Normal	Bronchovesicular	Rhonchi	Normal
COPD	None	Normal	- do -	Rhonchi/ Crackles	Normal

6. PROPHYLAXIS OF DVT

Low Risk
- < 40 years undergoing major surgery/ no other risk
- Minor surgery with no other risk
- Minor trauma or illness with history of DVT or PE

Early mobilisation

Medium Risk
- > 40 years undergoing major surgery/ ≥ 1 risk factor
- Major acute illness
- Major trauma
- Minor surgery/trauma illness if previous DVT/PE

Low dose subcutaneous heparin 5000 units

High Risk
- Fracture or major orthopaedic surgery
- Major pelvic/abdominal surgery
- Major surgery/trauma/ illness with previous DVT/PE
- Paraplegia
- Critical leg ischaemia, major leg amputation

Low molecular weight heparin Enoxaparin– 40 mg or 4000 units

Major Surgery > 30 minutes

7. SKIN MANIFESTATIONS IN SYSTEMIC DISEASES

Disease	Condition	Features
Erythema nodosum	IBD, sarcoidosis, sulfonamides, granulomatous disease	Tender ill-defined subcutaneous nodules usually on shins
Erythema multiformae	Sulfonamides, penicillin, *herpes simplex*, mycoplasma	Target lesions on extensor surfaces Major form–Stevens-Johnson syndrome
Erythema cc migrans	Lyme disease	Small papule which develops into spreading erythematous ring
Erythema ab igne	Chronic pancreatitis due to thermal injury –hot bag	Erythema at the site of thermal injury
Pyoderma gangrenosum	IBD, RA, liver disease, Wegener's, Myeloma	Nodulo-pustular ulcers with overhanging necrotic edge
Necrobiosis lipiodica	Diabetes mellitus	Waxy yellow-brown plaques on shin
Acanthosis nigricans	Underlying malignancy	Thickened hyperpigmented watery velvety skin
Dermatitis herpetiformis	Coeliac disease	Itchy blisters on elbow
Lupus pernio	Sarcoidosis	Bluish red swelling around nose or ear
Café-au-lait spots	Neurofibromatosis	Brownish macules > 5 in number
Adenoma sebaceum	Tuberous sclerosis	Reddish papules around nose
Ash leaf pigm	Tuberous sclerosis	Pale macules
Shagreen patch	Tuberous sclerosis	Firm flesh-coloured plaque on trunk
Granuloma annulare	Diabetes mellitus	Pinkish papules forming a ring
Collodoin patch	Dermatitis herpetiformis	Scaly purple red raised patches (Purple helitrope rash) on extensors of joints
Migratory necrolytic erythema	Glucagonoma	Burning geographic annular areas

8. DIFFERENTIAL DIAGNOSIS OF HEADACHE

Disease	Description of Headache	Treatment
Migraine	Episodic, severe, unilateral, +/– aura photophobia, phonophobia	Sumatriptan, Ergotamine Px – Pizotifen, Propranolol
Cluster headache	Episodes of periorbital pain lasting 4-12 weeks, blood shot eyes, facial flushing	Sumatriptan
Trigeminal neuralgia	Paroxysms of intense stabbing painlasting seconds triggered by washing, shaving, etc	Carbamazepine, Surgery
Giant cell arteritis	Malaise, tender scalp (Combing hair) jaw claudication when eating, amaurosis fugax	Steroids give dramatic improvement
Tension headache	Tight band not responding to analgesics	Relaxation therapy
Raised ICP	Early morning headache relieved by projectile vomiting, focal signs	Treat cause
Subarachnoid haemorrhage	Thunderclap headache associated with stiff neck and positive Kernig's sign	Surgery
Sinusitis	Dull constant pain over affected sinus, postnasal drip, tender overlying skin	Antibiotics, Antihistamine Analgesics
Meningitis	Fever, photophobia, neck stiffness, rash	Antibiotics

9. PAIN RELIEF IN LABOUR

Nitrous Oxide
- Can be administered throughout labour
- Self-administered and patient-controlled analgesia

Pethidine/ Meperidine
- Used in first stage–IM/IV
- Avoid within two hours of expected delivery –neonatal depression–Manage with antagonist – Naloxone

Morphine
- IM, stronger than pethidine, more adverse effects
- Parous woman in OP position and prolonged labour

Epidural
- Cervix must be 3 cm dilated, the patient is ambulant
- OP, breech, multiple pregnancy, forceps

Spinal
- The patient can move around
- Rotational forceps and caesarean section

Combined Spinal/Epidural: Combination of the above.

General Anaesthesia: For emergency C/S, e.g., foetal distress

Pudendal Block: Outlet manipulation like forceps in II stage

Paracervical Block
- Used from 5 cm dilatation
- Relieves pain of uterine contraction, not perineal pain

10. MANAGEMENT OF ENDOMETRIOSIS

Mild Endometriosis
- Duration of symptoms less than one-year– expectant management
- If duration greater than 1 year or if contra- ception required–COCP

Moderate Endometriosis: Conservative sur- gery, i.e., foci of endometriosis destroyed by laser/diathermy.

Severe Endometriosis: Radical surgery (Hys- terectomy) with estrogen replacement therapy if bilateral salpingo-oophorectomy has been done.

11. MANAGEMENT OF INFERTILITY

Azoospermia	: AID
Oligospermia	: AIH
Severe Oligospermia	: AIH/ ICSI
Problems of Sperm Deposition	: AIH
Unexplained Infertility	: GIFT
Failed GIFT	: ZIFT
Obstructive Oligospermia	: MESA/PESA
Anovulation	: Clomiphine
Tubal problems	: Surgery/ IVF
Hyperprolactinaemia	: Bromocriptine
Sperm antibodies	: Aspirin/ IVF

12. GUIDELINES FOR TREATMENT OF HYPERTENSION

- Initiate drug therapy in subjects with sustained systolic > 160 mm or sustained diastolic > 100 mm.
- If Systolic BP 140 to 159 mm and/or diastolic 90 to 99 mm, initiate therapy if features of target organ damage.
- In diabetics, initiate therapy if systolic >140 mm and diastolic > 90 mm.
- In the absence of any contraindications (allopurinol therapy) thiazide diuretics like Bendrofluazide are the preferred first-line agents.
- Once on thiazides, second-line drugs are either beta blockers or ACE inhibitors.
- Atenolol (cardioselective beta blocker) is the drug of choice in diabetics without proteinuria. However, they can mask symptoms of hypoglycaemia. They are contraindicated in asthma and PVD.
- The ACE inhibitors are the drug of choice in diabetics with proteinuria. They are relatively

ineffective in elderly and are contraindicated in renal artery stenosis.

- Angiotensin II receptor antagonist (Losartan) are indicated in patients who cannot tolerate ACEI.
- Arteliolar dilators like hydralazine and minoxidil are the preferred second-line drugs in PVD patients on thiazides.
- If the patient is on beta blocker, the preferred second-line drug is calcium channel blocker like Amblodipine.
- Emergency management of accelerated and malignant hypertension is by sodium nitroprusside.
- Drugs that can be used in pregnancy are methyl dopa, hydralazine, nifedipine and losartan.

13. GUIDELINES FOR PROPHYLAXIS IN INFECTIVE ENDOCARDITIS PATIENTS

Dental Procedures

- LA or no anaesthesia: Amoxicillin 3 g PO one hour before procedure. Clindamycin PO if penicillin allergy.

- GA with no special risk: Amoxicillin 1 g IV at induction + 500 mg PO 6 hours later OR Amoxicillin 3 g PO 4 hours before induction + 3 g PO after procedure.
- GA with special risk like prosthetic valve and previous endocarditis: Amoxicillin 1 g IV + Gentamycin 120 mg IV at induction + Amoxicillin 500 mg PO 6 hours later. If allergy to penicillin, you can use Vancomycin + Gentamicin or Tecoplanin + Gentamicin.

Upper Respiratory Procedures—
As above

Genitourinary Procedures

- Amoxicillin 1g IV + Gentamicin 120 mg IV at induction + Amoxicillin 500 mg PO 6 hours later. If allergy to penicillin, you can use Vancomycin + Gentamicin.

Gastrointestinal, Obstetric and Gynaecological Procedures

- Antibiotics indicated if prothetic valve or history of previous endocarditis.

14. DIAGNOSING CONGENITAL HEART DISEASE

Disease	Clinical Features	Radiography
ASD	Right ventricular heave, loud P2, fixed split S2, ESM in pulm area	Prominent pulmonary plethora
VSD	Prominent apex, cardiomegaly, thrill in left sternal edge, PSM	Prominent pulmonary artery
PDA	Continuous machinery murmur with thrill, collapsing pulse	Aorta + pulmonary artery prominent
Coarctation of aorta	Hypertension in UL, radiofemoral delay, murmur over spine– Suzman's sign, heaving apex	Notching, Dock sign, 3-sign
'Fallot's tetralogy	Cyanosis, squatting, clubbing, ESM in pulmonary area, soft P2	Boot shaped heart– Cor en sabot
Transposed vessels–TGA	Symptoms similar to TOF with signs of CCF	D-Transposition–Egg shaped heart
		L-Transposition–Convex Lt. Border
Ebstein's anomaly	Cyanosis, clubbing, triple rhythm, systolic and diastolic murmur	Straight upper left cardiac border
TAPVC	Cyanosis, clubbing, FTT	Snowman's sign or figure of 8, cottage leaf sign
Tricuspid atresia	Signs of RHF, right to left shunt	Box-shaped heart
PTA	FTT, pneumonias, heart failures	Right aortic arch, concave pulmonary artery

15. SIGNS IN VALVULAR HEART DISEASE

Feature *Disease*	*Apex/Pulse*	*Murmur*	*Miscellaneous*
Mitral Stenosis	Tapping Volume	Low-pitched rumbling MDM at apex	Opening snap
Mitral Regurgitation	Forceful/Volume Collapsing	High pitched PSM radiating to axilla	Soft S1, 3rd heart sound
Mit. Valve Prolapse	- do - Volume	Late systolic following the click	Mid-systolic click
Aortic stenosis	Heaving/ slow-rising – parvus et tardus	ESM at aortic area radiating to carotids	Systolic ejection click, reverse splitting of S2 S4
Aortic regurgitation	Forceful/ Bounding or collapsing	High-pitched early DM at left sternal edge in 4th space	Quinke's sign, pistol shot femorals
Tricuspid stenosis	Normal/ Volume	MDM at lower left sternal edge	Prominent a wave in JVP
Tricuspid regurgitation	Forceful/ Volume	Blowing PSM at tricuspid area	cv wave in JVP, pulsatile liver

16. MANAGEMENT OF TACHYARRHYTHMIAS

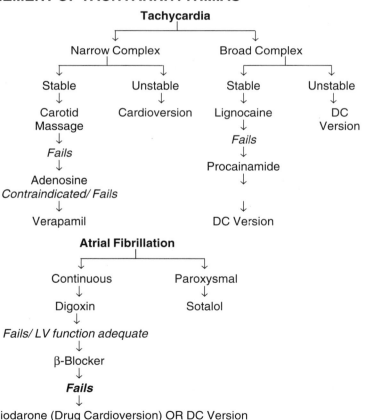

Tachycardia

Narrow Complex — Broad Complex

Narrow Complex:
- Stable → Carotid Massage → *Fails* → Adenosine → *Contraindicated/ Fails* → Verapamil
- Unstable → Cardioversion

Broad Complex:
- Stable → Lignocaine → *Fails* → Procainamide → DC Version
- Unstable → DC Version

Atrial Fibrillation

- Continuous → Digoxin → *Fails/ LV function adequate* → β-Blocker → ***Fails*** → Amiodarone (Drug Cardioversion) OR DC Version
- Paroxysmal → Sotalol

Ventricular Fibrillation → Defibrillation
Torsades de pointes → Stop anti-arrhythmics, Magnesium sulphate

17. TREATMENT OF BRADYCARDIA

If HR<40 or patient symptomatic

↓

Atropine

↓

Glucagon

↓

Temporary pacing

18. JUGULAR VENOUS PULSE/ PRESSURE (JVP)

Waveform

A wave   atrial systole

C wave   closure of tricuspid valve, normally not visible

X descent   fall in atrial pressure during ventricular systole

V wave   atrial filling against a closed tricuspid valve

Y descent   opening of tricuspid valve

1. Raised JVP with normal waveform—Fluid overload.
2. Raised JVP with absent pulsation—SVC obstruction.
3. A wave abnormalities.

   Absent : Atrial fibrillation

   Large : Pulmonary hypertension, PS

   Cannon : Complete heart block, ventricular arrhythmias/ ectopics, atrial flutter, single chamber ventricular pacing

4. X descent
   a. Deep: Constrictive pericarditis
5. V wave
   a. Large systolic v wave: Tricuspid regurgitation
6. Y descent
   a. Slow : Tricuspid stenosis
   b. Deep : Constrictive pericarditis.

19. ELECTROCARDIOGRAPHIC FINDINGS IN VARIOUS DISEASES

Normal Values

P Wave   : 0.08 sec, < 2 mm tall

P-R interval   : 0.12–0.20 seconds

QRS Complex : < 0.12 seconds

Q Wave   : < 0.04 seconds, < 2 mm deep

R-R interval   : 0.7–1.0 seconds

QT Interval   : 0.38–0.42

ST segment : Isoelectric

- *First Degree Heart Block:* One P per QRS complex, prolonged but constant PR interval.
- *Second Degree Heart Block Mobitz type II:* Constant PR interval with occasional drop of QRS.
- *Wenkebach block:* Progressive lengthening of PR followed by one non-conducted beat.
- *2:1 block:* One conducted atrial beat and two non-conducted beats giving twice as many P waves as QRS complexes.
- *Third Degree Heart Block:* No relationship between P waves and QRS complexes. Wide QRS complexes < 50/min.
- *RBBB:* QRS > 0.12 sec, 'RSR' pattern in V1, inverted T in V1–V3, deep S wave in V6.
- *LBBB:* QRS > 0.12 sec, 'M' pattern in V5, inverted T in lead I, AvL, V5–V6.
- *Bifascicular Block:* RBBB + left anterior bundle block.
- *Trifascicular Block:* Bifascicular + I degree heart block.
- *WPW syndrome:* Short PR interval, dominant R in V1.
- *Left Atrial Hypertrophy:* Bifid P waves – P.mitrale.
- *Right Atrial Hypertrophy:* Peaked P waves – P.pulmonale.
- *Left Ventricular Hypertrophy:* R wave in V6 > 25 mm, or SV1 +RV6 > 35 mm, inverted T waves in lead I, AvL, V5–V6, LAD.
- *Right Ventricular Hypertrophy:* R/S in V1 >1, T wave inversion in V1–V3, deep S in V6, RAD.
- *Pulmonary Embolism:* S1Q3T3 pattern, i.e., deep S in lead I, pathological Q in lead III and inverted T waves in lead III. Sinus

Tachycardia, RAD, RBBB, RV strain in V1-V3.

- *Digoxin toxicity:* ST depression and inverted T in V5 and V6—Reverse tick sign, ventricular ectopics, nodal bradycardia.
- *Hyperkalemia:* Tall peaked T waves, widened QRS complex, absent P–Sine wave appearance.
- *Hypokalemia:* Small T waves, prominent U waves.
- *Hypercalcaemia:* Shortened QT interval.
- *Hypocalcaemia:* Lengthened QT interval, small T waves.
- *Hypothermia:* J waves.
- Hypothyroidism, COPD, embolism, myocarditis, pericardial effusion, BBB–Low voltage QRS complex < 5 mm.
- *Myocarditis:* ST segment changes, T wave inversion, atrial Arrhythmias.

- *Acute pericarditis:* Saddle-shaped elevation of ST segment.
- *Angina:* Planar ST depression more than 0.5 mm.
- *Myocardial infarction:* Planar elevation of more than 1 mm.
  - Peaked T waves and ST elevation
  - T wave inverts, ST segment resolves
  - Pathological Q waves which usually persist.

Lead		Site of Infarct
II, III, AVF	:	Inferior
V1–V4	:	Anteroseptal
V4–V6, I, AVL	:	Anterolateral
Tall R and ST depression in V1–V2	:	Posterior
ST and T changes without Q waves	:	Non Q-wave infarcts–Subendocardial

20. DIFFERENTIATING ULCERATIVE COLITIS AND CROHN'S DISEASE

Feature	Ulcerative Colitis	Crohn's Disease
Clinical features	Profuse haemorrhage	Gross bleeding uncommon
	Perianal disease rare	Perianal disease common
	Small bowel not affected	May involve entire GI tract
Macroscopy	Extends proximally from rectum	Skip lesions
	No thickening of bowel wall	Thickened bowel wall, loss of haustrations
Microscopy	No granulomas	Granulomas
	Low inflammation	More inflammation
	Deeper ulcers	
	[hence named ulcerative]	Shallow ulcers
	Pseduopolyps.	
	Abcesses in crypts	Fibrosis
Extraintestinal manifestations	Sclerosing cholangitis	Erythema nodosum
	Pyoderma gangrenosum	Migratory polyarthritis
		Gallstones

21. INVESTIGATIONS IN BOWEL DISEASES

- Inflammatory bowel disease—
  - Acute   – CT scan
  - Chronic – Colonoscopy

- Colorectal tumours—Initially sigmoidoscopy followed by barium enema. Indications for colonoscopy are:
  - Inconclusive barium enema
  - Biopsy of lesion seen on barium enema.

22. INVESTIGATORY FINDINGS IN BLEEDING DISORDERS

Disorder	INR	APTT	TT	Platelets	BT
Heparin	↑	↑↑	↑↑	N	N
DIC	↑↑	↑↑	↑↑	↑	↑
Liver Disease	↑	↑	↑/N	↑/N	↑/N
Platelet defect	N	N	N	N	↑
Vitamin K def	↑↑	↑	N	N	N
Haemophilia	N	↑↑	N	N	N
v Willebrands	N	↑↑/ N	N	N	↑

23. INVESTIGATORY FINDINGS OF PLASMA IRON STUDIES

	MCV	Serum iron	TIBC	Serum Ferritin	Marrow iron	Iron in RBC
IDA	↓	↓	↑	↓	–	–
AOCD	↓/ N	↓	↓	↑	+	–/↓
Haemo-chroma-tosis	N	↓	↑/N	↑	↑	
Thala-ssaemia	↓↓↓	N	N	N	+	
Sidero-blastic	↓/↑	↑	N	↑	+	Ring

24. MANAGEMENT OF DIABETES MELLITUS

Drugs Available for NIDDM

- Sulphonylureas
  Gliclazide–Most commonly used, long acting
  Tolbutamide–Short acting, useful in elderly
- Biguanides
  Metformin–Used in obesity, may cause lactic acidosis
- Alpha glucosidase inhibitors
  Acarbose–Used in obese patients as an adjunct
- Rosglitazone–Reduces insulin resistance and decreases BP.

- Repaglanide–Stimulates insulin production at meal times.

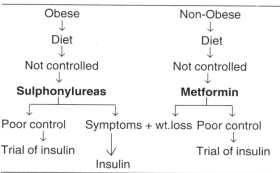

25. SLIDING SCALE INSULIN

Insulin Treated mild illness, e.g., Gastroenteritis

Maintain calorie intake–normal insulin to be continued

Insulin Treated moderate illness, e.g., pneumonia

Normal insulin + supplementary sliding scale of insulin QID

Insulin Treated severe illness, e.g., Myocardial infarction

IV soluble insulin by pump + IV dextrose

Diet and drug treated Moderate to Severe illness

If on metformin therapy—stop the drug

If on sulphonylureas and illness likely to be self limiting—continue drug treatment and supplement with subcutaneous insulin and sliding scale (moderate) or IV infusion (severe).

26. PROPHYLAXIS FOR MALARIA

High Risk	Includes all of Sub-Saharan Africa (Somalia, Ghana) except South Africa, India, South-east Asia, Indonesia and parts of China	Mefloquine 250 mg per week
Moderate Risk	Western Cambodia, Thailand, Myanmar, Papua New Guinea	Doxycycline 100 mg /day
Low Risk	Includes North Africa, Middle East, Central America and parts of South America	Chloroquine 300 mg/week or Proguanil 200 mg/day

27. VACCINATION ADVISE WHEN TRAVELLING

Africa	Meningitis, Typhoid, Tetanus, Polio, Hepatitis A ± Yellow fever
Asia	Meningitis, Typhoid, Tetanus, Polio, Hepatitis A
South America	Typhoid, Tetanus, Polio, Hepatitis A, ± Yellow fever

28. INCUBATION PERIOD OF COMMON DISEASES

Disease	Period	Disease	Period
Syphilis	9–90 days	Measles	7–21 days
Rubella	14–21 days	Mumps	14–21 days
Chickenpox	11–21 days	Hepatitis A	15–20 days
Cholera	3 hrs–5 days	Hepatitis B	50–180 days
Coxsackie	5–7 days	CJD	10–20 years

29. DIFFERENTIAL DIAGNOSIS OF ACUTE RED EYE

	Conjunctivitis	Iritis	Acute Glaucoma
Pain	±	++	+++
Red-ness	Conjunctival Injection	Ciliary Injection	Ciliary Injection
Photo-phobia	+	++	−
Blurred vision	−	+ due to aqueous precipitates	+ due to corneal oedema
Cornea	N	N	Hazy
Pupil	N	Miotic-spasm	mid-dilated
IOP	N	N	Increased
Pupils reaction	N	N or decre-ased no RAPD	Fixed pupils ± RAPD

30. PUPILLARY ABNORMALITIES

- Pinpoint pupils: Opioid abuse, pontine haemorrhage.
- Argyll Robertson pupil (Bilateral irregular small pupil reacting only to accommodation)– diabetes, neurosyphilis.
- Holmes: Adie's pupil (Dilated pupil with sluggish response to accommodation and light).

- Young women. Holmes-Adie syndrome— associated with absent ankle and knee jerks.
- Horner's syndrome, pupil (Miosis, ptosis, anhydrosis, enophthalmos, loss of ciliospinal reflex): PICA aneurysm, Pancoast tumour.
- Fixed dilated pupil with ptosis and ophthalmoplegia: III nerve palsy.

31. TREATMENT OF HYPERLIPIDAEMIA

Normal Values

Serum cholestrol	:	4- ≤ 6 mmol/l
Serum triglycerides	:	0.5–1.9 mmol/l

Disorder	Management
Hypercholestrolaemia	Statins
Hypertriglyceridaemia	Fibrates
Both are increased	Fibrates

32. RENAL TUBULAR ACIDOSIS

1. Type 1 (Distal)	Hypokalaemic, hyperchloraemic metabolic acidosis	Acute—correct hypokalaemia before acidosis
	• Lithium • Amphotericin	Chronic—-oral bicarbonates, potassium supplements
2. Type 2 (Proximal)	Hypokalaemic, hyperchloraemic metabolic acidosis	High doses of bicarbonates
	• Tetracycline • Acetazolamide	
3. Type IV	Hyperkalaemic metabolic acidosis	Fludrocortisone
	• Addison's • DM • ACE inhibitors • β-blockers • NSAIDs	

33. TREATMENT OF PARKINSONISM

1. Dopamine agonist, L-dopa and peripheral decarboxylase inhibitor, Carbidopa

2. For "on-off" phenomenon,
   - Early use of pergolide and bromocriptine prevents this
   - Slow release L-dopa
   - SC Apomorphine if severe
   - Entacapone increases the "on" time
3. For L-dopa's end of dose deterioration, Selegiline
4. For depression, Nortryptyline
5. For tremour, Mirtazapine and Procyclidine
6. Newer dopamine agonists
   - Cabergoline
   - Pramipexole
   - Entacapone.
   Adjuncts to L-dopa, dose of which can then be reduced.

34. TREATMENT OF MENINGITIS

Blind therapy	If you suspect a patient has meningitis and is outside hospital. IV/IM Benzyl penicillin
Empirical therapy	Select antibiotic to cover the most likely organism while awaiting culture reports
Pneumococcus	Cefotaxime +/– Vancomycin
Meningococcus	Benzyl penicillin
H.influenzae	Cefotaxime, Rifampicin
E.coli	Cefotaxime
Staph.aureus	Flucloxacillin
Listeria monocytogenes	Gentamicin + Ampicillin
M.tuberculosis	ATT
Cryptococcus neoformans	Amphotericin B + Flucytocine

35. DYSPHASIA

1. *Broca's (expressive):*
   Site of lesion: Infero-lateral dominant frontal lobe
   - Comprehension is intact
   - Poorly articulated and non-fluent speech
   - Errors of grammar and syntax
   - Reduced number of words used
   - Reading and writing impaired
2. *Wernicke's (receptive):*
   Site of lesion: Postero-superior dominant temporal lobe
   - Comprehension is impaired
   - Empty fluent speech with incorrect words (paraphasias) and nonsense words (neologisms)
   - He is oblivious of errors
   - Reading and writing is impaired
3. *Conduction aphasia:*
   Site of lesion: Perisylvian area with damage to arcuate fasciculus fibres
   - Inability to repeat phrases or words
   - Comprehension and fluency less so.
4. *Global dysphasia:*
   Site of lesion: Large areas in MCA territory
   - Features of both Broca's and Wernicke's

36. OPPORTUNISTIC INFECTIONS IN AIDS

Cryptococcal meningitis	Acute delirium
Non-bacterial thrombotic endocarditis	Acute hemiparesis
Chronic inflammatory demyelinating polyneuropathy	Progressive leg weakness
CNS lymphoma	Progressive hemiparesis
Chronic sensory polyneuropathy	Painful feet
Cerebral toxoplasmosis	Neurology + seizures Acute focal
Candidiasis	Dysphagia and oesophageal ulcers
Kaposi's sarcoma	Dusky lesions in oral mucosa

37. INVESTIGATION OF ENDOCRINE DISORDERS

1. *Dexamethasone suppression test*
   - Used for the diagnosis of Cushing's disease
   - Patient with Cushing's disease (excess

pituitary ACTH) will fail to suppress endogenous ACTH and thus cortisol production, when given a dose of synthetic steroid (dexamethasone), in contrast to normal subjects.

2. *Synacthen (Synthetic ACTH-en) test or short ACTH stimulation test*
   - Used for diagnosis of primary hypoadrenalism/Addison's disease
   - A healthy subject shows increased cortisol production (normal response) in contrast to addisonian patients with impaired or absent response
   - It can be confirmed, if necessary by a long ACTH stimulation test to exclude adrenal suppression by steroids.

3. *Water deprivation test*
   - Used to differentiate between cranial and nephrogenic diabetes insipidus
   - Vasopressin, desmopressin are antidiuretic hormones
   - A normal person will maintain plasma osmolality while concentrating urine during dehydration, unenhanced by desmopressin
   - In cranial DI, plasma osmolality rises while urine remains dilute, only concentrating after exogenous vasopressin administation
   - In nephrogenic DI, urine fails to concentrate even after vasopressin administation because of insensitivity of renal tubules to vasopressin.

4. *Clonidine suppression test or MIBG scan*
   - Used for diagnosis of pheochromocytoma

5. *Oral glucose tolerance test*
   - Used for diagnosis of acromegaly
   - Normally after administration of oral glucose, GH is suppressed
   - In acromegaly, there is no suppression of GH or the levels may rise.

6. *Insulin tolerance test*
   - Can be used for diagnosis of hypopituitarism
   - Normally on administration of IV insulin,

the resulting hypoglycemia stimulates increased production of both GH and cortisol, which fails to occur in hypopituitarism.

38. TREATMENT OF RHEUMATOLOGICAL CONDITIONS

1. **Rheumatoid Arthritis**
   a. NSAIDs , C.I in–asthma, active peptic ulcer
   b. NSAIDs + gastroprotective agent, PPI or misoprostol IF:
      - H/o peptic ulcer disease
      - Dyspepsia
      - Age > 70 years
      - On aspirin/steroids
      - Avoid NSAIDs if on warfarin.
   c. Steroids:
      - ↓ erosions when given in early disease
      - Place in treatment schema is controversial.
   d. DMARD's:
      - If 1 to 2 weeks trial of 3 NSAIDs fail to control pain
      - Synovitis for > 2 months
   e. Newer drugs:
      - Infliximab
      - Etanercept

2. **Osteoarthritis**
   a. Paracetamol, if pain does not improve NSAIDs
   b. Tricyclics for nocturnal pain
   c. Reduce weight
   d. Walking aid held in:
      - Contralateral hand in hip arthritis
      - Ipsilateral hand in knee arthritis
   e. Quadriceps exercises for knee arthritis.
   f. Joint replacement for end stage disease.

3. **Gout**
   a. NSAIDs
   b. Colchicine in patients with peptic ulceration

c. Allopurinol only if:
  * attacks are frequent and severe
  * associated renal impairment
  * not tolerating NSAIDs or colchicine.
d. Probenecid:
  * only in allopurinol allergic patients
  * C.I in renal failure, urate stones.

39. SYNCOPE

Vasovagal/ Cardio-inhibitory	• In response to pain, fear, standing for long due to reflex bradycardia peripheral vasodilation • Onset over seconds, Lasts < 2 min • Cannot occur if patient is recumbent
Postural hypotension/ Vaso-depressor	• Seen in elderly with impaired autonomic reflexes, can be drug induced • Head up tilt test distinguishes vasovagal from vasodepressor syncope, if symptoms are associated with BP drop > 30 mmHg→ Vasodepressor If associated with bradycardia → Vasovagal
Stokes-Adams attacks/cardiac syncope	• Caused by cardiac arrhythmias • Preceded by palpitations • Sudden LOC accompanied by pallor • Flushing as patient recovers
Drop attacks	• Seen in elderly women • Sudden attacks of weakness of legs • No warning, LOC or confusion
Carotid sinus syncope	• Due to excessive sensitivity of sinus to external pressure/ in elderly

40. DEVELOPMENTAL MILESTONES

6 weeks
  * *Gross motor:* Lifts chin occasionally when prone.
  * *Social:* Social smile.

2 months
  * *Gross motor:* Arms extend forward when prone.
  * *Fine motor:* Pulls at clothes.
  * *Speech:* Cooing sounds.

3 months
  * *Gross motor:* Moro's reflex gone.

4 months
  * *Gross motor:* Rolls from front to back.
  * *Fine motor:* Reaches, pulls objects to mouth.
  * *Speech:* Responds to human voice.

6 months
  * *Gross motor:* When prone, can put weight on hands.
  * *Fine motor:* Ulnar grasping.
  * *Speech:* Responds to name. Babbling starts.
  * *Social:* Stranger anxiety.

9 months
  * *Gross motor:* Pulls to stand.
  * *Fine motor:* Finger-thumb grasping.
  * *Speech:* 'Mamma, Dadda'.
  * *Social:* Separation anxiety.

12 months
  * *Gross motor:* Walks under support.
  * *Fine motor:* Pincer grasp. Throws. Babinski begins to disappear.
  * *Speech:* 2 words beyond 'Mamma, Dadda'.
  * *Social:* Drinks with cup.

15 months
  * *Gross motor:* Walks without support.
  * *Fine motor:* Draws line.
  * *Speech:* Jargon
  * *Social:* Points to needed items.

18 months
  * *Gross motor:* Climbs steps with support
  * *Fine motor:* Scribbling.
  * *Speech:* Says own name. 10 words.
  * *Social:* Uses spoon.

2 years
  * *Gross motor:* Runs. Kicks ball. Climbs 2 steps.
  * *Fine motor:* Undresses.
  * *Speech:* 2 word sentences, with pronouns. Favourite word is 'No'.
  * *Social:* Parallel play.

3 years
  * *Gross motor:* Rides tricycle.

- *Fine motor:* Copies a circle.
- *Speech:* Prepositions.
- *Social:* All dress/undress except buttons.

4 years
- *Gross motor:* Hop on 1 foot.
- *Fine motor:* Copies a cross.
- *Speech:* Tells story.
- *Social:* Cooperative play. Toilet trained. Buttons clothes.

5 years
- *Gross motor:* Skips. Catches ball.
- *Fine motor:* Copies a square, prints own name. Ties shoelaces.
- *Speech:* Alphabet. Future tense.
- *Social:* Oedipus complex.

6 years
- *Gross motor:* Rides bicycle.
- *Fine motor:* Copies a triangle.
- *Speech:* Begins reading.
- *Social:* Develops right vs. wrong sense.

Shape copying:
- Shapes are in alphabetical order: Circle (3 yr), Cross (4 yr), Square (5 yr), Triangle (6 yr), Rhomboid (8 yr), Cylinder (9 yr), Cube (11 yr).

41. IMMUNISATION SCHEDULE
3 days
- BCG

2 months
- DTP
- Live polio
- Hib

3 months
- DTP
- Live polio
- Hib

4 months
- DTP
- Live polio
- Hib

12-18 months
- MMR

3-5 years
- MMR
- Live polio booster
- Diphtheria booster
- Tetanus booster

10-14 years
- Rubella [girls]
- BCG [sometimes]

15-18 years
- Live polio booster, Diphtheria booster, Tetanus booster.

42. DIAGNOSTIC ANTIBODIES IN VARIOUS DISEASES

1. SLE
   - Antinuclear, Anti-Ro, Anti-La
2. Wegener's
   - cANCA
3. Goodpasture's
   - Anti-GBM
4. CREST
   - Anti-centromere
5. Diffuse scleroderma
   - Anti-nucleolus, Anti-topoisomerase
6. Polymyositis
   - Anti-Jo1
7. Churg-Strauss
   - pANCA
8. Autoimmune hepatitis type I
   - ANA, Anti-smooth muscle
9. Autoimmune hepatitis type II
   - Anti-liver/kidney microsomal
10. Primary biliary cirrhosis
    - Anti-mitochondrial
11. Sclerosing cholangitis
    - ANA, Smooth muscle antibody, ANCA
12. Coeliac disease
    - Anti-endomysial, Anti-gliadin antibodies

43. LOCALISING LESIONS IN THE BRAIN
Frontal Lobe
- Hemiparesis
- Personality change
- Broca's aphasia
- Positive grasp reflex
- Unilateral loss of smell
- Urinary incontinence.

Temporal Lobe
- Dysphasia
- Hypersexuality
- Contralateral upper quadrant hemianopia
- Acalculia
- Agraphia.

Parietal Lobe
- Hemisensory loss
- Asterognosis
- Decreased two-point discrimination
- Agraphaesthesia
- Dysphasia
- Sensory inattention
- Gerstmann's syndrome—Finger agnosia, right-left agnosia, dysgraphia, acalculia
- Contralateral lower quadrantanopia.

Occipital
- Contralateral homonymous hemianopia

Temporo-parietal left
- Wernicke's aphasia

Temporo-parieto-occipital junction
- Wernicke's + Broca's aphasia

Cerebello-pontine angle
- Ipsilateral deafness
- Nystagmus
- Decreased corneal reflex
- V and VII nerve palsy
- Ipsilateral cerebellar signs.

Cerebellum
- Intention tremour
- Dysarthria
- Past-pointing
- Dysdiadochokinesis
- Nystagmus
- Truncal ataxia

Midbrain
- Spastic weakness/paralysis in:
  - all four limbs or
  - limbs on the contralateral side of the body.
- Increased reflexes and muscle tone in limbs on the contralateral side or in all limbs (all limbs may be held in rigid extension, i.e., opisthotonus)

- Postural reaction deficits in limbs on the contralateral side or in all limbs
- Mental depression or coma
- Ipsilateral deficits of cranial nerve III (oculomotor):
  - ventrolateral strabismus
  - dilated pupil unresponsive to light, with normal vision
  - drooping of upper eyelid (ptosis).
- Hyperventilation:
  - ± Bilateral miosis
  - ± Obstinate progression/head pressing.

Pontomedullary lesions
- Weakness or paralysis in:
  - all four limbs or
  - limbs on the same side of the body as the lesion.
- Normal or increased reflexes and muscle tone in all limb(s)
- Postural reaction deficits in limbs on the same side as the lesion or in all limbs
- Multiple cranial nerve deficits:
  - Jaw paralysis, decreased facial sensation (cranial nerve V)
  - Depressed palpebral reflex (cranial nerves V, VII)
  - Facial paralysis (cranial nerve VII)
  - Head tilt, falling, rolling, nystagmus (cranial nerve VIII)
  - Pharyngeal/oesophageal/laryngeal paralysis (cranial nerves IX, X)
  - Tongue paralysis (cranial nerve XII).
- Irregular respiration
- Mental depression

Cervicothoracic syndrome (C6 through T2)
- Weakness/paralysis in:
  - all four limbs (i.e., tetraparesis/tetraplegia).
  - limbs on the same side of the body (i.e., hemiparesis/hemiplegia).
  - only one thoracic limb (i.e., monoparesis/monoplegia)
- Depressed reflexes and flaccid muscle tone

in thoracic limb(s), muscle atrophy after 1 to 2 weeks

- Normal/increased reflexes and muscle tone, without muscle atrophy, in pelvic limb(s)
- Postural reaction deficits in one thoracic limb, in limbs on the same side, or in all limbs
- Increased local sensitivity (hyperesthesia) at level of lesion
- Reduced sensitivity (hypesthesia) behind level of lesion
- Persistent scratching at one side of the shoulder/neck region
- Cutaneous trunci reflex depressed or absent (unilaterally or bilaterally)
- Horner's syndrome

Thoracolumbar syndrome (T3 to L3)

- Weakness or paralysis of pelvic limbs
- Pelvic limb reflexes normal or brisk (may seem clonus)
- No muscle atrophy in pelvic limbs
- Postural reaction deficits in pelvic limbs
- Reduced/absent cutaneous trunci reflex behind level of lesion
- Increased local sensitivity (hyperesthesia) at level of lesion
- Reduced sensitivity (hypesthesia) behind level of lesion

Lumbosacral distance (L4 to S3)

- Weakness/paralysis of pelvic limbs and tail
- Depressed pelvic limb reflexes and flaccid muscle tone
- Muscle atrophy in pelvic limbs, and/or hip muscles
- Postural reaction deficits in pelvic limbs
- Dilated anal sphincter
- Depressed bulbocavernosus reflex
- Reduced sensitivity (hypesthesia) in perineal area, pelvic limbs, or tail
- Urinary incontinence
- Faecal incontinence
- Root signature

Carotid system–Supplies anterior two-third of ipsilateral hemisphere + basal ganglion and produces

- Amaurosis fugax
- Aphasia
- Hemiparesis
- Hemisensory loss
- Hemianopic visual loss.

Vertebrobasilar system–Supplies the cerebellum, brainstem and posterior cerebral artery, and causes:

- Brainstem signs—nystagmus, diplopia, vertigo, vomiting, choking, dysarthria, ataxia
- Hemisensory loss
- Hemianopic visual loss, cortical blindness (Anton's syndrome)
- Transient global amnesia
- Tetraparesis.

44. CEREBRAL CIRCULATION

Features	Anterior Cerebral	Middle Cerebral	Posterior Cerebral
Contralateral hemiplegia	+ with milder hand symptoms and face spared	+	±
Hemisensory loss	+	+ mainly of face and arms	±
Dysphasia	–	+	–
Apraxia		+	– ,
Contralateral Hemianopia	–(Coma vigil state)	±	+

45. EPILEPSY
• Generalised

Type	Features	Management
Tonic-clonic/ grand mal	Sudden onset Limbs stiffen and jerk forcefully with LOC	Sodium valproate
Absence/ petit mal	Brief pauses Suddenly stops talking in mid sentence and then carries off where left off	Ethosuximidde

Type	Features	Management
Myoclonic	Thrown suddenly to ground or violently disobedient limb	Sodium valproate/ benzodiazapine
Atonic	Becomes flaccid	

- **Partial**

Type	Features	Management
Simple	No LOC	
Complex	Consciousness impaired, e.g., olfactory aura followed by automatism	Carbamazepine
Benign rolandic	Early morning seizures in young children	Carbamazepine
Infantile spasms	Jerks forward with arms flexed and hands extended, "salam attack"	Vigabatrin Sodium valproate

46. GLOMERULONEPHRITIS

Type	Electron Microscopy
Minimal change	Fusion of podocytes
Focal segmental glomerulosclerosis	Segmental areas of glomerulosclersis + ve IF for Ig M & C3
Mesangiocapillary	Double basement membrane or tram line effect
Type 1	Subendothelial deposits
Type 2	Intramembranous deposits
Membranous	If + ve for Ig G & C3 Subepithelial deposits
Poststreptococcal/ Proliferative	Subepithelial deposits ↑ ASOT ↑ C3
Rapidly progressive	Crescent formation

47. Hair Disorders

Telogen Effluvium: Excessive shedding of normal club hairs can be brought about by a number of stresses: parturition, febrile illness, psychological stress, crash diets and drugs. These factors may cause termination of the growing phase (anagen) of the hair follicles and transformation into the resting phase (telogen), causing a telogen fallout 2 to 4 months later. Treatment depends on determining the cause and correcting it. If a patient complains of hair breakage rather than the hair falling out at the roots, one may be dealing with a shaft problem. Microscopic examination of the actual shafts (hair mount) may be necessary to make the diagnosis. The most common cause of a hair shaft abnormality or hair fragility is trichorrhexis nodosa, with node-like swellings through which the shaft readily fractures. This usually appears as a result of trauma.

Trichotillomania

A compulsion to repetitively pull or pluck one's hair is trichotillomania. It gives rise to an unnatural pattern of hair loss. Clinical diagnosis can sometimes be quite difficult and may require a scalp biopsy for diagnostic confirmation. Examination of the distal hair shaft for bizarre twisting and fracture will increase the physician's index of suspicion. Fewer than 5 percent of such patients have deep-seated psychological disorders. Most cases resolve spontaneously. In severe cases, clomipramine may be prescribed.

Traction Alopecia

Traction alopecia occurs when hairs are constantly being pulled upon, usually by tightly braided hairstyles or elastic bands holding hairs together. This traumatises the hair follicles, and the hairs fall out before the end of their growth period. Traction alopecia is usually due to excessive tensional forces being exerted on hair shafts as a result of certain hair styling practices. It is seen more often in women, particularly East Indian and Black patients. Hair loss will be focal, depending on the way the hair is being pulled. Prolonged traction alopecia can lead to cicatrisation of the new hair follicle and permanent hair loss.

48. GUIDELINES FOR THE TREATMENT OF ASTHMA IN CHILDREN

Chronic Asthma

- In infrequent episodes, b2 agonists like Salbutamol are used as needed.
- In case of frequent episodes, Sodium cromoglycate or Nedocromil sodium + a bronchodilator are needed.
- Persistent asthma (daily symptoms), a trial of sodium cromoglycate + a bronchodilator is given as children are more susceptible to the side effects of steroids. If this does not control the symptoms, then inhaled steroids + intermittent bronchodilators are used.

Exercise-induced Asthma

- Cromolyn sodium is used both for prophylaxis and treatment in a known patient of exercise-induced asthma. If this is ineffective, it should be combined with a b2 agonist.
- For isolated and breakthrough exercise-induced asthma, inhaled b2 agonists are given.
- The indication for steroids, in children with exercise-induced asthma would be an underlying chronic asthma in the patient.

49. INVESTIGATION FOR PULMONARY EMBOLISM

This was one of the "always unsure" themes, but this is the rule I figured out.

In a patient with suspected pulmonary embolism, if he is stable, the investigation of choice would be V/Q Scan.

In an unstable patient, Spiral CT is preferred, over pulmonary angiography as it is non-invasive. However, if you're asked for the definitive investigation for this condition, it would be pulmonary angiography.

50. TUMOUR MARKERS

α Feto protein	• HCC
	• Germ cell tumour
	• Open neural tube defects
CA 125	• Ca ovary
CA 153	• Ca breast
	• Benign breast disease
CA 19-9	• Pancreatic Ca
	• Colorectal Ca
Carcinoembryonic antigen	• Colorectal Ca
HCG	• Choriocarcinoma
	• Pregnancy
	• Germ cell tumours
Neuron specific enolase	• Small cell Ca of lung
Placental alkaline phosphatase	• Seminoma
	• Ca ovary
	• Pregnancy
Prostate specific antigen	• Ca prostate

51. INVESTIGATION OF RENAL DISEASES

1. Suspected Renal Colic

- In any patient with suspected renal colic, first investigation is always a KUB X-ray.
- If the KUB is inconclusive, abdominal ultrasound is done because it is fast, cheap and there is no radiation risk as in IVU.
- In a patient with haematuria, IVU is preferred over abdominal USG as it would be useful in detecting any pathology distorting the collecting system and will also provide functional information of both the kidneys.
- In children less than 2 years, and in those with fever and vomiting, if the USG is inconclusive, you should proceed to do a Technitium renography.

2. Suspected Renal Infection

- In any patient with suspected renal infection, be it an adult or a child, the first investigation done is always an MSU.
- In infants, suprapubic aspiration is preferred as obtaining an MSU in them would be difficult.

- In children with recurrent UTI, an USG is done to detect reflux. If inconclusive an MCU is done which is the investigation of choice in children with recurrent UTI.
- In suspected pyelonephritis with abscess formation, immediate percutaneous nephrostomy is done.

52. INVESTIGATIONS IN BREAST DISEASE

- If a mass is present and malignancy has to be excluded–FNAC
- If there is no well-defined mass and malignancy has to be occluded–Sterotactic FNAC/ Biopsy
- For screening purposes–Mammography (not if breast tenderness is present)
- For ANDI (Fibroadenosis)–USG
- Breast implants–MRI.

53. DISORDERS OF CALCIUM METABOLISM

Disease	Calcium	Phosphorus	ALP	Vit D	PTH
Sarcoidosis	↑	←→	←→	↑	←→
Paget's disease	←→	←→	↑↑	←→	←→
Primary hyperparathyroidism	↑	↓	↑	↑	↑
Secondary Hyperparathyroidism	↓	↑	←→	←→	↑
Tertiary hyperparathyroidism	↑	↑	←→	←→	↑
Secondaries	↑	↑	↑	←→	←→
Osteomalacia	↓	↓	←→	↓	←→
Osteoporosis	←→	←→	←→	←→	←→

13 *Mock Exam No. 1*

> ◆ *This is unlike any other mock. I have deliberately selected few of the most confusing themes and included them in this one. Therefore, I recommend you to take this mock when you are well prepared, else you will be disappointed with your score!*

THEME 1

INVESTIGATION OF ACUTE ABDOMINAL PAIN

a. Serum amylase
b. Supine abdominal X-ray
c. β HCG
d. DPL
e. CRP
f. Gastrograffin enema
g. WBC count
h. Diagnostic laparoscopy
i. Immediate laparotomy
j. Abdominal USG
k. Erect CXR
l. CT abdomen

For each patient below, choose the investigation of first choice from the above list of options. Each option may be used once, more than once, or not at all.

1. A 25-year-old woman presents in a state of collapse. She has a painful tender rigid abdomen. Pulse is 120/min; BP 80/50 mm Hg. Bowel sounds are scanty.

2. A 52-year-old man presents with onset of severe abdominal pain over an hour. He has a history of episodic epigastric pain over the last three months. He is afebrile, tachycardic and normotensive. He has generalised tenderness with guarding and absent bowel sounds.

3. A 42-year-old obese woman complains of a 24-hour history of severe epigastric pain and profuse vomiting. On examination, she is tachycardic and mildly jaundiced. She has mild tenderness in the left upper quadrant and normal bowel sounds.

4. A 45-year-old builder fell from scaffolding to the ground this evening. He has landed on his left side and initially had pain in his left lower chest. He has now developed severe abdominal pain. He is becoming increasingly tachycardic and is hypotensive. His abdomen is tender with guarding and he is tender over his left 10th and 11th ribs.

THEME 2

INTERPRETATION OF HAEMATOLOGICAL RESULTS

a. CLL
b. AML
c. Rheumatoid arthritis
d. β-Thalassaemia minor
e. Folate deficiency
f. Old age
g. Cytotoxic drugs
h. Alcoholic liver disease
i. CML
j. Myelodysplasia
k. B_{12} deficiency
l. Iron deficiency

For each patient below, choose the single most likely diagnosis from the above list of options. Each option may be used once, more than once, or not at all.

5. A 40-year-old woman—Hb 9 gm/dl, MCV 82 fl, WCC 8.1* 10^9/litre, Platelets—450* 10^9, Serum ferritin 300 mg/litre.

6. A 60-year-old man with routine blood tests—Hb 10.8 gm/dl, MCV 87 fl, MCH 30 pg, WCC 18.4*10^9, Platelets 190*10^9, Direct antiglobulin test +.

7. A 55-year-old man with routine tests—Hb 13.8 gm/dl, MCV 106 fl, WCC 6.7* 10^9, Platelets 110*10^9, Blood film—target cells and hypersegmented neutrophils.

8. A 21-year-old woman booking visit to antenatal clinic—Hb 9.7 gm/dl, MCV 71 fl, MCH 27 pg, RBC count 6.7* 10^{12}, WCC 6.4* 10^9/litre, Platelets 310* 10^9, HbA$_2$—5%.

9. A 50-year-old man with long-standing epilepsy. Hb 10.1 gm/dl, MCV 115 fl, WCC 3.8* 10^9 (Lymphocytes 2.5, Neutrophils 1.3), Platelets 243 * 10^9.

10. A 75-year-old woman with investigations for fatigue. Hb 9.4 gm/dl, MCV 102 fl, WCC 4.5* 10^9/litre (Lymphocytes 1.8, Neutrophils 1.7, Monocytes 1, Myeloblasts 0.1), Platelets 190* 10^9.

THEME 3

MANAGEMENT OF DRUG DEPENDENCE

a. Gradual reducing course of Diazepam
b. Chlordiazepoxide
c. IV Vitamin B$_{12}$ and Thiamine
d. Group psychotherapy
e. Disulfiram
f. Hospital admission
g. Methadone
h. Needle exchange programme
i. Naloxone
j. Inform the police
k. Outpatient referral to drug dependency team
l. Chlormethiazole

For each patient below, choose management of first choice from the above list of options. Each option may be used once, more than once, or not at all.

11. A 30-year-old builder was admitted for an elective anterior cruciate ligament repair. He admits to drinking at least 60 units of alcohol per week and has no desire to stop. You are keen to prevent him from developing a withdrawal syndrome as this may impair his recovery.

12. A 70-year-old woman has taken 20 mg of temazepam at night for the last thirty years. She has begun to suffer with falls and has agreed that temazepam may be contributing to the falls.

13. A 63-year-old retired surgeon is admitted with a short history of bizarre behaviour. He claims that the GMC are investigating him for murder. He has evidence of a coarse tremour, horizontal nystagmus and an ataxic gait. His wife says that the story about the GMC is untrue but is worried about the amount of gin that her husband has drunk since retirement.

14. A 26-year-old heroin addict is worried because her partner has been diagnosed as having HIV infection. She is HIV negative. She feels, she cannot stop using heroin at present.

15. A 40-year-old man has become increasingly dependent on alcohol since his wife died last year. He admits that he has a problem and wishes to stop drinking. He does not wish to take antidepressants.

THEME 4

MANAGEMENT OF LOWER LIMB FRACTURES

a. Analgesia and active mobilization
b. Dynamic hip screw
c. Total hip replacement
d. Traction
e. External fixation
f. Hemiarthroplasty
g. ORIF
h. Below knee plaster
i. Bedrest only
j. Dynamic condylar screw
k. Above knee plaster
l. IM nail

For each patient below, choose the definitive management from the above list of options. Each option may be used once, more than once, or not at all.

16. An obese 32-year-old woman tripped on the kerv with eversion of her right foot. She has a displaced fracture of the medial malleolus and a fracture of her fibula above the level of her tibiofibular joint.

17. An 84-year-old man is admitted with a painful left hip after a fall at home. He has a fracture of his left inferior and superior pubic rami but his femur appears intact. He has pain on standing and no other significant medical history.

18. A 64-year-old woman with a history of osteoporosis is admitted with a displaced subcapital fracture of the right femoral neck. She has no other medical problems and is usually mobile without walking aids.

19. A 78-year-old woman is admitted with an intertrochantric fracture of her proximal femur. She has dementia and cardiac failure, which are well controlled. She lives in a nursing home and uses a Zimmer frame to walk short distances.

20. A 14-year-old boy fell from a stolen moped and sustained an open communited fracture of the distal third of his femur.

THEME 5

MANAGEMENT OF RAISED BLOOD PRESSURE

a. Lisinopril
b. Timetaphan camsilate
c. Imipramine followed by propanolol
d. Verapamil
e. Nifedipine
f. Propanolol
g. Sodium nitroprusside

Contd...

Contd...
h. Terazosin
i. Methyldopa
j. Hydralazine hydrochloride
k. Sotalol
l. Propanolol followed by phenoxybenzamine
m. Betaxolol
n. Digoxin
o. Glibenclamide
p. Phenoxybenzamine followed by propanolol

For of the patients described below, choose the single most useful medication from the list of options above. Each option may be used once, more than once, or not at all.

21. A frail 65-year-old man presents with difficulty in starting micturition associated with poor stream. He has no history of weight loss and denies any dysuria. On examination, a blood pressure of 130/90 mm Hg is found.

22. A 34-year-old known diabetic with chronic renal failure is examined and found to have a blood pressure of 150/100 mm Hg.

23. A 70-year-old woman complains of a chronic temporal headache associated with blurring of vision. She reports a history of seeing 'rings' of colour around lights, especially at night. Her blood pressure is found to be 135/90 mm Hg.

24. A 55-year-old company executive complains of palpitations and episodes of feeling dizzy. A 24-hour ECG tracing reveals episodes of a trial fibrillation which come and go at various times, lasting only 2 to 3 seconds.

25. A 45-year-old man has been treated for panic attacks by his GP for over six months without much improvement. He complains of excessive sweating, flushing and diarrhoea. On examination, he is found to have a blood pressure of 160/110 mm Hg. In the outpatients clinic the following day he is found to have glycosuria and a blood pressure of 130/80 mm Hg.

THEME 6

THE CLINICAL MANAGEMENT OF HYPERTENSION IN PREGNANCY

a. Magnesium hydroxide
b. Oral antihypertensives
c. Oral diuretic
d. Recheck blood pressure in seven days
e. Renal function tests
f. Retinoscopy
g. 24 hour urinary protein
h. A period of observation for blood pressure
i. Low-dose aspirin
j. Complete neurological examination
k. Foetal ultrasound
l. Immediate caesarean section
m. Induction of labour
n. Intravenous antihypertensive
o. Intravenous benzodiazepines

For each description below, choose the single most appropriate action from the above list of options. Each option may be used once, more than once, or not at all.

26. At 34 weeks, an 80-kg woman complains of persistent headaches and "flashing lights". BP is 155/100 mm Hg. Urinalysis is negative but she has digital oedema.

27. At 33 weeks, a 19-year-old primigavida is found to have BP of 145/100 mm Hg. At her first visit at 12 weeks, the BP was 145/90 mm Hg. She has no proteinuria, but she is found to have oedema to her knees.

28. At an ante-natal clinic visit at 38 weeks' gestation, a 38-year-old multigravida has BP of 140/95 mm Hg. She has no proteinuria and is otherwise well.

29. A 29-year-old woman has an uneventful first pregnancy to 31 weeks. She is then admitted as an emergency with epigastric pain. During the first 3 hours, her BP rises from 150/100 to 170/118 mm Hg. On dipstick, she is found to have 3+ proteinuria. The foetal cardioto-cogram is normal.

THEME 7

THE MANAGEMENT OF CHRONIC RENAL FAILURE

a. Aluminium hydroxide
b. Iron saccharin (Iron sucrose)
c. Insulin–increased dosage
d. Insulin–reduced dosage
e. Alpha-calcidol
f. Calcitriol
g. Calcium
h. Captopril
i. Diamorphine
j. Iron dextran
k. Frusemide
l. Renal dialysis
m. 25 Cholecalciferol
n. Metoprolol
o. Paracetamol
p. Recombinant erythropoietin
q. Calcium carbonate

For each description below, choose the single most appropriate management step from the above list of options. Each option may be used once, more than once, or not at all.

30. A 17-year-old youth with chronic renal failure has been noted to have a severe anaemia. The most cost effective first line treatment should be.

31. A 56-year-old man with diabetes mellitus and severe renal failure (serum creatinine 400 umol/l—and a blood glucose concentration of 59 mmol/l.

32. A 46-year-old woman with chronic renal failure is found to be severely anaemic. Iron therapy has been done without much success.

33. A 54-year-old woman with chronic renal failure presents with markedly swollen ankles.

34. A 34-year-old man with chronic renal failure is found to have a high phosphate concentration.

THEME 8

INVESTIGATION OF HOARSENESS

a. No investigation
b. Computed scan of the neck
c. Sputum for acid-fast bacilli
d. Cervical spine X-ray
e. Laryngoscopy
f. Bronchoscopy
g. Bronchoalveolar lavage
h. Chest X-ray
i. Lymph node biopsy
j. Treponemal haemagglutination assay

For each of the patients described below, choose the single most appropriate investigation from the list of options above. Each option may be used once, more than once, or not at all.

35. A 25-year-old man complains of a two-day history of hoarseness of voice. He denies any history of weight loss but admits to 4-year history of smoking.

36. A 13-year-old girl complains of a 2-day history of hoarseness of voice associated with dry cough. She feels feverish and on direct laryngoscopy, her vocal cords are grossly edematous.

37. A 34-year-old woman had a partial thyroidectomy 3 hours ago complains of mild hoarseness of voice. She had no history of phonation problems prior to surgery.

38. A 67-year-old man with a history of weight loss complains of hoarseness of voice. Computed tomography scan reveals an opacity in the right upper mediastinum. He denied any history of difficulty in breathing.

39. A 34-year-old IV drug user complains of a 4-month history of a productive cough. He has lost 10 kg in weight.

THEME 9

THE MANAGEMENT OF SUICIDE

a. Imipramine
b. Cognitive therapy

Contd...

Contd...
c. Coagulation profile
d. Detain under section II of the mental health act
e. Fluoxetine
f. Carbamazepine
g. Detain under section I of the mental health act
h. Admit and observe
i. Intensive psychiatric care
j. Electroconvulsive therapy (ECT)
k. Psychosurgery
l. Diazepam
m. Detain under section IV of the mental health act
n. No action

For each of the patients below, choose the single most appropriate treatment from the list of options above. Each option may be used once, more than once, or not at all.

40. A 34-year-old man starts punching people at the local tube station with no provocation. He is arrested by the police and asked to go for a mental health review. He disagrees strongly.

41. A known Schizophrenic goes missing from the local hospital. He is arrested by the police, but refuses to go back to hospital, despite the fact he has not finished the course of anti-psychotic medication prescribed by his doctor.

42. A 16-year-old boy refuses to go to church despite the constant insistence of his deeply religious mother. He had previously been a regular church-goer.

43. A 23-year-old woman complains of tearfulness and feeling low. However, denies any suicidal thoughts. She had her first child three days ago.

44. A 45-year-old man has been on anti-depressant therapy for six months. He continues to deteriorate and has had four serious suicidal attempts in the last ten days.

THEME 10

DIAGNOSIS OF SKIN PATHOLOGY

a. Pemphigus vulgaris
b. Pemphigoid
c. Porphyria cutanea tarda

Contd...

Contd...
d. Psoriasis
e. Impetigo
f. Pityriasis vesicolour
g. Acne rosacea
h. Erythema nodosum
i. Erythema multiforme
j. Erythema marginatum
k. Acne vulgaris
l. Erythema chronicum migrans
m. Erythema ab igne
n. Erythrodermic migraine
o. Toxic epidermal necrolysis

For each of the patients described below, choose the single most likely diagnosis from the list of options above. Each option may be used once, more than once, or not at all.

45. A 13-year-old boy complains of a non-pruritic rash characterised by papules and pustules effecting his face and upper chest. His voice has just started to deepen with sparse groin hair.

46. A 34-year-old man presents with a swollen erythematous nose. On examination, he is seen to have papules and telangiectasia in his face. Prior to this, he had experienced flushing after drinking alcohol and spicy food.

47. A 78-year-old man taking frusemide for nephrotic syndrome is seen in the dermatology clinic. He is found to have tense blisters covering the whole of his body save the oral mucosa. Skin biopsy is done and it reveals multiple linear IgG and C3 deposits along the basement membrane.

48. A 34-year-old woman presents with red lesions on her elbows and submammary areas. On examination, she is found to have extensive pitting and onycholysis of her nails.

49. A 32-year-old woman presents with flaccid blisters all over the body with extensive oral mucosa involvement. Skin biopsy reveals intercellular IgG with a 'crazy-paving' effect. She is being treated for migraine.

THEME 11

THE MANAGEMENT OF GENITAL PROLAPSE AND INCONTINENCE

a. Tension-free vaginal tape (TVT)
b. Vaginal pessary
c. Anterior colporrhaphy
d. Posterior colporrhaphy
e. Bilateral salpingo-oophrectomy
f. Pelvic floor exercises
g. Lose weight
h. Total abdominal hysterectomy
i. Oestrogen cream
j. Mirena coil (Progesterone containing IUCD)
k. Vaginopexy
l. Urodynamic studies
m. Bladder drill
n. Cystoscopy
o. Oxybutynin
p. Vaginal hysterectomy

For each of the patients described below, choose the single most appropriate treatment from the list of options below. Each option may be used once, more than once, or not at all.

50. A 56-year-old woman presents with a 2-month history of urinary incontinence. Because of her inconsistent history, you are unsure whether this is genuine stress incontinence or detrusor instability.

51. A 34-year-old woman with glaucoma presents with urinary incontinence. She is found to have detrusor instability. She dislikes surgery.

52. A 35-year-old woman presents with urinary incontinence. She is found to have genuine stress incontinence. She is put on conservative treatment without much success.

53. A 67-year-old woman presents with Grade II uterine prolapse. She also complains of urinary incontinence and is found to have a cystocoele.

54. A fit 65-year-old woman presents with uterine procidentia. She has five healthy children born from two different fathers.

THEME 12

ETHICAL PRACTICE OF MEDICINE IN THE UNITED KINGDOM

a. Reversal of the circumcision
b. Reversal of circumcision for catheter to be inserted and re-circumcising her
c. Trial of labour
d. Termination
e. Refusal of termination since it is illegal after 24 weeks for social reasons
f. Give her contraception
g. Withhold contraception
h. Call police and then give her the contraception
i. Inform mother and police immediately
j. Inform the general practitioner (GP)

For each of the scenarios described below, choose the single most appropriate action to take. Each option may be used once, more than once, or not at all.

55. A 22-year-old Somalian primigravida who doesn't speak English presents in labour. On vaginal examination you notice a very small introitus, barely enough to admit your little finger. A CTG is done and it shows a baseline rate of 100 beats/min. Your team decides, she needs an emergency caesarean section but because of the small introitus, you are unable to pass the catheter to proceed to theatre.

56. A 13-year-old girl demands the morning after pill. She says the condom she used with her 13-year-old boyfriend split in two, while having intercourse.

57. A tearful 19-year-old girl at 27 weeks of pregnancy requests a termination, saying her boyfriend has just left her and that she wouldn't want the baby to remind her of him. The boyfriend who is now in a jail is reported to have assaulted her during their stormy 2-year relationship.

THEME 13

THE DIFFERENTIAL DIAGNOSIS OF GENERALISED LYMPHADENOPATHY

a. Cytomegalovirus disease
b. Tuberculosis
c. Infectious mononucleosis
d. Syringobulbia
e. Toxoplasmosis
f. Sarcoidosis
g. HIV infection
h. Myeloma
i. Chronic granulomatous disease
j. Syringomyelia
k. Brucellosis
l. *Cryptococcus neoformans*

For each of the patients described below, choose the single most likely diagnosis from the list of options above. Each option may be used once, more than once, or not at all.

58. A 34-year-old sheep farmer from Cumbria presents with a 2-month history of an undulating fever, joint pain, weight loss and constipation. On further questioning, he is found to be depressed with marked generalised lymphadenopathy.

59. A 23-year-old university student complains of a sore throat, fever, and general malaise. On examination, numerous petechiae are seen on the palate.

60. A 33-year-old homosexual man presents with a 3-month history of a productive cough associated with two episodes of haemoptysis. He admits to losing 3 kg of weight. On examination, he is found to have generalised lymphadenopathy.

61. A 32-year-old man presents with confusion. A computed tomography scan of the head shows multiple ring enhancing lesions. He is being treated for HIV infection and on examination, generalised lymphadenopathy is found.

THEME 14

OVERDOSAGE MANAGEMENT

a. Acetylcysteine
b. Desferrioxamine
c. Dimercaprol
d. Ethanol
e. Flumazenil
f. Glucagon
g. Naloxone
h. Observation
i. Pralidoxime
j. Penicillamine
k. Sodium nitrite

For each of the scenarios described below, choose the single most appropriate action to take. Each option may be used once, more than once, or not at all.

62. A 50-year-old female is admitted unconscious after taking an overdose of an unknown substance. She has been depressed and anxious of late and has been prescribed some medication by the GP. Examination reveals a Glasgow coma scale of 10/15 and she responds and opens her eyes to pain. She has a pulse of 62 beats per minute regular, a blood pressure of 130/80 mm Hg and a respiratory rate of 20/minute with a saturation of 96 per cent.

63. A 70-year-old farmer is admitted acutely after ingesting an unknown overdose. Examination reveals a particularly anxious male who is sweaty and salivating. His temperature is 40°C and he has a blood pressure of 90/60 mm Hg with a pulse of 65 bpm.

64. A 6-year-old child is admitted after consuming her mother's ferrous sulphate tablets. She has had one haemetemesis.

65. A 52-year-old vagrant attends casualty with hyperventilation and vomiting. He confesses to having drunk methanol.

66. A 16-year-old girl is admitted after taking a paracetamol overdose with alcohol four hours previously. Her plasma paracetamol concentration is just below the nonagram concentration that would suggest treatment. Her plasma alcohol concentration is 120 mg/l.

THEME 15

DIFFERENTIAL DIAGNOSIS OF CHEST PAIN IN CHILDREN

a. Mitral insufficiency
b. Aortic stenosis
c. Pericarditis
d. Tricuspid incompetence
e. Costochondritic pain
f. Hiatus hernia
g. Pericardial tamponade
h. Reflux oesophagitis
i. Aortic insufficiency
j. Pleuritis

For each of the patient described below, choose the single most likely diagnosis. Each option may be used once, more than once, or not at all.

67. A 4-year-old boy wakes up frequently saying, 'It hurts here' while pointing to his chest. He was born prematurely but has done well otherwise. On examination, he has a 2/6 ejection systolic murmur between the left sternal border and the apex that radiates to the base and is accompanied by an apical S3.

68. A 7-year-old girl who had chickenpox four weeks ago complains of shortness of breath and a squeezing tightness in her midchest. She is anxious and refuses to lie down. Her heart rate is 110 beats per minute and blood pressure 110/80 mm Hg. Neck veins are distended.

69. A 14-year-old boy scout complains of exercise-induced sharp chest pain at the left lower sternal border that diminishes with resting. Palpation along the sternal edge replicates the symptoms.

70. A 17-year-old develops a tightening sensation in his mid, sternum during exercise. On examination the pulse rate is 180/minute and the blood pressure is 120/90 mm Hg. You hear a suprasternal notch thrill, an apical click, and a 3/6 ejection murmur at the right upper sternal border.

71. An 18-year-old girl has dull retrosternal pain and shortness of breath. On examination, she

has a heaving apical pulse, an apical systolic thrill and a short mid-diastolic rumbling murmur.

THEME 16

LOCALISATION OF NEUROLOGICAL DISORDER

a. Non-dominant frontal lobe
b. Dominant frontal lobe
c. Non-dominant temporal lobe
d. Dominant temporal lobe
e. Non-dominant parietal lobe
f. Dominant parietal lobe
g. Occipital lobes
h. Temporal-occipital-parietal (TOP) junction

For each of the scenarios described below, choose the single most appropriate option. Each option may be used once, more than once, or not at all.

72. A 45-year old stroke patient can clearly understand what someone says to him but he is unable to respond verbally to that person.

73. Although he can repeat phrases, the speech of a 52-year-old stroke patient is impaired and has difficulty understanding what someone says to him.

74. A well-educated stroke patient cannot add a column of four single digit numbers.

75. A 58-year-old stroke patient is unable to copy completely; a simple drawing of a clock face.

THEME 17

INVESTIGATIONS IN SUBSTANCE ABUSE

a. Dexamethasone suppression test
b. Electrocardiogram (ECG)
c. Electroencephalogram (EEG)
d. Full blood count
e. Gamma-glutamyl-transpeptidase (GGTP)
f. Genetic analysis

Contd...

Contd...
g. MRI brain
h. Serum toxicology screen
i. Thyroid function tests
j. *Treponema pallidum* haemagglutination assay (TPHA)
k. Urine drug screen

For each of the scenarios described below, choose the single most appropriate investigation of choice. Each option may be used once, more than once, or not at all.

76. A 32-year-old woman with bipolar affective disorder is brought to A and E department comatose. She is apyrexial and has no focal neurological deficit.

77. A 45-year-old man presents with low mood and tremour, worse first thing in the morning.

78. A 25-year-old nurse with a history of alcoholism; partner says that after an argument she took some medication after which she is behaving strangely, very agitated, profusely sweating, and with tremours and episodes of diarrhoea.

79. A 50-year-old patient says that he had brief spells of dizziness and palpitations since he has started his new medication. He also vomited twice and had trouble coming to the A and E because his vision is compounded with coloured haloes.

80. A 65-year-old man presents with progressive dementia, spastic paraparesis and seizures. He also has small irregular pupils that accommodate but do not react to light.

THEME 18

INVESTIGATIONS OF PAEDIATRIC ENDOCRINOLOGICAL AND METABOLIC DISORDERS

a. FBC
b. Serum electrolytes
c. Serum ADH

Contd...

Contd...

d. Serum GH
e. Phenylketones in urine
f. Guthrie's test
g. Galactose in urine
h. Serum ACTH
i. High serum blood glucose
j. Low blood glucose
k. Cystine in urine
l. Plasma cortisol

For each of the scenarios described below, choose the single most appropriate investigation of choice. Each option may be used once, more than once, or not at all.

81. A 1-month-old baby with poor feeding and lethargy. O/E umbilical hernia and enlarged tongue.

82. A newborn female with enlarged clitoris and fused labia.

83. A 13-year-old obese girl with asthma and eczema and amenorrhoea, BP 130/80 mm Hg.

84. A 1-month-old baby with vomiting, jaundice and hepatomegaly. Baby is worse after feeding.

85. An 8-year-old boy with short stature C/O thirst and passes huge volume of colourless urine.

THEME 19

DIFFERENTIAL DIAGNOSIS OF NEUROMUSCULAR DISEASE

a. Cerebrovascular accident
b. Guillain-Barré syndrome (GBS)
c. Amyotrophic lateral sclerosis (ALS)
d. Neurosyphilis
e. Duchenne's muscular dystrophy
f. Friedreich's ataxia
g. Myasthenia gravis
h. Transverse myelitis
i. Motor neurone disease
j. Syringomyelia

For each of the patients described below, choose the single likely diagnosis. Each option may be used once, more than once, or not at all.

86. A 39-year-old white man presents to his GP because of progressive muscle weakness of one week's duration. His medical history is unremarkable, although he reports having had an influenza-like episode two weeks ago. The GP notes a marked decrease in reflexes and loss of light touch and vibration sensation in the distal extremities.

87. A six-year-old black boy is brought to GP by his mother. She is concerned he is using his hands to pull himself up from the floor. The GP notes that the boy's calf muscles appear enlarged and his muscle strength is extremely impaired.

88. A 55-year-old man with no previous medical problem visits his GP because his arms have become progressively weaker over the past two months. The weakness and fatigue began first in one arm and developed later in the other. The GP notices hyper-reflexia, as well as generalised muscle weakness, in all four extremities. The man has no sensory dysfunction, and his gait is normal.

89. A 34-year-old woman presents with muscular weakness of three months' duration and says that she tires easily when she's trying to work. After she rests for a while, some of her strength returns. The GP notices bilateral facial weakness and asymmetric distribution of proximal limb weakness. Tendon reflexes are normal.

THEME 20

DIAGNOSIS OF PAEDIATRIC DISORDERS

a. Rubella
b. Landau-Barre syndrome
c. Landau-Kleffner syndrome
d. Cystinuria
e. Homocystinuria
f. Phenylketonuria

Contd...

Contd...
g. Hirschsprung's disease
h. Celiac disease
i. Fifth Disease
j. Measles
k. Infectious mononucleosis
l. Hypothyroidism
m. Cri-du-chat syndrome

For each of the patients described below, choose the single most likely diagnosis. Each option may be used once, more than once, or not at all.

90. A Chinese woman of 34 year presents to you with her 5-year-old son. She says that her child was speaking normally till about 3 year, thereafter he has been increasingly aloof and does not talk. O/E the child is mute. Auditory evoked response is normal B/L. The baby has Mongoloid features. There have been two episodes of generalised convulsions in the past not associated with fever. What is the most likely diagnosis?

91. A child presents to you with H/O convulsions.O/E white opacity is found in the eyes. The hair is thin and breaks easily. The urine biochemistry shows an abnormality for proteins.

92. A child presents with alternating diarrhoea and constipation, O/E abdominal distension is present. The child is in the 70th percentile of his weight for age.

93. A young adult man presents with flushed cheeks and rashes on his forearms. He c/o intermittent joint pain for the past two weeks. Cervical lymphadenopathy present. Monospot test is +.

94. An infant is brought to you with poor feeding. On examination, the muscle tone is decreased. The baby has a peculiar cry. He is a full-term baby delivered p/v. The mother is healthy and antenatal history is uneventful.

THEME 21

INVESTIGATIONS OF THE UNCONSCIOUS PATIENT

a. Blood cultures
b. Blood gases
c. Brainstem death tests
d. Carboxyhaemoglobin level
e. Computed tomography of head
f. Cardiac monitoring
g. Lumbar puncture
h. Serum glucose
i. Thyroid function tests
j. Toxicology screen
k. Urea and electrolytes

For each of the patients described below, choose the first investigation of choice. Each option may be used once, more than once, or not all.

95. A 47-year-old woman is found collapsed in her home. Examination reveals meningism and bilateral upgoing plantars.

96. A 67-year-old man with severe chronic obstructive pulmonary disease was brought to Casualty Department by an ambulance. His breathing and conscious level seems much worse with oxygen during the ambulance journey, although his oxygen saturation on pulse oximetry is 90%.

97. A middle-aged couple is found comatosed in their caravan by their teenaged son, who woke up in the middle of the night with nausea and vomiting. All three of them had been well before they went to sleep.

98. A 45-year-old man collapses in the ward. Examination reveals cardiorespiratory arrest.

99. A 56-year-old diabetic is found unresponsive at home by her neighbour. She is presently being treated for a urinary tract infection. There is no focal neurological deficit on examination.

THEME 22

TERATOGENICITY

a. Betamethasone	b. Norethisterone
c. Salbutamol	d. Ergometrine
e. Oxytocin	f. PG F2 alpha
g. Indomethacin	h. Oxytetracycline
i. Amoxycillin	j. Alcohol
k. Isotretinoin	l. Lithium
m. Valproic acid	n. Dilantin
o. Streptomycin	p. Thalidomide

For each of the anomalies described below, choose the most likely drug involved. Each option may be used once, more than once, or not at all.

100. Ebstein's anomaly.
101. Congenital deafness, CNS and heart defects.
102. Short palpebral fissure, long philtrum and midfacial hypoplasia.
103. Oligohydramnios.
104. Pulmonary oedema.
105. Virilisation of a female foetus.
106. Premature closure of ductus arteriosus.
107. Defective dentition of the foetus after 4th month.
108. Foetal hydantoin syndrome.
109. Neural tube defects.

THEME 23

DIAGNOSIS OF THYROID DISORDERS

a. Thyroglossal cyst	b. De Quervain's disease
c. Hypothyroidism	d. MEN Type I
e. Simple goitre	f. Hashimoto's thyroiditis
g. Graves' disease	h. MEN Type II A
i. Papillary carcinoma	j. Lymphoma
k. Follicular carcinoma	l. MEN Type II B

For each of the patients described below, choose the single most likely diagnosis. Each option may be used once, more than once, or not at all.

110. A 26-year-old man presents with hypertension, bone pains, prominent mucosal neuromas involving lips, tongue, and inner aspect of the eyelids. His uncle had the same problems.
111. A 43-year-old woman presents with weight loss despite good appetite, constipation, frontal headaches and metrorrhagia. Also complains of recurrent dyspepsia and peptic ulcers. Her abdominal radiography shows renal stones.
112. A 30-year-old woman presents with weight gain, constipation, lethargy, and flaky rash. She prefers to stay indoors even in warm weather.
113. A 19-year-old student presents with a neck swelling. On examination, swelling moves up with swallowing and protrusion of the tongue.
114. A 49-year-old woman presents with goitre. On examination, thyroid is firm and rubbery. Thyroid microsomal antibodies are positive in high titre.

THEME 24

MANAGEMENT OF BLOOD CONDITIONS

a. Oral ferrous sulphate
b. Folic acid
c. Oral prednisolone
d. Venesection
e. Venesection followed by hydroxyurea
f. Vitamin K
g. Heparin
h. Protamine sulphate
i. DDAVP
j. Tranexamic acid
k. NSAIDs
l. IV morphine
m. SC diamorphine with cyclizine
n. TENS
o. Phentolamine

For each of the patients described below, choose the single most appropriate management. Each option may be used once, more than once, or not at all.

115. A 55-year-old man presented in A and E

with chest pain of two hours duration and suspected MI. He has been well yet has developed night sweats and lost 8 kg in last three months. He doesn't smoke nor has past history of chest problems. His Hb came out 22 g/dl, PCV 0.58, WBC 20* 10^9/L and platelets 600* 10^9/L.

116. A 29-year-old woman has had a D and C for long standing menorrhagia. She is taken back to the theatre yet no abnormality can be found. She says that she had been having problems in the past with bleeding after dental extractions. Surprisingly upon ordering her PT, APTT and platelet count, all turn out normal.

117. A 72-year-old man presented to medical OPD with dyspnoea, wheezing, fever and cough productive of sputum. Initial investigations are: Hb 23 g/dl, PCV 0.62, a mild neutrophilia and platelets 200* 10^9/L. His son says that he has been smoking all his life and keeps on getting bouts of bronchitis but is otherwise well.

118. A 19-year-old Afro-Carribean female presented to A and E with pains in her left leg, right hip and back. She has had been on an all night rave club.

THEME 25

TREATMENT IN EYE CONDITIONS

a. Pilocarpine drops
b. Tetracycline ointment + sulfadimethoxine
c. Peripheral iridectomy
d. Pressure on the eyeball
e. ECCE
f. ICCE
g. Tetracycline ointment + ciprofloxacin
h. Scleral buckling
i. 1% tropicamide
j. 1% cyclopentolate
k. Corticosteroids

For each of the patients described below, choose the single most appropriate treatment.

Each option may be used once, more than once, or not at all.

119. A 54-year-old myopic develops flashes of light and then sudden loss of vision.

120. A 54-year-old hypertensive p/w sudden loss of vision and on fundoscopy there is pale retina with cherry red spot at fovea.

121. A 29-year-old man presents with meiosis and photophobia. The ophthalmologist prescribes a drug, so that he may not develop synechiae as a sequel to this presentation.

122. An 8-year-old African boy complains of grittiness and lacrimation in eyes. His siblings also have this problem.

123. A 47-year-old male with mild headache. Has changed his spectacles thrice in one year. There is mild cupping and sickle-shaped scotomata in both eyes.

THEME 26

ORAL HYPOGLYCAEMIC THERAPY: INDICATIONS AND CONTRA-INDICATIONS

a. Glibenclamide
b. Orlistat-Xenical
c. Metformin
d. Acarbose
e. Gliclazide
f. Rosglitazone
g. Repaglinide
h. Netaglinide
i. Guar gum
j. Chlorpropamide
k. Pravastatin

For each of the patients described below, choose the most likely choice of drug. Each option may be used once, more than once, or not at all.

124. A 77-year-old man with a BMI 34 kg /M2 complains of feeling increasingly lethargic. He has suffered with type 2 diabetes treated with diet only for two years and his HbA_{1c} measures 9%.

125. The most appropriate drug for an 83-year-old lady, with diet treated type 2 diabetes, most recent HbA_{1c} 8.9% and BMI 26 kg / M2. She lives on her own and complains of osmotic symptoms.

126. A 42-year-old man with type 2 diabetes and obesity (BMI 39 kg/M2). His glycaemic control is moderate with HbA$_{1c}$ 8% and no osmotic symptoms. He has successfully lost 3.6 kg in weight over the last two months and is on a low-fat diet, with a noticeable improvement in his home glucose monitoring.

127. A 66-year-old man intolerant of metformin with HbA$_{1c}$ 10.6% on glibenclamide 15 mg daily.

128. A 51-year-old man with type 2 diabetes for five years. BMI 36 kg/M2, HbA$_{1c}$ 9.9% complaining of thirst and lethargy. Present medication glicalzide 160 mg twice daily, metformin 2 grams daily.

THEME 27

GYNAECOMASTIA

a. Acromegaly
b. Anorexia nervosa
c. Congenital adrenal hyperplasia
d. Delayed puberty
e. Fragile X syndrome
f. Kallmann's syndrome
g. Klinefelter's syndrome
h. LH secreting pituitary tumour
i. Prolactinoma
j. Small cell cancer
k. Testicular carcinoma

For each of the patients described below, choose the single most likely diagnosis. Each option may be used once, more than once, or not at all.

129. A 28-year-old male presents with reduced shaving frequency. He is tall, has absent pubic and axillary hair and has gynaecomastia.

130. A 16-year-old male is referred with poor development. He is noted to be rather short and to have had a repair of a cleft palate. He has absent pubic and axillary hair, with delayed development of the genitalia.

131. A 16-year-old male is seen in the clinic. His parents complain that he is prone to outbursts, has poor academic performance and he attends the remedial class in school. He has normal secondary sexual characteristics and large testes.

132. A 25-year-old male smoker complains of painful breasts. He is noted to have mild and tender gynaecomastia. He has a normal right testis but the left is not palpable.

133. A 15-year-old male is referred with concerns regarding his development. He is thin with diffuse lanugo hair over the body, but absent secondary sexual characteristics.

THEME 28

BLOOD SUPPLY TO THE BRAIN

a. Basilar artery
b. Anterior cerebral artery
c. Superior cerebral artery
d. Posterior cerebral artery
e. Anterior communicating artery
f. Middle cerebral artery
g. Circle of Willis
h. Posterior communicating artery
i. Anterior inferior cerebellar artery
j. Spinal artery
k. Posterior inferior cerebellar artery

For each of the areas described below, choose the artery supplying. Each option may be used once, more than once, or not at all.

134. Broca's area of speech.

135. Trigeminal nerve nucleus in the medulla oblongata.

136. Visual cortex.

137. Leg area in the motor cortex.

138. Anterior aspect of the pons.

THEME 29

MANAGEMENT OF ARRHYTHMIAS

a. Carotid sinus massage
b. Adenosine
c. Lignocaine

Contd...

Contd...
d. Sotalol
e. Emergency DC version
f. Amiodarone
g. Digoxin
h. CaCl$_2$
i. Disopyramide
j. Elective DC cardioversion
k. Flecainide

For each of the patients described below, choose the single most appropriate management from the above list of options. Each option may be used once, more than once, or not at all.

139. 50-year-old man was admitted with ac ant MI. Two hours after thrombolysis with TPA he suddenly c/o feeling faint. O/E pulse is 145/min, BP 100/40 mm Hg. Cardiac monitor shows long run of VT.

140. A young woman 31 weeks pregnant presents in the A and E complaining of dizziness. O/E her ECG shows re-entrant tachycardia. She had one such episode in the past, which resolved spontaneously and she is not taking any medication.

141. A 30-year-old woman with history of palpitations for the past six months. Her ECG shows a shortened PR interval and delta waves. Holter monitor shows evidence of paroxysmal SVT.

142. A 65-year-old man with renal failure being treated with CAPD presents with abdominal pain for the last two days. O/E his temperature 99.8°F. He has also noted that the dialisate is cloudy after exchange. He suddenly deteriorates with broad complex tachycardia. The BP is 75/40 mm Hg.

143. A 70-year-old male collapsed on surgical ward following a left hemicolectomy. He has a very weak carotid pulse, BP cannot be recorded. Cardiac monitor shows broad complex tachycardia, the rate is 160/min.

THEME 30

DIAGNOSIS OF FRACTURES

a. Anterior displaced radial head
b. Posterior displaced radial head
c. Subluxation of MCP joint of thumb with abduction
d. Thenar eminence swelling, palmar bruising and inability to move thumb
e. Pain in the area between extensor and abductor pollices longus tendons

For each of the abnormalities below, choose the most likely description from the above list of options. Each option may be used once, more than once or not at all.

144. Colles's fracture.
145. Smith's fracture.
146. Fracture of scaphoid bone.
147. Bennett's fracture.
148. Game keeper's thumb.

THEME 31

DIAGNOSIS OF CHROMOSOMAL DISORDERS

a. Cri-du-chat syndrome
b. Turner's syndrome
c. Down's syndrome
d. Edward's syndrome
e. Patau's syndrome
f. Klinefelter's syndrome
g. Noonan's syndrome
h. Marfan's syndrome
i. Kartagener's syndrome
j. Kallmann's syndrome

For each of the patients described below, choose the single most likely diagnosis from the above list of options. Each option may be used once, more than once, or not at all.

149. Abnormal ear and facies, flared fingers, growth deficiency, rocker bottom feet.
150. Short stature, webbed neck, normal intelligence, cubitus valgus and infertility.

151. Cleft lip and palate, polydactyly, scalp defects, mental deficiency, microphthalmia.
152. Microcephaly, dysmorphic features, mental retardation, abnormal cry.
153. Mental deficiency, hypotonia, duodenal atresia, simian crease, Brushfield's spots on iris, Mongoloid facies.

THEME 32

DIAGNOSIS OF RESPIRATORY DISORDERS

a. Acute Type 1 Respiratory failure
b. Acute Type 2 Respiratory failure
c. Chronic Type 1 Respiratory failure
d. Chronic Type 2 Respiratory failure
e. Metabolic acidosis
f. Metabolic alkalosis
g. Lactic Acidosis
h. Hyperventilation syndrome
i. Mitochondrial myopathy
j. Normal finding

For each set of values described below, choose the single most likely diagnosis from the above list of options. Each option may be used once, more than once, or not at all.

154. $P O_2 = 9,$ $P CO_2 = 7,$
    $pH = 7.4,$ $HCO_3 = 32.$
155. $P O_2 = 9,$ $P CO_2 = 5,$
    $pH = 7.4,$ $HCO_3 = 25.$
156. $P O_2 = 7.5,$ $P CO_2 = 4.0,$
    $pH = 7.6,$ $HCO_3 = 24.$
157. $P O_2 = 8,$ $P CO_2 = 8,$
    $pH = 7.2,$ $HCO_3 = 22.$
158. $P O_2 = 12,$ $P CO_2 = 2,$
    $pH = 7.8,$ $HCO_3 = 22.$

Note: Normal values are:

$P O_2 = 12\text{-}15 \text{ kPa},$
$P CO_2 = 4.4\text{-}6.1 \text{ kPa},$
$pH = 7.4,$
$HCO_3 = 21\text{-}27.5 \text{ mmol/L}$

THEME 33

PRINCIPLES OF THE DUTIES OF A DOCTOR REGISTERED WITH THE GENERAL MEDICAL COUNCIL

a. Make the care of your patient your first concern.
b. Treat every patient politely and considerately.
c. Respect patients' dignity and privacy.
d. Listen to patients and respect their views.
e. Give patients information in a way they can understand.
f. Respect the right of patients to be fully involved in decisions about their care.
g. Keep your professional knowledge and skills up-to-date.
h. Recognise the limits of your professional competence.
i. Be honest and trustworthy.
j. Respect and protect confidential information.
k. Make sure that your personal beliefs do not prejudice your patients' care.
l. Act quickly to protect patients from risk if you have good reason to believe that your colleague may not be fit to practice.
m. Avoid abusing your position as a doctor.
n. Work with colleagues in the ways that best serve patients' interests.

For each of the patients described below, choose the single most appropriate action from the above list of options. Each option may be used once, more than once, or not at all.

159. A 23-year-old Indian woman requests a female doctor to perform a pelvic exam.
160. A 55-year-old man who is being admitted for a total knee replacement states that he is a Jehovah's witness and therefore refuses any blood products.
161. A 16-year-old girl informs you that she may be pregnant, and her parents are unaware.
162. A 28-year-old man is offered the choice of whether he would like to receive interferon injections for multiple sclerosis.
163. A 65-year-old diabetic sees you for a neurological option and asks if you would renew his insulin prescription as a favour.

164. There is a lunch-time teaching session, but a patient on the ward is experiencing chest pain.
165. Your patient reports feeling of depression. You seek a psychiatric opinion.
166. You asked a patient to undress to examine the abdomen. You remember to cover the patient's groin.
167. You are asked to examine a patient at his bedside. You remember to pull the curtain around the bed to ensure privacy.
168. You see an overworked colleague struggle with his duties. You intervene and offer assistance.

THEME 34

DIAGNOSIS OF ARRHYTHMIAS

a. Atrial flutter
b. Atrial fibrillation
c. Ventricular tachycardia
d. Ventricular extrasystoles (ectopics)
e. Heart block
f. Sinus tachycardia
g. Sinus bradycardia
h. Supraventricular tachycardia
i. Blood loss
j. Wenckebach's phenomenon

For each of the patients described below, choose the single most likely diagnosis from the above list of options. Each option may be used once, more than once, or not at all.

169. A 65-year-old man, post myocardial infarction is found to have a regular pulse, with a rate of 50 beats/min.
170. A 50-year-old man with palpitations is treated with a carotid massage. He now has no other complaints.
171. Following a road traffic accident, a 25-year-old man is brought to the A and E. He is found to have a pulse rate of 120 beats/min and blood pressure of 90/50 mm Hg.

172. A 65-year-old man is found to have an irregular pulse, with a rate of 110 beats/min.
173. A 23-year-old footballer is examined by his GP and found to have a pulse rate of 50 beats/min. He is otherwise well.
174. A 50-year-old man, post myocardial infarction in ITU is found to have a pounding heartbeat which then disappeared spontaneously. The patient remains conscious.

THEME 35

MANAGEMENT OF HEART FAILURE

a. ACE inhibitors
b. Digoxin
c. Aortic valve replacement
d. Thiazide diuretics
e. Heart transplant
f. IV furosemide
g. Nitrates (oral)
h. Nitrates (IV)
i. Thiamine (IV)
j. Pericardiocentesis

For each of the patients described below, choose the single most appropriate management from the above list of options. Each option may be used once, more than once, or not at all.

175. A 15-year-old boy is examined and found to have severe congestive cardiac failure.
176. A 40-year-old man with cardiac failure is found to have a palpable thrill in the right second intercostal space, which radiates to the neck.
177. A 50-year-old man with suspected heart failure has a blood pressure of 90/60 mm Hg and pulse rate of 110 beats/min. Chest X-ray shows globular heart.
178. A 50-year-old suspected alcoholic has biventricular cardiac failure. He has deranged liver function tests.
179. A 60-year-old female in cardiac failure wants long-term treatment for her conditions. Echocardiography shows global hypokinesia and loss of contractility.

THEME 36

DIARRHOEA AND WEIGHT LOSS

a. IBD
b. Tuberculous enterocolitis
c. Cytomegalovirus (CMV) infection
d. Celiac disease
e. Tropical sprue
f. Hyperthyroidism
g. Amyloidosis
h. Intestinal lymphoma
i. Whipple's disease
j. Chronic pancreatitis

For each of the patients described below, choose the single likely diagnosis from the above list of options. Each option may be used once, more than once or not at all.

180. A 48-year-old man presents with watery stools 4 to 6 times a day, he also has abdominal cramps, flatulence and borborygmi. He has lost 20 £ over the last 8 months. He is of Irish descent.

181. A thirty-year-old HIV positive man with a 3 week history of intermittent bloody diarrhoea, urgency, abdominal pain and malaise. Repeated stool examinations negative for ova and parasites including multiple stool cultures for enteric pathogens.

182. A 50-year-old man with diarrhoea and migratory arthralgias for the last 6 months, he has lost 20 £ in weight and relatives describe a decline in mental acuity.

183. A 28-year-old man with diarrhoea and crampy abdominal pain of the right lower abdomen for the last eight weeks, he also complains of fever, anorexia and weight loss. He has not responded to antituberculous therapy for the last three weeks.

184. A 63-year-old woman with rheumatoid arthritis for the last 20 years presents with weight loss, foul smelling diarrhoea, easy bruising and peripheral oedema. On examination, she has waxy skin plaques, especially in the axillary folds.

THEME 37

VERTIGO

a. Benign positional vertigo
b. Vestibular neuronitis
c. Meniere's disease
d. Migraine
e. Multiple sclerosis
f. Alcohol
g. TIA
h. Complex partial seizures
i. Posterior fossa tumours

For each of the patients described below, choose the single most likely diagnosis from the above list of options. Each option may be used once, more than once or not at all.

185. A 50-year-old woman with paroxysmal attacks of giddiness lasting 25 to 30 seconds. They occur on sitting up or lying down, looking up or looking down, particularly with the head rotated to the left. The attacks persist for about one month and have occurred three times over the last two years.

186. A 68-year-old man with a two-week history of occipital headache, nausea and ataxia. He has intense vertigo on movement of the head in any direction. Examination reveals gaze evoked nystagmus to the left and ataxia of the left-sided limbs. CXR reveals a hilar mass.

187. A 14-year-old boy with sudden vertigo and vomiting three days after contracting an upper respiratory infection. His hearing is normal.

188. A 60-year-old woman with a history of bursting sensation in the head followed by a roaring noise in the right ear. She has episodes of intense vertigo, which are reduced by lying still with the right ear uppermost.

189. A 54-year-old hypertensive, diabetic with a history of sudden onset rotatory feelings accompanied by slurred speech and unsteadiness while walking. The episode lasted for 25 minutes.

THEME 38

CONFUSION

a. Hyponatremia
b. Hypoglycaemia
c. Hypothyroidism
d. Hyperthyroidism
e. Hypercapnoeic encephalopathy
f. Hepatic encephalopathy
g. Uremic encephalopathy
h. Subacute combined degeneration of cord
i. Wernicke's encephalopathy
j. Hypertensive encephalopathy
k. *Herpes simplex encephalitis*

For each of the patients described below, choose the single most likely diagnosis from the above list of options. Each option may be used once, more than once, or not at all.

190. A 72-year-old man on chlorpropamide for diabetes mellitus presents with confusion, after an attack of gastroenteritis.

191. A 68-year-old vegan presenting with confusion, disorientation and ataxia. Examination reveals pallor and a tinge of icterus.

192. A 48-year-old widower with a history of peptic ulcer disease with vomiting after meals for the past two weeks. He is found in a drowsy inebriated state in his flat by the neighbour. Examination reveals ataxic gait with dysconjugate eye movements and gaze evoked nystagmus in all directions.

193. A 40-year-old man admitted with a history of confusion for one day. His wife says that he has had fever for the past 48 hours. Examination reveals a temperature of 39°C. No neck stiffness but very poor recent memory. CSF reveals 50000/mm³ cells with 90% lymphocytes and 20 RBC's/mm³. CSF protein is 80 mg/dl and glucose 90 mg/dl with RBS of 130 mg/dl.

194. A 56-year-old chronic smoker presenting with progressive dyspnoea, anasarca and confusion. Examination reveals bounding pulses. Papilloedema and asterixis.

THEME 39

HEADACHE

a. Tension headache
b. Migraine
c. Cluster headache
d. Encephalitis
e. Subarachnoid haemorrhage
f. Intracranial tumour
g. Temporal arteritis
h. Meningitis
i. Glaucoma
j. *Pseudotumour cerebrii*

For each of the patients described below, choose the single most likely diagnosis from the above list of options. Each option may be used once, more than once, or not at all.

195. A middle-aged man with recurrent severe nocturnal headaches accompanied by eye pain—watering from the eyes and nasal congestion. The pain lasts about two hours and returns the next night. The pain recurs for about a week and then disappears for months.

196. A 15-year-old girl with headaches for the last 15 days. She now presents with very severe headache for one day and on examination has a complete left ophthalmoplegia.

197. A 32-year-old HIV+ve woman with progressive headache for the past two months. Examination reveals papilloedema.

198. A 35-year-old obese woman on the O.C. pill presents with progressive headache for the last three months. She gives history of visual obscuration and examination reveals an enlarged blind spot, papilloedema and impaired visual acuity.

199. A 17-year-old male with severe headache altered sensorium and vomiting. He has had fever, cough and a rash for the last four days.

200. A 26-year-old man comes with complaints of headache, pain in the eye. On examination, there is cupping of his optic disc.

14 *Answers to Mock Exam No. 1*

◆ *When attempting the EMQ's you will see that more than knowing why the answer to a particular question is 'this', you will need to know why the answer is not 'that'. I have tried to do just that in explaining these themes.*

THEME 1

INVESTIGATION OF ACUTE ABDOMINAL PAIN

1. B HCG

When investigating acute abdominal pain/collapse in a woman of reproductive age group, the first investigation should always be a urine HCG test to confirm/rule out pregnancy. This woman could be suffering from an ectopic pregnancy. If the HCG is negative, twisted ovarian cyst could be a possibility and diagnostic lap should be performed.

2. Erect CXR

The history of episodic epigastric pain suggests an acid peptic disease. The present symptoms and signs could be due to perforation of an ulcer and erect CXR would reveal gas under the diaphragm.

3. Serum amylase

This seems to be a case of acute pancreatitis. Serum amylase, though not very specific for this condition, is the first investigation performed before an USG abdomen.

4. Immediate laparotomy

The features are those of a ruptured spleen and an immediate laparotomy is warranted.

THEME 2

INTERPRETATION OF HAEMATO-LOGICAL RESULTS

5. Rheumatoid arthritis (RA)

The features are suggestive of a normocytic and normochromic anaemia and the ferritin level is within normal limits. This is anaemia of chronic disease, which occurs in RA.

6. CLL

Warm autoimmune haemolytic anaemia (AHA) presents with a positive antiglobulin test and is a common association with CLL.

7. Alcoholic liver disease

An MCV of less than 110 fl is suggestive of alcoholic liver disease in a patient with macrocytic anaemia as in this patient. Target cells are seen in alcoholic liver disease and sickle cell disease.

8. β-thalassaemia minor

Microcytic hypochromic anaemia with HbA_2 more than 2%.

9. Folate deficiency

Phenytoin therapy in epilepsy often leads to folate deficiency as in this patient with macrocytic anaemia.

10. Myelodysplasia

Anaemia, neutropenia, monocytosis and blasts are diagnostic.

THEME 3

MANAGEMENT OF DRUG DEPENDENCE

11. Chlordiazepoxide

Diazepam and Chlordiazepoxide are used to prevent withdrawal symptoms in alcoholics.

Chlormethiazole is not used anymore as it causes dependency and respiratory depression.

12. Gradual reducing course of Diazepam

Temazepam is a short-acting benzodiazepine, so withdrawal is harder. Hence, you should change to long-acting b'diazepines like diazepam and gradually reduce its dose by 2 mg/week.

13. IV Vitamin B_{12} and Thiamine

These features are suggestive of Korsakoff's psychosis (confabulation) that occurs in Wernicke's encephalopathy (ataxia, nystagmus, ophthalmoplegia).

14. Needle exchange programme

Since she cannot stop using heroin, which would be ideal, the next choice would be a needle exchange programme. If her boyfriend had to be forcing her to take heroin, the choice would be to 'Inform the police'.

15. Group psychotherapy

Since he admits that his drinking is a problem and has a desire to stop, drugs are not required.

THEME 4

MANAGEMENT OF LOWER LIMB FRACTURES

16. ORIF (Open reduction with internal fixation)

Fractures of the ankle usually require operative treatment if there is significant disruption of the joint or if there is instability.

Displaced stable fractures can be treated by closed reduction.

17. Analgesia and active mobilization

Pubic ramus fractures rarely require operative treatment except if there is pelvic instability or associated displaced acetabular fracture.

18. Total hip replacement

A subcapital fracture of the femoral neck may be associated with damage to the joint capsule, resulting in impairment of the blood supply of the femoral head and subsequent avascular necrosis.

19. Dynamic hip screw

The management of an intertrochantric fracture is to use a sliding (dynamic) hip screw or an intramedullary nail with a screw through the fracture into the femoral head.

20. Traction

Conservative treatment with traction is preferred in open or distal fractures and in children.

THEME 5

MANAGEMENT OF RAISED BLOOD PRESSURE

21. Terazosin

This man has features suggestive of a BPH and alpha-blockers are used as they would both control the BP as well as they contract the detrusor and relaxes the internal meatus thereby relieving him of his micturition problems.

22. Lisinopril

The ACE inhibitors are the drugs of choice in diabetic patients with renovascular hypertension. Regular monitoring of renal function is required as they can cause renal artery stenosis.

23. Betaxolol

This selective β-blocker is the drug of choice in chronic simple glaucoma, which this patient is suffering from.

24. Sotalol

This is the first line drug in paroxysmal atrial fibrillation.

25. Methyldopa

Pregnancy-induced hypertension (PIH) is treated by methyldopa.

THEME 6

THE CLINICAL MANAGEMENT OF HYPERTENSION IN PREGNANCY

26. Oral antihypertensives

The obese women are more prone to develop pregnancy-induced hypertension (PIH). Proteinuria is often the last feature to develop in PIH. The flashing lights could be due to retinal involvement.

27. Recheck blood pressure in seven days

This patient is an unlikely candidate for PIH as her BP has remained steadily high from the first trimester. She could be having essential hypertension before she was pregnant. Drug treatment would not be required as she is asymptomatic, with a BP less than 170/110 mm Hg (indications for anti-HTN therapy).

28. A period of observation for blood pressure

Here again the patient is asymptomatic and has mild hypertension. As she is of 38 weeks' gestation, a period of observation for blood pressure should precede an induction of labour.

29. Induction of labour

Since it has been three hours from the time of admission, an IV antihypertensive was probably started and still the BP rose to 170/118 mm Hg. This is a sign of impending eclampsia, the only cure for which is immediate delivery.

THEME 7

THE MANAGEMENT OF CHRONIC RENAL FAILURE

30. Iron saccharin (Iron sucrose)

Since they have asked the 'most cost effective' first line management, iron saccharin would be the answer as erythropoietin is expensive and not of proven benefit.

Iron saccharin has better absorption than iron dextran.

31. Renal dialysis

A serum creatinine greater than 350 umol/l in non-diabetics and greater than 250 umol/l is an indication for renal dialysis.

32. Recombinant erythropoietin

This is the best drug for the treatment of anaemia in CRF, which occurs largely due to erythropoietin deficiency.

33. Frusemide

Loop diuretics treat oedema of CRF.

34. Calcium carbonate

It is used in hyperphosphatemia as it is a phosphate binder.

THEME 8

INVESTIGATION OF HOARSENESS

35. No investigation

Since there is no history of fever or weight loss, this is probably a viral laryngitis. The 2-day history rules out smoking as a probable cause.

36. No investigation

This is a case of bacterial laryngitis and since direct laryngoscopy has already been done, no further investigations are required. Antibiotics are indicated.

37. No investigation

Mild hoarseness of the voice is common after thyroidectomy and requires no investigation. If it persists, a laryngoscopy is required.

38. Laryngoscopy

The opacities in the mediastinum could be lymph nodes with the primary in the larynx; hence a laryngoscopy should be done to rule out laryngeal CA.

39. Sputum for acid-fast bacilli

This could be an opportunistic tuberculous infection in a patient with HIV infection.

THEME 9

THE MANAGEMENT OF SUICIDE

40. Admit and observe

Section 136—detained for 72 hours—for the purpose of psychiatric assessment of those in public places thought by the police to be mentally ill and in need of a place of safety.

41. Admit and observe

Reason the same as above.

42.   No action

He has the right to refuse to go to the church.

43.   Cognitive therapy

Postpartum blues are common and should be treated by cognitive therapy. Postpartum depression is treated by fluoxetine and postpartum psychosis by electroconvulsive therapy (ECT).

44.   Electroconvulsive therapy (ECT)

Repeated suicidal attempts are an indication for ECT.

THEME 10

DIAGNOSIS OF SKIN PATHOLOGY

45.   Acne vulgaris

It is an inflammatory disorder of the pilosebaceous follicle common in teenagers and affecting the face, neck, upper chest and back.

46.   Acne rosacea

Facial flushing, inflammatory papules and pustules affecting the nose, forehead and cheeks, and triggered by alcohol. The swollen erythematous nose could be a rhinophyma, which is a frequent association.

47.   Pemphigoid

The IgG and C3 deposits in pemphigoid are seen along the basement membrane, whereas in pemphigus they are seen within the epidermis. Tense blisters are characteristic.

48.   Psoriasis

Flexural lesions are characteristic and psoriasis is associated with pitting and destruction of the nails.

49.   Pemphigus vulgaris

Intercellular (within the epidermis) deposits of IgG and 'flaccid' blisters are diagnostic.

THEME 11

THE MANAGEMENT OF GENITAL PROLAPSE AND INCONTINENCE

50.   Urodynamic studies

Studies of intravesical pressure are useful to differentiate stress incontinence from detrusor instability.

51.   Bladder drill (Exercise not drilling!)

Glaucoma could be worsened by anticholinergic therapy, so bladder training exercises are recommended in this patient.

52.   Tension-free vaginal tape (TVT)

In genuine stress incontinence, failure of conservative treatment (pelvic floor exercises and physiotherapy) is an indication for tension-free vaginal tape.

53.   Anterior colporrhaphy

Anterior colporrhaphy with Kelly's stitch is the management of low-grade prolapse with cystocele.

54.   Vaginal hysterectomy

Since she has completed her family and has a procidentia, a hysterectomy would be ideal. Vaginal is preferred as it has fewer complications.

THEME 12

ETHICAL PRACTICE OF MEDICINE IN THE UNITED KINGDOM

55.   Reversal of the circumcision

Female circumcision is commonly practiced in African countries. Hence, a reversal of circumcision would be required to pass the catheter. The second choice is not appropriate because circumcision is illegal in the UK.

56.   Give her contraception

If she is above 12 years, she is a major and has the right to ask for a pill without consent from her parents.

57.   Termination

Termination in the UK is illegal after 24 weeks but may be done if continuation would cause:

- Risk to the mother's life

- Grave or permanent injury to the mother's physical or mental health

- Risk of the child, if born, being seriously handicapped.

THEME 13

THE DIFFERENTIAL DIAGNOSIS OF GENERALISED LYMPHADENOPATHY

58. Brucellosis
59. Infectious mononucleosis
60. Tuberculosis
61. Toxoplasmosis

THEME 14

OVERDOSAGE MANAGEMENT

62. Observation

Since her vitals are stable and from the features it is unable to identify the drug involved, a period of observation would be required.

63. Pralidoxime

Hypersecretion from glands, hyperthermia and hypotension are characteristic of OP poisoning. In addition, he is a farmer. Pralidoxime should be administered along with atropine.

64. Desferrioxamine

It is an iron-chelating agent.

65. Ethanol

Ethanol is the antidote for methanol poisoning.

66. Acetylcysteine

Antidote for paracetamol. Methionine is an alternative.

THEME 15

DIFFERENTIAL DIAGNOSIS OF CHEST PAIN IN CHILDREN

67. Reflux esophagitis

The pain at night is due to gastric contents regurgitating into his oesophagus. Ejection systolic murmurs are common in children and are known as innocent murmurs. S3 are also common in children.

68. Pericarditis

The preceding viral infection, aggravation of pain on lying, tachycardia and high JVP suggest this condition in this girl.

69. Costochondritic pain

Exercise-induced pain aggravated by palpation is characteristic of costochondritis.

70. Aortic stenosis
71. Mitral insufficiency

The heaving apex and apical thrill suggest a volume overload and hence mitral insufficiency. The diastolic murmur could be due to an associated MS.

THEME 16

LOCALISATION OF NEUROLOGICAL DISORDER

72. Dominant frontal lobe

Broca's aphasia is due to a lesion in the dominant (usually left) frontal lobe—inferior frontal gyrus where the speech motor area (Broca's area) is situated.

73. TOP Junction

A lesion in the angular gyrus, which is located in this area, disrupts the communication between the motor and sensory speech area. Hence, both understanding and speech is impaired. Since the arcuate fasciculus is not involved, repetition is preserved.

74. Dominant parietal lobe

A lesion in this part produces the Gertsmann's syndrome characterised by acalculia, finger agnosia, right-left agnosia and dysgraphia.

75. Non-dominant parietal lobe

Spatial disorientation is a feature of non-dominant parietal lobe lesion.

THEME 17

INVESTIGATIONS IN SUBSTANCE ABUSE

76. Serum toxicology screen

Lithium is the drug of choice in bipolar affective disorder and it is associated with a narrow therapeutic index. Toxic symptoms, such as drowsiness, blurred vision, coarse tremour, ataxia and dysarthria, may occur.

77.   Gamma-glutamyl-transpeptidase (GGTP)

These are symptoms of alcohol withdrawal and a GGTP level would be recommended.

78.   Thyroid function tests

These symptoms are suggestive of hyperthyroidism. Amiodarone and iodine are drugs that cause hyperthyroidism, but it is unlikely that the lady has taken these. In any case, thyroid function tests are warranted.

79.   Electrocardiogram (ECG)

The symptoms are suggestive of digoxin toxicity and an ECG would show characteristic changes. For more information see ECG in PLAB-1 revision aid chapter.

80. *Treponema pallidum* haemagglutination assay (TPHA)

The features are characteristic of neurosyphilis. The pupil is known as Argyll Robertson pupil.

THEME 18

INVESTIGATIONS OF PAEDIATRIC ENDOCRINOLOGICAL AND METABOLIC DISORDERS

81.   Guthrie's test

It is the heel prick test done in newborns to estimate thyroid hormone levels. The features are suggestive of hypothyroidism.

82.   Serum ACTH

Enlarged clitoris and fused labia are suggestive of congenital adrenal hyperplasia and a serum ACTH is confirmative.

83.   Plasma cortisol

There are two possibilities in this case: obesity and amenorrhoea are suggestive of Cushing's, whereas the mention of asthma and eczema suggests secondary hypoadrenalism due to steroid therapy. A plasma cortisol will differentiate.

84.   Galactose in urine

An inborn error of carbohydrate metabolism, galactosemia presents with progressive hepatosplenomegaly, cataracts and renal tubular defects. Worsening status after feeding is seen due to acidosis caused by accumulation of Gal-1-phosphate.

85.   Serum ADH

Presence of short stature and large amounts of dilute urine is suggestive of diabetes insipidus.

THEME 19

DIFFERENTIAL DIAGNOSIS OF NEUROMUSCULAR DISEASE

86.   Guillain-Barré syndrome (GBS)

Progressive muscle weakness following a viral illness is indicative of this condition. Involvement of dorsal column is common.

87.   Duchenne's muscular dystrophy

Hypertrophy of calf muscles and using hands to pull him up (Gowers' sign +) is diagnostic.

88.   Amyotrophic lateral sclerosis (ALS)

The features of progressive spastic tetraparesis or paraparesis with a mix of LMN and UMN signs is suggestive.

89.   Myasthenia gravis

Easy fatigability and regaining of power after a while of rest are features of myasthenia gravis. Proximal limb muscles and facial muscles are also involved.

THEME 20

DIAGNOSIS OF PAEDIATRIC DISORDERS

90.   Landau-Kleffner syndrome

91.   Homocystinuria

92.   Hirschsprung's disease

93.   Fifth disease

Also known as Slapped Cheek syndrome or Erythema infectiosum, this disease presents with flushed cheeks, rashes and cervical lymphadenopathy. False positive monospot test is invariably positive.

94. Hypothyroidism

Cri-du-chat syndrome is an alternative but in that case there would be other features like CVS abnormalities, microcephaly, wide-spaced eyes and moon face. There would be no hypotonia.

THEME 21

THE INVESTIGATIONS OF UNCONSCIOUS PATIENT

95. CT Head

Signs of meningism and upgoing plantars are suggestive of a subarachnoid bleed.

96. Blood gases

This patient has an exacerbation of his COPD. Since carbon dioxide is accumulated and provides with the respiratory drive, administering oxygen will negate this effect and aggravate his condition.

97. Carboxyhaemoglobin level

They were well before they went to sleep which rules out any drug overdose and the need for toxicology screen. The event happening in a caravan would suggest carbon monoxide poisoning.

98. Cardiac monitoring

Cardiac monitoring should accompany aggressive cardiopulmonary resuscitation.

99. Serum glucose

The first investigation for loss of consciousness in a diabetic should always be serum glucose measurement.

THEME 22

TERATOGENICITY

100. Lithium
101. Isotretinoin
102. Alcohol
103. Indomethacin
104. Salbutamol
105. Norethisterone
106. Indomethacin
107. Oxytetracycline
108. Dilantin
109. Valproic acid

THEME 23

DIAGNOSIS OF THYROID DISORDERS

110. MEN Type II B

Adrenal, thyroid, parathyroid and mucocutaneous neuromas are diagnostic.

111. MEN Type I

Involvement of the parathyroid, pituitary, pancreas, adrenal and thyroid glands.

112. Hypothyroidism
113. Thyroglossal cyst

Movement of the swelling on protrusion of tongue rules out a thyroid mass. A thyroglossal cyst moves on protrusion of the tongue because of its attachment to the hyoid bone.

114. Hashimoto's thyroiditis

Usually presents in women of middle age with a firm and rubber thyroid. Thyroid microsomal antibodies are present in a very high titre.

THEME 24

MANAGEMENT OF BLOOD CONDITIONS

115. Venesection followed by hydroxyurea

Features are suggestive of primary polycythaemia vera the treatment of which is repeated venesection and chemotherapy with hydroxyurea to control thrombocytosis.

116. NSAIDs

NSAIDs, such as mefenamic acid, are the drugs of choice in dysfunctional uterine bleeding. Tranexaminic acid is not used frequently as it may cause excess bleeding itself.

117. Venesection

This is a case of secondary polycythaemia due to chronic bronchitis and hypoxia. Venesection will provide symptomatic relief. Chemotherapy is not required.

118. TENS

Transcutaneous electric nerve stimulation (TENS) is useful in reducing dorsal horn cell response, which is causing symptoms in this girl.

THEME 25

TREATMENT IN EYE CONDITIONS

119. Scleral buckling

This is the definitive management in retinal detachment where the retina is secured back in place. Retinal detachment is more common in myopics.

120. Pressure on the eyeball

The immediate management of central retinal artery occlusion (CRAO) is pressure on the eye, which might assist in dislodging the embolus. This has to be done within one hour of onset. Firm pressure is applied until the patient feels pain, and then released.

121. 1% cyclopentolate

This mydriatic agent, by dilating the pupil prevents the formation of synechiae.

122. Tetracycline ointment + sulfadimethoxine

Trachoma is common in hot, dry and dusty climate and is treated by the above antibiotics.

123. Pilocarpine drops

Chronic simple glaucoma is managed by beta-blockers and pilocarpine, which reduce the resistance to the outflow of aqueous.

THEME 26

ORAL HYPOGLYCAEMIC THERAPY: INDICATIONS AND CONTRA-INDICATIONS

124. Metformin

Type II diabetes with obesity is treated by Biguanides, if dietary measures fail.

125. Gliclazide

Preferred in elderly because it is short acting and hence rarely causes hypoglycaemia.

126. Orlistat-Xenical

Xenical (orlistat) is a lipase inhibitor for obesity management that acts by inhibiting the absorption of dietary fats. Since his blood glucose is under control, his only problem would be to control his weight.

127. Rosglitazone

The NICE recommends its use an alternate to insulin only if metformin with a sulfonyl urea is not working or not tolerated.

128. Rosglitazone.

As above.

THEME 27

GYNAECOMASTIA

129. Klinefelter's syndrome

Male phenotype with reduced/absent pubic hair and increased arm span characterises this chromosomal disorder.

130. Kallmann's syndrome

Isolated hypogonadism. More than half of the patients have associated somatic stigmata, most commonly, nerve deafness, colour blindness, mid-line cranio-facial deformities, such as cleft palate or harelip, and renal abnormalities.

131. Fragile X syndrome

Also known as Martin-Bell syndrome, it is a significant cause of male mental retardation and presents with a large testis and facial asymmetry.

132. Testicular carcinoma

Since the left testis is not palpable, this could be an undescended testis, which has undergone a malignant change that commonly cause gynaeco-mastia.

133. Anorexia nervosa

Diffuse lanugo hair over the body and absent secondary sexual characteristics are suggestive.

THEME 28

BLOOD SUPPLY TO THE BRAIN

134. Middle cerebral artery

135. Basilar artery
136. Posterior cerebral artery
137. Anterior cerebral artery
138. Middle cerebral artery

THEME 29

MANAGEMENT OF ARRHYTHMIAS

139. Lignocaine
    Long run of VT, if the patient is not in severe hemodynamic distress, is initially managed by lignocaine.
140. Carotid sinus massage
    The first management in re-entrant tachycardia, which is a type of supraventricular tachycardia, is a carotid massage.
141. Sotalol
    WPW syndrome with paroxysmal SVT.
142. $CaCl_2$
    This patient is in renal failure with hyperkalemia and should be given calcium chloride or gluconate.
143. Emergency DC version
    Severe hemodynamic instability.

THEME 30

DIAGNOSIS OF FRACTURES

144. Anterior displaced radial head
    Dinner fork deformity.
145. Posterior displaced radial head
    Garden-spade deformity.
146. Pain in the area between extensor and abductor pollices longus tendons
    Pain in the anatomical snuff box.
147. Thenar eminence swelling, palmar bruising and inability to move thumb
    Fracture dislocation of carpometacarpal joint.
148. Subluxation of MCP joint of thumb with abduction.

THEME 31

DIAGNOSIS OF CHROMOSOMAL DISORDERS

149. Edward's syndrome
150. Turner's syndrome
151. Patau's syndrome
152. Cri-du-chat syndrome
153. Down's syndrome

THEME 32

DIAGNOSIS OF RESPIRATORY DISORDERS

154. Chronic Type 2 Respiratory failure
    Hypoxia, hypercapnoea and since pH is maintained, the condition is a chronic one.
155. Chronic Type 1 Respiratory failure
    Hypoxia, normal pCO_2 and pH.
156. Acute Type 1 Respiratory failure
    Hypoxia with alkalosis.
157. Acute Type 2 Respiratory failure
    Hypoxia, hypercapnoea with acidosis.
158. Hyperventilation syndrome
    Alkalosis with low pCO_2—diagnostic.

THEME 33

PRINCIPLES OF THE DUTIES OF A DOCTOR REGISTERED WITH THE GENERAL MEDICAL COUNCIL

159. Listen to patients and respect their views.
160. Make sure that your personal beliefs do not prejudice your patients' care.
161. Respect and protect confidential information.
162. Respect the right of patients to be fully involved in decisions about their care.
163. Recognise the limits of your professional competence.

164. Make the care of your patient your first concern.

165. Work with colleagues in the ways that best serve patients' interests.

166. Respect patients' dignity and privacy.

167. Respect patients' dignity and privacy.

168. Act quickly to protect patients from risk if you have good reason to believe that your colleague may not be fit to practice.

THEME 34

DIAGNOSIS OF ARRHYTHMIAS

169. Sinus bradycardia.

170. Supraventricular tachycardia.

171. Blood loss.

172. Atrial fibrillation.

173. Sinus bradycardia.

174. Ventricular extrasystoles.

THEME 35

MANAGEMENT OF HEART FAILURE

175. Digoxin

The CCF is managed by inotropes like digoxin and amrinone.

176. Aortic valve replacement.

This patient has aortic regurgitation.

177. Pericardiocentesis

Globular heart is suggestive of pericardial effusion as are hypotension and tachycardia.

178. Thiamine (IV)

These are features of wet beri beri caused by thiamine deficiency.

179. Heart transplant

The ACE inhibitors are preferred in patients with global hypokinesia and loss of contractility but should not be used in elderly people for long term as they may cause renal impairment.

THEME 36

DIARRHOEA AND WEIGHT LOSS

180. Celiac disease

People of Northern European origin have an HLA predisposition to hypersensitivity to wheat proteins. Diarrhoea, steatorrhoea, weight loss and abdominal pain are common.

181. Cytomegalovirus (CMV) infection

Immunocompromised + inflammatory colitis + negative microscopic exam + negative cultures for standard enteric pathogens—CMV.

182. Whipple's disease

Malabsorption, arthritis and dementia are the characteristic features of Whipple's disease.

183. Crohn's disease

The symptoms are suggestive of tuberculosis but since the patient has shown no improvement to ATT, the next diagnostic possibility would be Crohn's which is common in twenties.

184. Amyloidosis

Secondary amyloidosis is common in chronic inflammations, such as RA, and tends to present with these symptoms. There may also be involvement of kidneys, liver and spleen.

THEME 37

VERTIGO

185. Benign positional vertigo

Repeated attacks of vertigo related to positional change, lasting for more than 30 seconds are characteristic. It is common after head injury.

186. Posterior fossa tumours

Features if raised ICP + ataxia, nystagmus and vertigo are suggestive of posterior fossa involvement. These could be secondaries from the primary in the lung.

187. Vestibular neuronitis

Sudden onset of vertigo following a viral infection is suggestive.

188. Meniere's disease

Attacks that occur in clusters and consist of vertigo lasting for up to 12 hours, nausea, vomiting, unilateral or bilateral tinnitus and progressive sensorineural hearing loss.

189. TIA

Vertebrobasilar TIA in a hypertensive, which lasts for less than 24 hours.

THEME 38

CONFUSION

190. Hypoglycaemia

Chlorpropamide is a long-acting drug known to cause hypoglycaemia and in this case, the infection has precipitated the attack.

191. Subacute combined degeneration of cord.

Vegetarians are prone to develop B_{12} deficiency, which leads to this condition.

192. Wernicke's encephalopathy

Drowsiness, ataxia, confusion, nystagmus and ophthalmoplegia are characteristic of this condition. His peptic ulcer disease could be due to alcohol consumption, too.

193. *Herpes simplex encephalitis*

The CSF findings are suggestive of viral infection. Lack of neck stiffness rules out meningitis.

194. Hypercapnoeic encephalopathy

The COPD patients are prone to CO_2 retention and this presents with the above features.

THEME 39

HEADACHE

195. Cluster headache

Pain occurs once or twice every 24 hours and each episode lasts for 2 to 3 hours. Clusters last 4 to 12 weeks. The pain then disappears for months. It presents with rapid onset of periorbital pain, which is unilateral with watering, lid swelling and rhinorrhoea.

196. Intracranial tumour

Probably, a tumour of the brainstem, which has caused the ophthalmoplegia.

197. Meningitis

Immunocompromised state predisposes to opportunistic infections such as cryptococcus.

198. *Pseudotumour cerebrii*

Also known as benign intracranial hypertension, this condition is more common in obese women and those on OC pills. It presents with features of raised ICP without any obvious cause for it.

199. Encephalitis

Altered sensorium suggests parenchymal involvement.

200. Glaucoma.

15 Mock Exam No. 2

> ◆ *Again, find here, some of the most mind-boggling themes and see how good your preparation is... let's say pass mark is 144. All the best !*

THEME 1

TREAMENT OF PNEUMONIA

a. Erythromycin
b. Tobramycin + Carbenicillin
c. Ciprofloxacin
d. Beta 2 agonist
e. Co-trimoxazole
f. Benzyl Penicillin
g. Cefotaxime
h. Rifampicin + Isoniazid

For each of the patient described below, choose the single most appropriate treatment from the above list of options. Each option may be used once, more than once, or not at all.

1. A 20-year-old woman presents with a week's history of fever, rigors and productive rusty cough. CXR shows right lower lobe consolidation.

2. A 50-year-old man presents with shortness of breath and dry cough CXR shows widespread pulmonary shadowing. He takes azathioprine for resistant rheumatoid arthritis.

3. A 60-year-old diabetic presents with productive cough and malaise. CXR shows right upper lobe consolidation and hilar lymphadenopathy.

4. A 12-year-old boy with cystic fibrosis presents with chest infection. He also suffers from mild renal failure.

5. A 40-year-old mental patient with dry cough and confusion. Blood tests reveal lymphopenia and hyponatremia. The CXR shows right lobar shadowing.

THEME 2

DIAGNOSIS OF UPPER RESPIRATORY INFECTIONS

a. Epiglottitis
b. Pneumonia
c. Croup
d. Bronchiolitis
e. Glandular Fever
f. Sinusitis
g. Influenza

For each of the patient described below, choose the single most appropriate diagnosis from the above list of options. Each option may be used once, more than once, or not at all.

6. A 2-year-old boy presents with 3-day history of noisy breathing on inspiration and a barking cough worse at night. He has low-grade fever and is hoarse.

7. A 3-year-old girl presents with fever and stridor. She is in severe respiratory distress and is drooling saliva.

8. An 18-year-old man presents with fever, trismus and stridor. His breathing becomes laboured with use of accessory muscles and is cyanotic. He initially presented to his GP with a sore throat a few days back.

9. A 2-year-old boy presents with cough and wheeze. Other members of the family are also suffering from URTI. On examination, he has flaring of the nostrils and audible expiratory wheezes.

10. A 2-year-old boy presents with chronic cough. The CXR reveals bronchiectasis. He also suffers from steatorrhoea

THEME 3

CAUSES OF BREATHLESSNESS

a. Goodpasture's syndrome
b. Acute myocardial infarct
c. Extrinsic allergic alveolitis (EAA)
d. Histoplasmosis
e. Cystic fibrosis
f. Churg-Strauss syndrome
g. Cryptogenic fibrosing alveolitis
h. Allergic bronchopulmonary aspergillosis (ABPA)
i. Pneumothorax

For each of the patients described below, choose the single most likely diagnosis from the above list of options. Each option may be used once, more than once, or not at all.

11. A 32-year-old farmer presented with worsening cough, breathlessness and flu- like symptoms, which he had each winter for three years. The CXR shows fine miliary shadows.

12. A 30-year-old man presented with breathlessness at rest, cough and haemoptysis, all of which he has had for a few days. He is cyanosed with bilateral inspiratory/expiratory wheeze. The PEFR is normal. Blood test showed high creatinine.

13. A 65-year-old man presents with pneumonia, which he had for three weeks. It was resistant to antibiotics. He had asthmatic bronchitis for more than 50 years. The CXR shows consolidation of right upper zone and perihilar consolidation.

14. A 45-year-old man with progressive burning pains in the sole of his left foot, bilateral cramps in both calves and left foot drop. He is a known asthmatic and suffers from recurrent sinusitis. The FBC shows eosinophilia.

THEME 4

INTERPRETATION OF ECG FINDINGS

a. Hyperkalemia   *ex not in BL.*
b. Digoxin toxicity   *digitalis usw too high heart ti.*
c. Pericarditis   *infla. or heart s/c*
d. Sick sinus syndrome
e. Hypokalemia
f. Myocardial infarction (MI)
g. WPW syndrome *wolf-parkinson-white - irregular heart b.*
h. Hypothyroidism
i. Complete heart block

For each of the patients described below, choose the single most likely diagnosis from the above list of options. Each option may be used once, more than once, or not at all.

15. A patient's ECG shows prolonged PR interval, ventricular ectopics and bradycardia.

16. A 50-year-old man presents with fever and chest pain. He has a history of angina and his ECG reveals concave elevation of straight segment in Lead II, V5 and V6.

17. A 65-year-old man is tired and nauseous. On examination, his ECG shows deep Q waves, elevated ST segment and T wave inversion.

18. An old woman suffers repeated drop attacks. ECG reveals, LVH, LAD, atrial ectopics and atrial tachycardia.

19. A 40-year-old woman is drowsy and confused. ECG findings: profound bradycardia, absent P waves, Q waves, tall T waves and a long QT interval.

THEME 5

IMMEDIATE MANAGEMENT OF MENINGITIS

a. Treat immediate contacts
b. Urinary catheter

Contd...

Contd...

c. IV sodium bicarbonate
d. IV 20% dextrose
e. High-dose steroids
f. Lumbar puncture
g. Acyclovir — *ANTIVIRAL DRUG USED FOR HERPES*
h. Cranial CT scan
i. Antipyretics — *DRUG REDUCES TEMP.*
j. High-dose steroids
k. IV plasma expansion
l. Thick and thin blood films

For each of the patients described below, choose the single most likely management from the above list of options. Each option may be used once, more than once, or not at all.

20. A 45-year-old executive visited western Africa at short notice for four days. Twenty-four hours after returning home, he has fever, rigors and stiff neck and shoulders. On examination, he has excoriated urticarial lesions on his ankles and mild jaundice.

21. A 20-year-old woman who is known to have AIDS has a 3-week history of increasing vomiting, headache and weight loss. On examination, she is confused with papilloedema and bradycardia.

22. A 6-year-old girl who has never been immunised has been treated with ampicillin for otitis media. After four days, she is more unwell with fever, headache, photophobia, neck stiffness, but no alteration in consciousness.

23. A previously fit college student is brought by his friend unconscious. On arrival at the A&E he has weak pulse, tachycardia and a spreading rash. His college doctor has given him IM penicillin.

24. A school boy developed fever, neck stiffness and photophobia with petechial rash. Antibiotics were given for suspected meningococcal meningitis. He is now stable.

THEME 6

DIAGNOSIS OF MUSCLE WEAKNESS

18. SLE *SYSTEMIC LUPUS ERYTHMATOSIS.*
19. Dermatomyositis *CONNECTIVE TISSUE DISEASE RELATED TO POLYMYOSITIS.*
20. Polymyalgia rheumatica
21. MS
22. Charcot-Marie-Tooth disease *HEREDITARY SENSORI MOTOR NEUROPATHY.*
23. Motor neuron disease
24. Subacute combined degeneration
25. Poliomyelitis
26. Bell's palsy
27. GBS *GUILLIAN BARRÉ SYNDROME*
28. Syringomyelia *x CYST OR CAVITY FORMS IN THE SPINAL CORD.*

For each of the patients described below, choose the single most likely diagnosis from the above list of options. Each option may be used once, more than once, or not at all.

25. A 30-year-old man presents with palsy of his right side of his face including his forehead. His otological examination and other cranial nerves are normal.

26. A 43-year-old man presents with paraesthesiae, which rapidly develop, to flaccid paralysis of lower limbs. This was preceded by an URTI a week back. The CSF examination shows very high protein but no white cells.

27. A 50-year-old woman presents with a purple rash on her cheeks and eyelids and symmetrical proximal muscle weakness.

28. A 45-year-old man presents with diplopia on lateral gaze, nystagmus, paraesthesiae and muscle weakness. The CSF examination reveals oligoclonal bands and an increase in IgG.

29. A 20-year-old woman presents with flaccid paralysis of legs with loss of reflexes. She reports recovering from a mild URTI but then developing meningitis. The CSF shows protein and lymphocytes.

THEME 7

INTERPRETATION OF THYROID FUNCTION TESTS

a. Graves' disease *GOITER (ENL. THYR)*
b. Pregnancy
c. Hypothyroidism
d. Anaplastic carcinoma *THYR CANCER*
e. Non-toxic goitre
f. Thyroid-binding globulin deficiency
g. Riedel's thyroiditis *CHRONIC FORM OF ROCK HARD.*
h. Nephrotic syndrome *KIDNEY DISEASE LEAK PROTEIN*
i. Subacute thyroiditis
j. Hashimoto's thyroiditis *MOST COMMON BODY PROD. ANTI BODIES THAT ATTACK THY.*

For each of the patients described below, choose the single most likely diagnosis from the above list of options. Each option may be used once, more than once, or not at all.

30. Normal TSH, free T_4 and T_3. Decreased serum total T_4. *THYROID SECRETING HORMONE STIMULATING.*
31. Normal T_3 and T_4 in a patient with neck mass.
32. Elevated serum T_4 and increased radioactive iodine uptake.
33. Elevated serum T_4 and low T_3 resin uptake.
34. Elevated serum T_4 and low radioactive iodine uptake.

THEME 8

TREATMENT OF DIABETIC COMPLICATIONS

a. Sugary drink
b. Insulin sliding scale, heparin and 0.9% normal saline
c. Insulin sliding scale, heparin and 0.45% normal saline
d. 50 ml of 50% dextrose
e. Insulin sliding scale, 0.9% NS and potassium replacement
f. Chest X-ray
g. Measure C-peptide levels
h. Insulin sliding scale, 0.45% NS and potassium replacement.

For each of the patients described below, choose the single most likely management from

the above list of options. Each option may be used once, more than once, or not at all.

35. A 50-year-old man presents with sweating, agitation and tachycardia. His wife is a diabetic and he has had a history of Munchausen's syndrome. *FAKING ILLNESS FOR ATTENTION*

36. A 65-year-old woman is brought to the A and E in an unconscious state. His glucose is 35 mmol/l, pH 7.2, $PaCO_2$ 2, serum Na 140, K 3, Cl 100 and HCO_3 5 mmol/l.

37. A 79-year-old man is noted to have glucose level of 37 mmol/l and Na of 163 mmol/l. He has no prior history of DM and has been on IV fluids for a week. His other medications include dexamethazone, metronidazole and cefuroxime.

38. A 40-year-old diabetic is started on propranolol for stage fear. He collapses after a day shooting but has not changed his insulin regime.

39. A 55-year-old diabetic presents with coma. He is febrile with diminished breath sounds on auscultation and also has warm extremities. His glucose is 20 mmol/l WBC count is 22* 1,000,000/l with increased neutrophils.

THEME 9

ERYTHROPOIETIN LEVELS *HORMONE MANU. IN KIDNEYS.*

a. Haemophilia A
b. Renal failure
c. Anaemia of chronic disease
d. Thalassaemia major *↑ DEFECTIVE GENES - ANAEMIA ETC*
e. Congenital spherocytosis *missshapen BLOOD CELLS → ↑ Anaemia etc*
f. Secondary polycythaemia
g. Thalassaemia minor *↓2*
h. von Willebrand's disease *BLOOD PLATELET DISEASE*
i. G6PD deficiency
j. Primary polycythaemia
k. Aplastic anaemia

For each of the patients described below, choose the single most likely diagnosis from the above list of options. Each option may be used once, more than once, or not at all.

40. Low erythropoietin levels with good response to exogenous erythropoietin.
41. Elevated erythropoietin with a poor response to exogenous erythropoietin.
42. Extremely high plasma erythropoietin levels.
43. Low or absent erythropoietin levels.
44. Normal or slightly elevated erythropoietin levels with a variable response to exogenous erythropoietin.

THEME 10

DIAGNOSIS OF ANAEMIA

a. Sickle cell trait
b. Sickle cell disease
c. Aplastic anaemia nutritional anaemia
d. Iron deficiency anaemia
e. Sideroblastic anaemia
f. Thalassaemia major
g. G6PD deficiency
h. Thalassaemia minor
i. Pernicious anaemia
j. Vitamin B_{12} deficiency

For each of the patients described below, choose the single most likely diagnosis from the above list of options. Each option may be used once, more than once, or not at all.

45. A Jamaican boy presents to the A&E with episodes of chest pain associated with pallor. He also has jaundice.
46. A 24-year-old Greek man presents with rapid anaemia and jaundice following treatment for malaria. He is noted to have Heinz bodies.
47. A 36-year-old woman presents with dyspnoea, paraesthesia and sore red tongue. Her blood film shows an MCV of > 110 fl, low Hb, and hypersegmented polymorphs.
48. A 60-year-old woman post-gastrectomy presents with macrocytic anaemia. She drinks alcohol regularly.
49. A 5-month-old baby boy presents with severe anaemia and failure to thrive. His blood film shows target cells, microcytic hypochromic RBC. HbF persists.

THEME 11

INTERPRETATION OF HAEMATOLOGICAL RESULTS

a. Factor 7 deficiency
b. von Willebrand's disease
c. Phospholipid excess
d. Platelet deficiency
e. Liver disease
f. Heparin
g. Calcium deficiency
h. Factor 5 deficiency
i. Factor 9 deficiency
j. Increased tissue thromboplastin
k. Normal finding
l. Fibrinogen deficiency

For each of the patients described below, choose the single most likely diagnosis from the above list of options. Each option may be used once, more than once, or not at all.

50. PT, APTT and TT are prolonged but BT is normal.
51. PT -13 secs, APTT- 40 secs, TT- 12 secs, BT- prolonged.
52. PT- 11secs, APTT- 48 secs, TT- 13 secs, BT- prolonged.
53. PT- prolonged, APTT- prolonged, TT and BT are normal. Factors 2, 5 and 10 are normal. The patient also has mild pruritis.

THEME 12

DIAGNOSIS OF RHEUMATOLOGICAL CONDITIONS

a. Behcet's disease
b. Henoch-Schonlein purpura
c. Goodpasture's syndrome
d. Microscopic polyangiitis
e. Wegener's granulomatosis
f. Kawasaki's disease
g. Takayasu's arteritis
h. Polyarteritis nodosa (PAN)
i. Giant cell arteritis
j. Cryoglobulinemia
k. Churg-Strauss syndrome

For each of the patients described below, choose the single most likely diagnosis from the above list of options. Each option may be used once, more than once, or not at all.

54. A 26-year-old man presented with fever, myalgia and abdominal pain. His temperature was 38.8°C, BP 190/110 mm hg and pulse 120/min. He had tender abdomen with guarding and bowel sounds were absent.

55. A 67-year-old man presented with acute loss of vision in his left eye, which was transient, temporal headache for about four months. His optic disc was swollen with flame-shaped haemorrhages at 7 o'clock position. Eye movements were full and painless.

56. A 33-year-old woman presented with worsening headache, nausea, painful neck and fever. A year ago she had developed pain in her legs on jogging. Her BP was 190/105 mm Hg, femoral pulses were weak with a radio femoral delay and abdominal bruit was heard.

57. A college student presented with severe chest pain, temperature was 38.8°C, BP 100/60 mm Hg and pulse 120/min. There was conjunctival congestion, polymorphous rash and palpable lymphadenopathy.

THEME 13

MANAGEMENT OF JOINT PAIN

a. Methotexate
b. Sulphasalazine
c. Paracetamol
d. Colchicine
e. Allopurinol
f. Oral NSAIDs
g. Behavioural therapy
h. Antidepressant
i. Gold
j. Joint replacement
k. Oral NSAIDs with gastric protection
l. Joint aspiration and blood culture

For each of the patients described below, choose the single most likely management from the above list of options. Each option may be used once, more than once, or not at all.

58. A 75-year-old man with heart disease complains of stiff painful hands, neck, knees and feet. Heberden's nodes are also seen.

59. A 65-year-old independent woman complains of increasing pain in her left knee and episodes of joint "giving way". She is no longer able to climb stairs. Valgus deformity with obvious instability is also noted.

60. A 45-year-old man with long-standing rheumatoid arthritis presents with a red swollen inflamed right knee and swinging fever.

61. An old woman who drinks 40 units of alcohol/week presents with fifth episode of red hot ankle. Aspiration of the joint has revealed negatively birefringent crystals.

62. A 22-year-old student with ankylosing spondylitis has increasing back pain and early morning stiffness. He is not on any medication.

THEME 14

DIAGNOSIS OF RASH

a. Impetigo
b. Varicella
c. Measles
d. Epstein-Barr virus (EBV)
e. Meningitis
f. Scabies
g. Erythema toxicum
h. *Roseola infantum*
i. *Herpes simplex* virus
j. Psoriasis
k. Pityriasis rosea
l. Kawasaki's disease

For each of the patients described below, choose the single most likely diagnosis from the above list of options. Each option may be used once, more than once, or not at all.

63. A 11-month-old girl is admitted with fever for two days. Though her fever subsides, on discharge she develops a generalised erythematous rash.

64. A teenage girl with sore throat and fever is found to have cervical lymphadenopathy. She is given ampicillin and gets a generalised rash.

65. An infant with fever and desquamating rash of fingertips also has oedematous lips.

66. A young boy with fever, headache, neck stiffness and photophobia is found to have a generalised non-blanching skin rash.

THEME 15

DIAGNOSIS OF SEXUALLY TRANSMITTED DISEASES (STD)

a. *Candida albicans*
b. *Haemophilus ducreyi*
c. *Syphilis*
d. *Herpes simplex* virus
e. *Gonorrhoea*
f. *Human papilloma virus*
g. *Klebsiella granulomatis*
h. *Chlamydia trachomatis*
i. *Gardenella*
j. *Trichomonas vaginalis*
k. *Phthirus pubis*
l. *Chlamydia pneumoniae*

For each of the patients described below, choose the single most likely diagnosis from the above list of options. Each option may be used once, more than once, or not at all.

67. A 40-year-old woman presents with solitary painless genital ulcer with a hard, indurated base. Dark ground microscopy of fluid from the lesion is diagnostic.

68. A young homosexual man presents with proctalgia and bloody anal discharge. Gram staining of the anal discharge shows gram negative intracellular diplococci.

69. A 20-year-old man presents with multiple painful ulcers and suppurative inguinal lymph nodes. The edges of the ulcers are ragged and undermined.

70. A 40-year-old man presents with large groin nodes and a penile ulcer. The nodes are present on either side of the inguinal ligament.

71. A 38-year-old man presents with painless genital ulcers. The ulcer edge is rolled and scrapings demonstrate Donovan bodies.

THEME 16

DIAGNOSIS OF RENAL PATHOLOGY

a. Minimal change nephropathy
b. Cystinuria
c. Medullary sponge kidney
d. Renal artery stenosis
e. Renal vein thrombosis
f. Idiopathic hypercalciuria
g. Diabetic nephropathy
h. Renal tubular acidosis
i. Acute interstitial nephritis
j. Bartter's syndrome
k. Lupus nephritis
l. Hypertensive nephropathy

For each of the patients described below, choose the single most likely diagnosis from the above list of options. Each option may be used once, more than once, or not at all.

72. A 70-year-old diabetic woman on indomethacin and glibenclamide was investigated for hyperkalemia. Blood tests showed evidence of renal impairment, hyperkalemia and hyperchloremia.

73. A 30-year-old woman presented with BP of 190/110 mm Hg and impaired renal function. Urine microscopy showed scanty red cells and granular casts. Linear IgG on glomerular basement membrane.

74. A 20-year-old carpenter was started on flucloxacillin for an infected wound. Urine was positive for blood and protein. Abdominal USG showed normal kidneys with no evidence of obstruction. Blood tests done three days later showed evidence of renal failure.

75. A middle-aged man presented with renal colic

with similar episodes in the past, which were sometimes associated with passing small stones. Abdominal X-ray showed calcified opacities in both the kidneys. All other relevant tests were normal.

76. A 25-year-old woman presented with renal colic. She was previously fit and had no family history of renal problems. Blood tests were all normal but urinary calcium was elevated.

80. A 9-year-old girl with a 12-hour history of nausea and central abdominal pain now radiating to the right iliac fossa has urinary frequency.

81. An infant had severe urine infection complicated by *E. coli* septicaemia a month back. He is on prophylactic antibiotics though his urine is now sterile. The USG abdomen during the acute phase was normal.

THEME 17

INVESTIGATION OF URINARY TRACT INFECTION (UTI)

a. Urodynamics
b. Suprapubic aspiration of urine for culture
c. Abdominal X-ray
d. Isotope renal scan
e. IVU
f. MSU
g. Laparotomy
h. Lumbosacral spine X-ray
i. Serum creatinine
j. Urinary glucose
k. MCU

For each of the patients described below, choose the single most appropriate management from the above list of options. Each option may be used once, more than once, or not at all.

77. A teenage girl had pseudomonas UTI and her BP is 140/95 mm Hg on repeated measurements. She has a past history of recurrent UTI and an abdominal USG at age three was normal.

78. A week old girl has developed fever and jaundice and is not feeding well. A bag of urine specimen showed red and white cells and a culture of mixed organisms. Abdominal examination is normal.

79. A 5-year-old boy has history of diurnal and nocturnal enuresis and soiling. Abdominal examination is normal. He had a series of orthopaedic operations for his deformed foot. Urine culture is positive for Proteus.

THEME 18

INVESTIGATION OF BREAST DISEASE

a. Ductography
b. FNAC *Fine Needle Aspiration Cytology*
c. MRI
d. CT scan
e. Family history
f. Stereotactic cone biopsy
g. Wide excision
h. USG
i. Mammography

For each of the patients described below, choose the single most appropriate investigation from the above list of options. Each option may be used once, more than once, or not at all.

82. A 30-year-old woman had a mammography done showing diffuse calcifications. She wants to know for sure that she has no malignancy.

83. A 60-year-old woman has a mass in the upper quadrant of her right breast. The skin is pulled in and there is no axillary involvement.

84. A 25-year-old woman presents with diffuse nodular breast swelling, which seems to increase in size during her periods. There is no axillary involvement and it disappears after her menses.

85. A 28-year-old woman presenting with a mass in the right upper quadrant of her right breast has a discrete 2 cm mass, which is mobile, non-tender and doesn't involve the axilla. She is scared of needles.

THEME 19

INVESTIGATION OF ISCHAEMIC LIMB

a. Coagulation profile
b. USG
c. Venography
d. Digital subtraction angiography
e. ECG
f. ABPI
g. V/Q scan
h. Duplex scan
i. Femoral arteriography
j. None of the above

For each of the patients described below, choose the single most appropriate investigation from the above list of options. Each option may be used once, more than once, or not at all.

86. A 45-year-old woman is brought to the A&E breathless and complaining of chest pain. She has a 2-month history of leg pain.
87. A 59-year-old man complains of intermittent pain in right toe on walking which sometimes also looks white.
88. A 34-year-old man complains of pain in the calves only while walking, but not on rest.
89. A 40-year-old man complains of pain in the calves at rest.

THEME 20

TREATMENT OF POST -OPERATIVE PAIN

a. IM Pethidine
b. IV Pethidine
c. Aspirin tablets
d. Patient-controlled analgesia with morphine
e. Carbamazepine
f. Diamorphine
g. Epidural analgesia
h. Paracetamol
i. Diclofenac suppositories
j. Dihydrocodeine
k. Intercostal nerve block

For each of the patients described below, choose the single most appropriate management from the above list of options. Each option may be used once, more than once, or not at all.

90. A 60-year-old man with analgesia following a partial thyroidectomy.
91. A 30-year-old man requires analgesia following an exploratory laparotomy and splenectomy.
92. A 50-year-old woman with terminal metastatic breast carcinoma requires long-term analgesia following radical mastectomy.
93. A 56-year-old man complains of phantom limb pain following below knee amputation.
94. A 25-year-old woman underwent excision of sebaceous cyst under LA. She uses salbutamol inhaler on a regular basis.

THEME 21

INVESTIGATION OF AORTIC ANEURYSM

a. Abdominal X-ray
b. Abdominal USG
c. Barium swallow
d. Coronary angiography
e. Spiral CT scan
f. Barium meal
g. ECHO
h. Chest X-ray
i. Transesophageal echo
j. Lower limb angiography
k. CT head
l. Endoscopic studies

For each of the patients described below, choose the single most appropriate management from the above list of options. Each option may be used once, more than once, or not at all.

95. An obese 36-year-old man complains of retrosternal pain associated with water bash.
96. A man presents with abdominal pain radiating to the back. He is found to have a pulsatile mass in the abdomen associated with pain, though is haemodynamically stable.
97. A 57-year-old man wants to know about the extension of AAA to the renal artery before his surgery for repair of the aneurysm.

98. A 60-year-old man is being prepared for the repair of an aortic aneurysm. His exercise ECG reveals ischaemia. There is claudication of the legs.

THEME 22

CAUSES OF BACK PAIN

a. Osteoarthritis
b. Rheumatoid arthritis
c. Spinal stenosis
d. Reiter's disease
e. Osteomyelitis
f. Lupus
g. Secondary prostate disease
h. Multiple myeloma
i. Ankylosing spondylitis
j. Lumbar prolapse and sciatica
k. Paget's disease
l. Sarcoidosis

For each of the patients described below, choose the single most likely diagnosis from the above list of options. Each option may be used once, more than once, or not at all

99. A 20-year-old man comes with lower back pain radiating to back of his legs. He has an elevated ESR with square vertebrae on X-ray.

100. 2. A 50-year-old woman presents with backache and has a higher ESR with normochromic and normocytic anaemia.

101. A 65-year-old man presents with lumbar spine bone pain and pain in his hips. He is noted to have elevated serum alkaline phosphatase of 1000 IU/l, calcium and phosphate levels are normal. He is also hard of hearing.

102. A 35-year-old lady complains of sudden back pain. On examination, she has pain from buttock to her ankle and sensory loss over the sole of her foot and calf.

103. An old woman presents with back pain radiating down both legs. The pain is aggravated by walking and relieved by resting or leaning forward. She has limited straight leg raising and absent ankle reflexes.

THEME 23

TREATMENT OF INTESTINAL OBSTRUCTION

a. Proximal loop colostomy
b. Right hemicolectomy
c. Anterior resection
d. Sigmoid colectomy
e. Explorative laparotomy with Hartmann's procedure
f. Urgent herniorrhaphy
g. Nasogastric aspiration and fluid replacement
h. Abdominal perineal resection with end colostomy
i. Subtotal colectomy and ileorectal anastomosis
j. Transverse colectomy

For each of the patients described below, choose the single most likely treatment from the above list of options. Each option may be used once, more than once, or not at all.

104. An 80-year-old man presents with abdominal distension and pain. Sigmoidoscopy and barium enema confirm an obstructing carcinoma of the rectosigmoid.

105. A 56-year-old man complains of constant groin pain associated with nausea and vomiting. He has positive cough impulse with a tender tense lump, which is not reducible.

106. A 60-year-old man presents with vomiting, fever and intense left iliac fossa pain. Has rigid distended abdomen with rebound tenderness on the left. Erect chest X-ray reveals free air under the diaphragm.

107. A 73-year-old man presents with bowel obstruction and pain in the rectum. Rectal examination and biopsy confirm an obstructing carcinoma of rectum.

108. A 60-year-old man presents with abdominal pain in the right iliac fossa and distension. The X-ray shows a single distended loop

of bowel of 12 cm in diameter with convexity under the left hemidiaphragm.

THEME 24

DIAGNOSIS OF AMENORRHOEA

a. Bulimia
b. Menopause
c. Anorexia nervosa
d. Hypothyroidism
e. Prolactinoma
f. Pregnancy
g. Turner's syndrome
h. Hyperthyroidism
i. Androgen insensitivity
j. Intrauterine synechiae
k. Premature ovarian failure
l. PCOS
m. Hypogonadal hypogonadism

For each of the patients described below, choose the single most likely diagnosis from the above list of options. Each option may be used once, more than once, or not at all.

109. An 18-year-old girl with secondary amenorrhoea is reported to be binge eating. She has a BMI of 16 and is concerned that she is fat and goes to the gym frequently.

110. A 20-year-old dancer presents with secondary amenorrhoea. She is 1 m 65 cm tall and weighs 46 kg.

111. A 35-year-old woman presents with a 7-month history of amenorrhoea. She also complains of hot flushes, night sweats and mood swings.

112. A 17-year-old girl presents with an 8-month history of secondary amenorrhoea, prior to this her periods were irregular since menarche at the age of 12. Her BMI is 32.

113. A 30-year-old woman presents with a 7-month history of secondary amenorrhoea. She admits to a weight loss of 6 kg despite having good appetite.

THEME 25

MANAGEMENT OF MENOPAUSAL SYMPTOMS

a. Vaginal oestrogens
b. Clonidine
c. Psychological support
d. Raloxifene
e. Combined HRT
f. Referral to psychiatrist
g. Hypnotic preparations
h. Oestrogen only HRT
i. Vaginal lubricants
j. Regular exercise

For each of the patients described below, choose the single most likely management from the above list of options. Each option may be used once, more than once, or not at all.

114. A 45-year-old woman who has had a total abdominal hysterectomy and bilateral salpingo-oophorectomy for fibroids complains of hot flushes, night sweats and mood swings. She has no other medical problems.

115. A married 55-year-old woman who has a family history of breast cancer has been experiencing discomfort for a few hours following intercourse for last month. She is worried about using hormones.

116. A 70-year-old woman has experienced burning micturition intermittently for the last few months. The MSU cultures have been persistently negative. She is otherwise well and would like her symptoms to be resolved.

117. A 60-year-old woman whose periods stopped five years back has become increasingly depressed. She now feels life is no longer worth living and threatens suicide.

118. A 55-year-old woman who attained menopause two years back, now complains hot flushes and mood swings. She has a family history of breast and endometrial carcinoma.

THEME 26

CHOICE OF CONTRACEPTION

a. OC pills	b. Rhythm method
c. Bilateral tubal ligation	d. Barrier method
e. Postcoital pill	f. IUCD
g. Condom and OC pills	h. Vasectomy
i. Douching	j. Injectables

For each of the patients described below, choose the single most preferred method of contraception from the above list of options. Each option may be used once, more than once or not at all.

119. A married 23-year-old woman with recent glandular fever would like a form of contraception as she would like to postpone starting family for a year.
120. An 18-year-old girl would like to start having sexual relationships.
121. A 28-year-old woman living with her boyfriend asks for advice regarding contraception.
122. A married 35-year-old obese mother of three with varicose veins and a 20-cigarette per day smoking habit would like a form of contraception.
123. A married 25-year-old nulliparous woman would like to postpone having a family for two years.

THEME 27

PAIN RELIEF

a. Paracetamol	b. Topical Ketoprofen
c. Tramadol	d. Morphine
e. Diclofenac	f. Nitrous oxide
g. Ibuprofen	h. Diamorphine
i. Pethidine	j. Co-proxomol
k. Carbamazepine	l. Aspirin

For each of the patients described below, choose the single most appropriate drug from the above list of options. Each option may be used once, more than once, or not at all.

124. A 25-year-old man has dislocated his terminal phalanx of his right finger in a fight. There doesn't appear to be fracture and you wish to give him analgesia to allow reduction.
125. A 19-year-old boy has a dental extraction and is complaining of pain.
126. A 70year-old man has an acutely painful, red and swollen left knee. He has recently been started on frussemide by his GP.
127. A 50-year-old woman has bone pain from metastatic breast disease. Simple analgesia has been infective.
128. A 40-year-old man has been admitted with an acutely painful abdomen. He has epigastric tenderness and his amylase is elevated.

THEME 28

DRUG OF CHOICE IN INFECTIONS

a. Metronidazole	b. Amoxycillin
c. Co-amoxiclav	d. Ciprofloxacin
e. Benzyl penicillin	
f. 2 or more antibiotics together	
g. Cefotaxime	h. Gentamycin
i. Trimethoprim	j. Erythromycin
k. None	l. Doxycycline

For each of the patients described below, choose the single most appropriate drug from the above list of options. Each option may be used once, more than once, or not at all.

129. A 60-year-old male smoker presents with dyspnoea, dry cough and fever. He is unwell, tachycardic and cyanosed.
130. A 36-year-old man complains of severe burning while passing urine. He also has a penile discharge which shows gram-negative organisms on Gram stain.
131. A 3-year-old child presents with acute fever, drowsiness, stridor and drooling. He looks shocked and unwell.
132. A 45-year-old man has cough, fever and

mild dyspnoea. He has reduced air entry and is dull to percussion at the left lung base. He is neither systemically unwell nor hypoxic. He has a documented penicillin allergy.

133. A 20-year-old student develops bloody diarrhoea after eating a reheated mutton dish.

THEME 29

PREVENTION AND TREATMENT OF THROMBOTIC DISEASE

a. Thrombolytics
b. IV heparin
c. Aspirin
d. Phenindione
e. Compression stockings
f. Early mobilization
g. SC unfractionated heparin
h. Warfarin (INR 2-3)
i. Warfarin (INR 3-4.5)
j. SC LMW heparin

For each of the patients described below, choose the single most appropriate drug from the above list of options. Each option may be used once, more than once, or not at all.

134. A 30-year-old woman is 16 weeks' pregnant and develops a painful swollen leg. A femoral vein thrombosis is diagnosed with Doppler USG. She had already been started on IV heparin.

135. A 53-year-old man is admitted for an elective total hip replacement. He has history of peptic ulcer disease and takes lansoprazole. How will you prevent thrombosis occurring in him?

136. A 24-year-old woman has had four spontaneous abortions, two DVT's and suffers from migraine. Blood tests confirm antiphospholipid antibodies.

THEME 30

FITNESS TO DRIVE

a. Banned from driving
b. Should not drive for 1 month
c. Should not drive for 3 months
d. Should not drive for 1 year
e. Should not drive for 2 months
f. Must not drive for 2 years
g. Must not drive for 3 years
h. May drive but must inform DVLA
i. Must not drive for 6 weeks
j. Must not drive for 48 hours

For each of the patients described below, choose the single most appropriate drug from the above list of options. Each option may be used once, more than once, or not at all.

137. A 25-year-old woman has DM and takes insulin. She has had a number of hypoglycemic attacks without warning.

138. A 36-year-old man has had a single episode of unexplained syncope without convulsions.

139. A 50-year-old woman has had a stroke. Her hemiplegia has resolved and she has normal visual fields.

140. A 39-year-old man has had two grand mal seizures and is now on phenytoin. When may he drive if he remains fit free?

THEME 31

INVESTIGATION OF SYNCOPE

a. EEG
b. Exercise ECG
c. Holter monitoring
d. Carotid arteriography
e. CT scan head
f. Echo
g. Head-up tilts
h. Ambulatory EEG

For each of the patients described below, choose the single most appropriate investigation from the above list of options. Each option may be used once, more than once, or not at all.

141. A 10-year-old girl loses consciousness after a period of prolonged standing. She becomes pale but regains consciousness within a few seconds.
142. An elderly woman reports history of LOC on five occasions. Each time she regains consciousness after a few minutes.
143. A 60-year-old woman presents with history of sudden weakness of lower limbs and falling. No LOC.
144. A 63-year-old woman complains of dizziness and blackouts. On examination her pulse is 50/min.

THEME 32

CHOICE OF ANTIPSYCHOTIC DRUG

a.	Clozapine	b.	Haloperidol
c.	Chlorpromazine	d.	Fluphenazine
e.	Trifluoperazine	f.	Promazine
g.	Sulpiride	h.	Sertindole
i.	Resperidone	j.	Trazodone

For each of the patients described below, choose the single most appropriate drug from the above list of options. Each option may be used once, more than once, or not at all

145. For florid positive symptoms of schizophrenia.
146. Prophylactic antipsychotic.
147. Sedative antipsychotic.
148. Antipsychotic used in acute episodes.
149. Preferred antipsychotic in pregnancy.
150. For negative symptoms of schizophrenia.
151. Antipsychotic for the elderly.
152. Intractable schizophrenia.

THEME 33

DIAGNOSIS OF ABDOMINAL PAIN

a.	Acute cholecystitis	b.	Acute pancreatitis
c.	Acute appendicitis	d.	Peptic ulcer

Contd...

Contd...

e.	Duodenal ulcer	f.	Biliary colic
g.	Nonulcer dyspepsia	h.	Duodenitis
i.	Hepatitis	j.	Faecal impaction

For each patient described below, choose the single most likely diagnosis from the above list of options. Each option may be used once, more than once, or not at all.

153. A 40-year-old investment broker comes to the A and E with severe upper abdominal pain. His breath smells of alcohol. He is pale and sweaty with board-like rigidity.
154. A 38-year-old man points to his epigastrium with complaints of severe pain. The pain is worse at night and taking food relieves him. His serum amylase is slightly elevated.
155. A 42-year-old marketing executive presents with acute epigastric pain. The pain is continuous and it has been increasing in intensity over the past few days with radiation to right hypochondrium.
156. A 50-year-old cook presents with nausea and acute abdominal pain boring through to the back. The epigastrium is very tender. He has had three similar episodes in the past 18 months with a normal barium meal.
157. A 43-year-old Cypriot female comes with right upper abdominal pain of four hours duration. She is also nauseous.

THEME 34

DIAGNOSIS OF DIARRHOEA

a.	Laxative abuse
b.	Campylobacter infection
c.	Ulcerative colitis
d.	Crohn's disease
e.	Giardiasis
f.	Collagenous colitis
g.	Glucagonoma
h.	Adenocarcinoma of pancreas
i.	Carcinoid syndrome
j.	Coeliac disease

For each patient described below, choose the single most likely diagnosis from the above list of options. Each option may be used once, more than once, or not at all.

158. A healthy 20-year-old man presented with a 6-week h/o bloody diarrhoea, crampy abdominal pain and fever. Proctosigmoidoscopy shows bleeding and friable mucosa.

159. A previously fit 24-year-old man presented with acute bloody diarrhoea, crampy abdominal pain and low-grade fever. His symptoms resolved spontaneously in a week.

160. A 55-year-old woman presented with a six-year history of recurrent non-bloody diarrhoea. All investigations were normal apart from a raised ESR and eosinophilic band in the sub-epithelial layer on colonic biopsy.

161. An 18-year-old emaciated lady presents with chronic watery diarrhoea. Stool electrolyte studies show an osmotic gap. She is also hypokalemic.

162. A 50-year-old diabetic woman presents with weight loss, anaemia and diarrhoea. She is noted to have migratory necrolytic erythema.

THEME 35

DIAGNOSIS OF LIVER CONDITIONS

a. HCC
b. Wilson's disease
c. Haemochromatosis
d. Primary biliary cirrhosis (PBC)
e. Sclerosing cholangitis
f. Budd-Chiari syndrome
g. Veno-occlusive disease
h. Chronic active hepatitis
i. Haemolytic jaundice
j. Alcoholic hepatitis

For each patient described below, choose the single most likely diagnosis from the above list of options. Each option may be used once, more than once, or not at all.

163. A 55-year-old woman presents with hepatomegaly and dark skin pigmentation. She admits to heavy drinking and she is noted to have glycosuria.

164. A 33-year-old woman on OC pills and Prozac presents with right upper quadrant pain and ascites. She has hepatomegaly and liver scintiscan shows maximal uptake in the caudate lobe alone.

165. A 25-year-old man presents with tremour and dysarthria. On examination, greenish pigment is seen in the corneo scleral junction.

166. A 47-year-old woman has melanotic skin pigmentation, pruritis, hepatomegaly and dark urine. She develops jaundice five years after onset of the above features.

167. A 39-year-old man presents with jaundice, fever, mouth ulceration, blood and mucus per rectum and pyoderma gangrenosum.

THEME 36

INVESTIGATIONS OF ABDOMINAL PAIN

a. ERCP
b. HIDA
c. PTC
d. CT scan
e. Pregnancy test
f. Erect CXR
g. USG abdomen
h. KUB X-ray
i. Diagnostic laparoscopy
j. Immediate operation

For each patient described below, choose the single most useful investigation from the above list of options. Each option may be used once, more than once, or not at all.

168. A 50-year-old obese woman presents with acute upper abdominal pain, pyearexia, tachycardia tenderness in the right upper abdomen. The CXR reveals no free peritoneal gas. The USG is inconclusive.

169. A 90-year-old woman suffering from rheumatoid arthritis presents with severe epigastric pain and vomiting. She also complains of shoulder tip pain.

170. A 25-year-old woman presents to the A&E with a sudden onset left iliac fossa pain. She is pale and has a pulse of 120 with BP of 105/65 mm Hg. She is tender at the left iliac fossa.

171. A fit 18-year-old man presents with a 12 hour history of central abdominal pain localising to right iliac fossa. He is pyrexial with tenderness at the same area.

THEME 37

IMMEDIATE MANAGEMENT OF HEAD INJURY

a. Observe and discharge later
b. Urgent CT scan
c. Emergency burr holes
d. Lumbar puncture
e. IV mannitol
f. Consult neurosurgeon
g. 50 ml of 50% dextrose
h. Discharge after check skull X-ray
i. Pyrimethamine + Sulfadiazine
j. Naloxone

For each patient described below, choose the single most appropriate management from the above list of options. Each option may be used once, more than once, or not at all.

172. A 35-year-old man is brought to the A&E after a drunken brawl, unconscious. His breathing becomes progressively deeper and then shallower despite initial resuscitation. His pupils constrict and then become fixed and dilated. A CT scan has been done.

173. A 40-year-old IV drug abuser is brought to the A&E with severe headache and confusion. A CT scan shows multiple ring enhancing lesions.

174. An 18-year-old boy is brought to the A&E

following an RTA with rhinorroea and peri orbital edema. His GCS is 5.

175. A 45-year-old man involved in RTA is brought to the A&E with a bruise in the left temporal area. His GCS is 11.

176. A 25-year-old man is brought to the A&E with his left pupil dilated. His blood glucose is 5 mmol/l and smells of alcohol. The neurosurgeon is not available at that moment.

THEME 38

DIAGNOSIS OF DEMENTIA

a. Alcoholic dementia
b. Pick's disease
c. Parkinsonism
d. HIV
e. Toxin-induced dementia
f. Head trauma
g. Alzheimer's dementia
h. Space occupying lesion
i. Huntington's chorea
j. Creutzfeldt-Jakob disease
k. Vascular dementia
l. Substance-induced dementia

For each patient described below, choose the single most likely diagnosis from the above list of options. Each option may be used once, more than once, or not at all.

177. A 32-year-old woman presents with memory loss, poor concentration and inability to recognise household objects. She has a right hand involuntary writing movements with a strong family history of similar complaints.

178. A 60-year-old man with no previous history is brought to the A&E by his wife who says he has progressively become forgetful, tends to loose his temper and is emotionally labile. There is no history of infectious disease or trauma.

179. A 72-year-old man presents with weakness in his arm and leg (recovered in a few days)

and short term memory loss. He has an extensor plantar response. He had similar episode two years ago and became unable to speak fluently. He is on anti-tubercular therapy.

180. A 46-year-old man presents with difficulty in initiating movement and general slowness in all his activities. He is put on dopaminergic drugs by his GP but shows no response.

181. A 44-year-old woman comes with complaints of poor memory, talking to strangers and making inappropriate comments in public.

THEME 39

INVESTIGATION OF CONFUSION

a.	Urea and electrolytes	b.	MSU
c.	Chest X-ray	d.	CT scan
e.	ECG	f.	Full blood count
g.	Stool culture	h.	Blood glucose
i.	Thyroid function tests	j.	USG abdomen
k.	Blood culture		

For each patient described below, choose the single most likely investigation from the above list of options. Each option may be used once, more than once, or not at all.

182. A very old woman presents with poor mobility and recent history of falls. She has deteriorated over the past two weeks with fluctuating confusion. On examination she has mild hemiparesis.

183. A 70-year-old man with known Alzheimer's disease became suddenly more confused yesterday. When seen in the A&E, his BP was 90/60 mm Hg and pulse 40/min and regular.

184. A 65-year-old man had recently been started on tablets by his GP. He is brought to the A&E by his wife with sudden aggressive behaviour, confusion and drowsiness. Prior

to starting the tablets, he was complaining of losing weight and thirst.

185. An 84-year-old woman in a nursing home has been constipated for a week. Over the past few days, she has become increasingly confused and incontinent.

THEME 40

EYE DISEASES

a. Malignant melanoma of eye
b. Holmes-Aides pupil
c. Proliferative retinopathy
d. Toxic amblyopia
e. Methanol poisoning
f. Psychogenic
g. CMV retinopathy
h. Syphilis
i. Senile macular degeneration
j. Cortical blindness
k. Retinitis pigmentosa
l. Retinoblastoma
m. Optic neuritis

For each of the patients described below, choose the single most likely diagnosis from the above options. Each option may be used once, more than once, or not at all.

186. A 34-year-old man with a long history of smoking and alcohol presents with blurring of vision. His wife has noted that he cannot differentiate between red and green colours now.

187. A 32-year-old male with some blurring of vision and pain on eye movements.

188. A soldier returned from Vietnam now complains of some visual problems. On fundoscopy, there are pale areas with haemorrhages below the fovea.

189. A 38-year-old male with meiosis and irregular pupils. His pupils respond to accommodation but not to light

190. A 65-year-old woman blind on testing but

denies that there is any problem with her eyesight.

191. A 14-year-old boy says he cannot see properly in night. There are black particles near fundus.

THEME 41

ADVERSE EFFECTS OF ANTI-CANCER DRUGS

a. Haemorrhagic cystitis	b. Seizures
c. Pancreatitis	d. Pulmonary fibrosis
e. Visceral fibrosis	f. GI ulceration
g. Peripheral neuropathy	h. Bone marrow
i. Cardiotoxicity	suppression
j. Hepatotoxicity	k. Vomiting

For each of the drugs, choose the single most likely adverse effect from the above options. Each option may be used once, more than once, or not at all.

192. Vinblastine

193. Vincristine

194. Cyclophosphamide

195. Actinomycin D

196. L-asparaginase

197. Melphalan

THEME 42

RESPIRATORY DISEASES

a. Cystic fibrosis
b. ARDS
c. Tuberculosis
d. Cor pulmonale
e. Bronchial adenocarcinoma
f. Squamous cell carcinoma
g. Large cell carcinoma
h. Kartagner's syndrome
i. Hypertrophic pulmonary osteoarthropathy
j. Pulmonary oedema
k. Oat cell carcinoma

For each of the patients described below, choose the single most likely diagnosis from the above options. Each option may be used once, more than once, or not at all.

198. A 57-year-old p/w wt loss and hyponatremia. The CXR had paratracheal lymphadenopathy.

199. A 46-years-old smoker p/w dull pain in wrist and ankles. He is cachexic and also complains of chest pain and dyspnoea.

200. A 45-year-old smoker with weight loss and haemoptysis. He is clubbed and has reduced breath sounds in left upper zone of chest. The CXR confirms left upper lobe collapse.

16 *Answers to Mock Exam No. 2*

> ◆ *You need to get 124 of the answers right, right? But you would also want to know why the ones you have answered wrong are so… find out the reason here.*

THEME 1

TREATMENT OF PNEUMONIA

1. Benzyl penicillin

   The most common cause of community acquired pneumonia is *Streptococcus pneumoniae*. First line drug for this condition is benzyl penicillin.

2. Co-trimoxazole

   In an immunocompromised patient with the given clinical features, the most suggestive organism is *Pneumocystis carinii*.

3. Rifampicin + Isoniazid

   The clinical picture in this immunocompromised patient is classical of pulmonary tuberculosis.

4. Ciprofloxacin

   The most common organism causing pneumonia in cystic fibrosis patient is *Pseudomonas*. Drug of choice for this would be the answer (b), but for this patient with renal impairment Aminogycosides are contraindicated, hence the answer is (c).

5. Erythromycin

   The causative organism is *Mycoplasma*.

THEME 2

DIAGNOSIS OF UPPER RESPIRATORY INFECTIONS

6. Croup

   The causative organism is RSV. Low-grade fever and barking cough is most suggestive of this condition.

7. Epiglottitis

   The causative organism is a bacterium, *H.influenzae*. Stridor and drooling of saliva caused by the swollen epiglottis is suggestive of this.

8. Glandular fever

   Infectious mononucleosis always presents with a sore throat initially followed by respiratory difficulty caused by the enlargement of the lymph nodes in the Waldeyer's ring.

9. Bronchiolitis

   Bronchiolitis is caused by respiratory syncitial virus and presents with cough and outflow obstruction. It is treated by nebulised ribivarin.

10. Sinusitis

    In this cystic fibrosis patient, immotile cilia are responsible for sinusitis.

THEME 3

CAUSES OF BREATHLESSNESS

11. Extrinsic allergic alveolitis (EAA)

Episodic symptoms in a farmer with fine miliary shadows on chest X-ray are suggestive of this. It cannot be cryptogenic fibrosing alveolitis as it is always progressive.

12. Goodpasture's syndrome

This syndrome is characterised by both pulmonary and renal involvement as it affects the basement membrane.

13. Allergic bronchopulmonary aspergillosis (ABPA)

Aspergillosis is common in asthmatic patients Usually, affects the upper lobe and since it is a fungal infection, it will not respond to antibiotics.

14. Churg-Strauss syndrome

This condition consists of the characteristic tetrad of rhinitis, asthma, eosinophilia and systemic vasculitis and is treated by steroids.

THEME 4

INTERPRETATION OF ECG FINDINGS

15. Digoxin toxicity.

16. Pericarditis.

17. Myocardial infarction (MI).

18. Sick sinus syndrome.

19. Hypokalemia.

THEME 5

IMMEDIATE MANAGEMENT OF MENINGITIS

20. Thick and thin blood films

This patient has malaria as he was not able to take chemoprophylaxis and all the clinical features suggest the same.

21. Cranial CT scan

In an AIDS patient, the most common CNS infection is by Toxoplasma. Characteristic ring-shaped contrast enhancing lesions are seen on CT.

22. Lumbar puncture

The most common cause of community, acquired meningitis in children under 14 years of age who have never been vaccinated is *H. influenzae.*

23. IV plasma expansion

Clinical features are suggestive of *Meningococcus,* but since the patient is haemodynamically unstable and has received penicillin, he requires plasma expansion.

24. Treat immediate contacts.

THEME 6

DIAGNOSIS OF MUSCLE WEAKNESS

25. Bell's palsy

Idiopathic isolated LMN facial nerve palsy.

26. GBS

The LMN palsy preceded by an URTI with albumino-cytological dissociation in the CSF is characteristic of this condition.

27. Dermatomyositis

Heliotrope rash with symmetrical proximal muscle weakness.

28. MS

Oligoclonal bands in the CSF is pathognomonic.

29. Poliomyelitis

Acute flaccid paralysis with the given CSF findings goes in favour of this diagnosis.

THEME 7

INTERPRETATION OF THYROID FUNCTION TESTS

30. Thyroid-binding globulin deficiency

Total T_4 includes TBG bound T_4 and free T_4. Since free T_4 levels (active form) are normal, features of hypothyroidism are not seen even though total T_4 is low.

31. Non-toxic goitre

His goitre is not producing any hormones and hence the T_3 and T_4 levels are normal.

32. Graves' disease

Increased T_4 and increased uptake of radio-active iodine is characteristic of hyperthyroidism.

33. Pregnancy

In pregnancy, TBG levels are raised leading to raised serum T_4 levels with normal free T_4.

34. Subacute thyroiditis

This is characterised by raised T_4 levels and no uptake on scan.

THEME 8

TREATMENT OF DIABETIC COMPLICATIONS

35. Measure C-peptide levels

Hypoglycemic features are due to self-administration of insulin injection with which his wife is being treated in this patient with a history of Munchausen's syndrome.

36. Insulin sliding scale, potassium and 0.9 % NS

In this patient of diabetic ketoacidosis, insulin sliding scale is required since he is hyperglycemic. Potassium replacement is required to correct his hypokalemia. Normal saline will do because his sodium level is normal.

37. Insulin sliding scale, heparin and 0.45% NS

This patient has non-ketotic hyperosmolar coma. Since the sodium is high, half normal saline is preferred. Hyperosmolarity leads to dehydration, which is a procoagulant, state for which heparin is required.

38. 50 ml of 50 % dextrose

Beta-blockers decrease hypoglycemic aware-ness. Hypoglycemic coma requires IV glucose. Sugary drinks are given for mild hypoglycemic symptoms.

39. Chest X-ray

This patient has pneumonia.

THEME 9

ERYTHROPOIETIN LEVELS

40. Renal failure

Kidneys fail to produce adequate erythropoietin, which can be corrected by exogenous administration.

41. Aplastic anaemia

In aplastic anaemia, there is bone marrow failure, which leads to severe anaemia, and consequent high erythropoietin levels, which is refractory to even exogenous administration of erythropoietin.

42. Secondary polycythaemia

Secondary polycythaemia can either be due to an appropriate increase in red cells in response to anoxia, or to an inappropriate increase associated with tumours.

43. Primary polycythaemia

Due to polycythaemia, there is a negative feedback, which suppresses erythropoietin levels.

44. Anaemia of chronic disease

The decreased release of iron from the bone marrow to the developing erythroblasts results in variable response to erythropoietin.

THEME 10

DIAGNOSIS OF ANAEMIA

45. Sickle cell disease

This is common in African countries. This boy is having the hand and foot syndrome seen in sickle cell disease. In sickle cell trait anaemia is not present.

46. G6PD deficiency

Heinz bodies in a patient of Mediterranean origin following drug treatment are characteristic of this condition.

47. Pernicious anaemia

Macrocytic blood picture with paraesthesia and sore tongue is seen in pernicious anaemia.

48. Vitamin B_{12} deficiency

In a patient of gastrectomy, there is loss of vitamin B_{12} binding proteins leading to deficiency.

49. Thalassaemia major

Microcytic hypochromic anaemia in a child with persistence of HbF is pathognomonic of thalassaemia major.

THEME 11

INTERPRETATION OF HAEMATOLOGICAL RESULTS

50. Heparin.

51. Platelet deficiency.

52. von Willebrand's disease.

53. Liver disease.

THEME 12

DIAGNOSIS OF RHEUMATOLOGICAL CONDITIONS

54. Polyarteritis nodosa (PAN)

55. Giant cell arteritis.

56. Takayasu's arteritis.

57. Kawasaki's disease.

THEME 13

MANAGEMENT OF JOINT PAIN

58. Colchicine.

59. Joint replacement.

60. Joint aspiration and blood culture.

61. Allopurinol.

62. Oral NSAIDs.

THEME 14

DIAGNOSIS OF RASH

63. *Roseola infantum.*

Synonyms are *Exanthem subitum*, fourth disease or three-day fever. Common in infants who present with high fever, whose peak is followed by a macular rash.

64. Epstein-Barr virus (EBV)

Infectious mononucleosis is characterised by sore throat followed by fever and lymphadenopathy. Rashes may be seen, especially with ampicillin, but this does not indicate life-long ampicillin allergy.

65. Kawasaki's disease

Rash involving the fingertips and oedema is characteristic of this disease. Cervical lymphadenopathy is common.

66. Meningitis

THEME 15

DIAGNOSIS OF STD

67. Syphilis

68. Gonorrhoea

69. *Chlamydia trachomatis*

70. *Haemophilus ducreyi*

71. *Klebsiella granulomatis*

THEME 16

DIAGNOSIS OF RENAL PATHOLOGY

72. Renal tubular acidosis (RTA), type 4

Hyperkalemic, hyperchloraemic metabolic acidosis. Seen in diabetic patients and also with NSAIDs administration.

73. Lupus nephritis

Lupus causes membranous glomerulonephritis with proteinuria and granular casts.

74. Acute interstitial nephritis

Other drugs include penicillin, frusemide, NSAIDs or infection.

75. Medullary sponge kidney

This condition characterised by dilatation of collecting ducts and cyst formation presents with renal colic and haematuria. Small calculi form within the cysts and diagnosis is made by IVU.

76. Idiopathic hypercalciuria

These patients have normal blood tests but an elevated urinary calcium excretion.

THEME 17

INVESTIGATION OF UTI

77. Isotope renal scan

To rule out renal scarring caused by recurrent UTI, scan is essential which also provides information on renal function.

78. Suprapubic aspiration of urine for culture

A week old girl cannot be asked to provide an MSU. A bag of urine with mixed organisms indicates contamination.

79. Lumbosacral spine X-ray

Club foot is associated with spina bifida, which may be the cause of his bowel and bladder disturbances. To rule out this, the above investigation is required.

80. Laparotomy

Acute appendicitis. Retro-colic appendix causes frequency.

81. MCU

In a male infant with UTI, always rule out VUR after the acute phase is resolved.

THEME 18

INVESTIGATION OF BREAST DISEASE

82. FNAC

Cytological examination is the definitive investigation to rule out malignancy.

83. FNAC

84. USG

The investigation of choice for fibroadenosis or diffuse lumps is USG as a distinct lump is required for FNAC.

85. Mammography

Mammography is usually done for non-palpable lumps, but in this case since the patient is scared of needles, it is preferred.

THEME 19

INVESTIGATION OF ISCHAEMIC LIMB

86. V/Q scan

The patient probably had DVT, which has led to pulmonary embolism, the first line investigation for which is V/Q scan and definitive is pulmonary angiography.

87. ABPI

Intermittent pain and white toe are signs of critical ischaemia, which can be ruled out by ABPI.

88. Duplex scan

The patient is mostly in the initial stages of arterial disease, which can be confirmed by duplex scan.

89. Femoral arteriography

Rest pain is a surgical emergency. Arteriography is required to localise the site of lesion.

THEME 20

TREATMENT OF POST-OPERATIVE PAIN

90. Dihydrocodeine

To prevent cough in this patient and also provide analgesia, this drug is preferred.

91. Patient-controlled analgesia with morphine.
Most ideal analgesic in this patient

92. Diamorphine
It is twice as effective as morphine and is given orally which will be useful in this patient as it is required on a long-term basis.

93. Carbamazepine

94. Paracetamol
Aspirin cannot be used as she is an asthmatic.

THEME 21

INVESTIGATION OF AORTIC ANEURYSM

95. Endoscopic studies
Clinical features are in favour of GORD.

96. Transesophageal echo
Investigation of choice for dissecting aneurysm.

97. Spiral CT scan
To know the extension of aneurysm, involvement of branches and also for selection of graft size.

98. Coronary angiography
Pre-operatively to rule out cardiac involvement as this patient has claudication of legs.

THEME 22

CAUSES OF BACK PAIN

99. Ankylosing spondylitis
This condition usually starts in the twenties in males, who present with sacroiliac pain, and show the characteristic square-shaped 'bamboo spine' on radiology due to calcification of the intervertebral ligaments.

100. Multiple myeloma (MM)

The MM characteristically presents with backache, high ESR and anaemia due to increased plasma cells in the bone marrow.

101. Paget's disease (of bone)
The disease causes pain and enlargement of skull, femur, clavicle and tibia—sabre tibia. Associated features are CCF and nerve deafness due to bone overgrowth. An alkaline phosphatase of >1000 is characteristic.

102. Lumbar prolapse and sciatica
The sudden onset of the pain and the radiation (sciatica) is suggestive. Sensory loss is due to compression of the nerve roots supplying the dermatomes of the foot and calf.

103. Spinal stenosis
Pain worse on walking with aching and heaviness is known as spinal claudication. This condition usually presents with a negative SLR contrary to the case here.

THEME 23

TREATMENT OF INTESTINAL OBSTRUCTION

104. Subtotal colectomy and ileorectal anastomosis
Hartmann's procedure could be an alternative but not chosen for two reasons; firstly, the instructions ask you to choose the 'single most likely treatment' and not 'immediate management'. Hartmann's procedure is not a definitive cure. Secondly, the choice is 'Explorative laparatomy with Hartmann's procedure' which is done in acute cases of suspected intestinal obstruction where the site of obstruction is not known.

105. Urgent herniorrhaphy
This is a case of strangulated inguinal hernia.

106. Explorative laparotomy with Hartmann's procedure

Here is an acute case with the site of involvement not known, though it could probably be a case of diverticulitis with perforation. The definitive management of any GI perforation is surgical. Immediate management could be nasogastric aspiration and fluid replacement.

107. Anterior resection

A 73-year-old man cannot withstand an APR and anterior resection is always a better alternative if there is a choice.

108. Right hemicolectomy

A case of obstructed *Caecal volvulus*. The distended loop is called the 'Omega loop sign' where the twisted caecum gets lifted up.

THEME 24

DIAGNOSIS OF AMENORRHOEA

109. Anorexia nervosa

This condition is differentiated from bulimia by a BMI of <17. Binge eating is present in both conditions but in bulimia, the patient uses mechanisms to overcome the fattening affect of binges, such as induced vomiting, and laxative and diuretic abuse.

110. Anorexia nervosa

As above, with a BMI of < 17 and no episodes of induced vomiting and/or laxative abuse.

111. Premature ovarian failure

The symptoms are those of menopause, and since the lady is only 35 years old, a premature failure of ovaries has led to these manifestations.

112. PCOS

The PCOS is characterised by amenorrhoea/ oligomenorrhoea, hirsutism and obesity.

113. Hyperthyroidism

Menstrual problems are common in thyroid disorders.

THEME 25

MANAGEMENT OF MENOPAUSAL SYMPTOMS

114. Oestrogen only HRT

The HRT is the first line management of menopausal symptoms. Only patients with a uterus need progestogen therapy to protect them from the endometrial cancer-inducing effect of oestrogen.

115. Vaginal lubricants

This female is probably suffering from atrophic vaginitis and vaginal oestrogens should be preferred, but since she does not want to use any hormonal preparations, we prescribe her lubricants.

116. Vaginal oestrogens

They are the preferred treatment for urethral syndrome.

117. Referral to psychiatrist

You could start her on some anti-depressants, but since she is threatening suicide, a psychiatric referral is required.

118. Raloxifene

This selective estrogen (or oestrogen) receptor modulator (SERM) protects bones while reducing the risk of breast and endometrial cancer.

THEME 26

CHOICE OF CONTRACEPTION

119. Barrier method

The OC pills would be ideal in this lady but infectious mononucleosis is a contraindication to OC pills.

120. Condom and OC pills

She would probably be having multiple sexual partners, so condoms should also be used to protect against STD's.

121. OC pills

A stable single relationship does not demand the use of barrier methods.

122. IUCD

Smoking, obesity and arterial or venous disease are a few of many contraindications to OC pills.

123. OC pills

The IUCDs cannot be used in nulliparous women.

THEME 27

PAIN RELIEF

124. Nitrous oxide

Correction of a dislocation is always done under GA.

125. Paracetamol

Simple analgesics like paracetamol are preferred for mild pain.

126. Ibuprofen

The NSAIDs are the first line drugs for gout. Ibuprofen is preferred over Diclofenac as it is more potent and causes less gastric irritation.

127. Diamorphine

Opiates are used when simple analgesia has proved ineffective. Oral diamorphine is used as this patient requires long-term analgesia.

128. Pethidine

Morphine is contraindicated in acute pancreatitis because it causes spasm of the sphincter of oddi, which could aggravate his condition. Pethidine, though less potent, does not have this adverse effect.

THEME 28

DRUG OF CHOICE IN INFECTIONS

129. Amoxycillin

This patient probably has an exacerbation of his chronic bronchitis and apart from other emergency measures like bronchodilators, steroids and oxygen, amoxycillin is given.

130. Benzyl penicillin

Penile discharge is indicative of urethritis and hence this patient has gonococcal infection.

131. Cefotaxime

This is the drug of choice in acute epiglottitis, which is caused by *Haemophilis influenzae*.

132. Erythromycin

Probably a case of *Streptococcal pneumoniae*, erythromycin is preferred in cases of penicillin allergy.

133. Ciprofloxacin

Bacillary dysentery is treated by ciprofloxacin, as it covers a wide spectrum of organisms.

THEME 29

PREVENTION AND TREATMENT OF THROMBOTIC DISEASE

134. Warfarin (INR 2-3)

Treatment of DVT initially involves giving IV heparin and then starting warfarin. Warfarin (INR 3-4.5) is given in conditions mentioned in Q.136.

135. SC LMW heparin

The LMW heparin is preferable to ordinary heparin in major orthopaedic surgery as it causes less bleeding, less incidence of DVT and pulmonary embolism, and has the convenience of a once daily subcutaneous administration.

136. Warfarin (INR 3-4.5)

Indications of Warfarin (INR 3-4.5):
- Antiphospholipid syndrome
- Prosthetic heart valve
- Cornary artery graft thrombosis
- Recurrence of venous thrombosis while on warfarin.

Note: • LMW heparin: Molecular weight–2000-8000 daltons

- Unfractionated Heparin: 13000 daltons
- Low-dose Heparin: 5000 daltons, e.g., dalteparin, tinzaparin.

THEME 30

FITNESS TO DRIVE

137. Banned from driving

Hypoglycaemic attacks without warning precludes driving.

138. Should not drive for 1 year

These patients should be restrained from driving for at least one year if free from further episodes. They must inform the DVLA.

139. Should not drive for 3 months

Patients with TIA/stroke must not drive for one year, but in this case since the hemiplegia is resolved, driving can be allowed after three months of symptom-free period.

140. Should not drive for 1 year

All epileptics must inform DVLA. They can drive if they remain symptom free for 1 year.

Note: DVLA—Driver and Vehicle Licensing Authority

THEME 31

INVESTIGATION OF SYNCOPE

141. Head-up tilts

Head-up tilt tests distinguish vasovagal (cardioinhibitory) from postural (vasodepressor) syncope. If positive symptoms are associated with a BP drop of >30 mm Hg, then it is postural syncope. If it is associated with bradycardia, then it is vasovagal syncope. Treatment of postural syncope is by beta-blockers and vasovagal syncope is by pacing.

142. Carotid arteriography

The diagnosis is TIA. In elderly patients TIA in the posterior cerebral circulation or vertebro-basilar insufficiency can present with LOC. Arteriography or Doppler of carotids and vertebral arteries may show the extent and severity of the disease.

143. CT scan head

Diagnosis is that of 'Drop attacks' which can be differentiated from stroke by the retainment of consciousness. Drop attacks occur largely in women over 60. They are presumed to be due to brainstem involvement, but may occur due to hippocampal involvement, too.

144. Holter monitoring

Cardiac syncope or Stokes-Adams attacks are important causes of recurrent episodes of LOC in elderly. A 24-hour ambulatory Holter ECG monitoring is recommended.

THEME 32

CHOICE OF ANTIPSYCHOTIC DRUG

145. Sulpiride

Highly selective D2 receptor antagonists are less likely to produce extrapyramidal disorders.

146. Fluphenazine

Used as a long-term prophylactic to prevent relapse as a depot injection.

147. Chlorpromazine.

148. Haloperidol.

149. Haloperidol.

150. Sertindole

Particularly for the negative symptoms, it is associated with QT interval prolongation.

151. Promazine

Promazine or thioridazine is useful in elderly when it is desirable to reduce the risk of extrapyramidal and anti-cholinergic side effects.

152. Clozapine

It is used in patients who have failed to respond to at least two conventional anti-psychotic drugs.

THEME 33

DIAGNOSIS OF ABDOMINAL PAIN

153. Peptic ulcer

People with stress-related jobs are likely to suffer from peptic ulcer as in this case. Pale, sweaty condition and board-like rigidity are characteristics of perforated viscus.

154. Duodenal ulcer

Pain that is worse at night—hunger pains occur in duodenal ulcers. Serum amylase may be elevated in peptic ulcers, but not to the level seen in pancreatitis.

155. Acute cholecystitis

The differential diagnosis here could be acute pancreatitis, but in that condition, the pain is constant, whereas in cholecystitis, the pain is gradually progressive.

156. Acute pancreatitis

Epigastric pain radiating to the back accompanied by nausea and vomiting are characteristics of pancreatitis.

157. Biliary colic

Sickle cell disease is more common in the Mediterranean region and these patients are prone to develop gallstones.

THEME 34

DIAGNOSIS OF DIARRHOEA

158. Ulcerative colitis

159. Campylobacter infection

This is a self-limiting infection that presents with bloody diarrhoea.

160. Collagenous colitis

Eosinophilic bands in the sub-epithelial layer are characteristics.

161. Laxative abuse

Osmotic gap on electrolyte studies is seen in laxative abuse.

162. Glucagonoma

This condition presents with weight loss, diabetes and the characteristic migratory necrolytic erythema.

THEME 35

DIAGNOSIS OF LIVER CONDITIONS

163. Haemochromatosis.

164. Budd-Chiari syndrome.

165. Wilson's disease.

166. Primary biliary cirrhosis (PBC).

167. Sclerosing cholangitis.

Note: Refer to Hepatology Revision Aid.

THEME 36

INVESTIGATIONS OF ABDOMINAL PAIN

168. ERCP

The USG is the first line of investigation in acute cholecystitis. If this fails, as in this case, and there is a strong suspicion, The ERCP is the best choice to confirm the diagnosis and its cause.

169. Erect CXR

The NSAIDs that are the initial choice of therapy in rheumatoid arthritis are known to cause acid peptic disease, and hence perforation of the GI tract. Shoulder tip pain is due to diaphragmatic irritation.

170. Diagnostic laparoscopy

A pregnancy test is definitely recommended but the instruction says—choose the single most useful investigation which in this case would be diagnostic lap, which would be diagnostic as well as therapeutic.

171. Immediate operation

Appendicitis requires immediate surgery.

THEME 37

IMMEDIATE MANAGEMENT OF HEAD INJURY

172. IV Mannitol

Since the CT scan has been done and no positive findings have been mentioned, it must be normal. Progressive respiratory depression is suggestive of cerebral oedema and hence mannitol is recommended.

173. Pyrimethamine + sulfadiazine

Multiple ring enhancing lesions are suggestive of toxoplasmosis in this patient with a probable HIV infection.

174. Consult neurosurgeon

The features are suggestive of fracture of anterior cranial fossa, and with a GCS of 5 immediate neurosurgical consultation is warranted.

175. Discharge after check skull X-ray

176. Emergency burr holes

In alcoholics with unconsciousness the first possibility to be considered is hypoglycaemia, but the blood glucose is normal here, the next possibility is that of a subdural bleed.

THEME 38

DIAGNOSIS OF DEMENTIA

177. Huntington's chorea

178. Alzheimer's dementia

179. Vascular dementia

Patients with vascular dementia or multi-infarct dementia suffer from step-like progression over months or years with each subsequent infarct.

180. Parkinsonism

Dopaminergic drugs are acted upon by peripheral decarboxylase and hence show no response. When combined with a decarboxylase inhibitor like carbidopa, the combination becomes useful.

181. Pick's disease

Patients with Pick's disease characteristically become extrovert and lose inhibition. Other features are same as Alzheimer's dementia.

THEME 39

INVESTIGATION OF CONFUSION

182. CT scan.

183. ECG

The first investigation of choice in a patient with bradycardia is ECG.

184. Blood glucose

Hypoglycaemia.

185. MSU

Constipation in this lady could be due to faecal impaction. This constipation could be the cause of urinary retention and hence UTI which in turn has caused incontinence and delirium.

THEME 40

EYE DISEASES

186. Toxic amblyopia

The patient with a history of smoking and alcohol with blurring of vision and colour blindness is suggestive of secondary optic atrophy.

187. Optic neuritis.

188. CMV retinopathy

Haemorrhages below the fovea are characteristic.

189. Syphilis

Argyll Robertson pupil.

190. Cortical blindness

Widespread bilateral occipital lobe damage by tumour, trauma or infarction causes this condition of cortical blindness also known as Anton's syndrome.

191. Retinitis pigmentosa

Night blindness and particles resembling bone corpuscles are the features of this incurable disease.

THEME 41

ADVERSE EFFECTS OF ANTI-CANCER DRUGS

192. Bone marrow suppression.

193. Peripheral neuropathy.

194. Haemorrhagic cystitis.

195. Vomiting.

196. Hepatotoxicity.

197. Pulmonary fibrosis.

THEME 42

RESPIRATORY DISEASES

198. Oat cell carcinoma

Small cell carcinoma of the lung, also known as oat cell carcinoma, presents with extrapulmonary manifestations like SIADH.

199. Hypertrophic pulmonary osteoarthropathy (HPOA)

Another extra-articular manifestation and the final stage of clubbing.

200. Squamous cell carcinoma (SCC)

The SCC is more common in smokers.

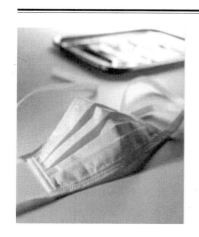

Section *Three*

Plab Part 2—The OSCE

17 *Introduction*

◆ *Like in the introduction to the Part 1 exam, I have described here the format of the exam, what happens on the actual day of the exam and the scoring pattern.*

Part 2 of the PLAB test is also known as the Objective Structured Clinical Examination or the OSCE. The aim of the OSCE is to test your clinical and communication skills. It is designed such that the examiner just observes you putting these skills into practice.

EXPECTED STANDARD
A Pass in the Part 2 will exhibit that the successful candidate has the ability to practice safely as a senior house officer (SHO) grade in a first engagement in a United Kingdom hospital. This is the standard laid down by the General Medical Council for granting limited registration.

ELIGIBILITY FOR OSCE
- You may apply for Part 2 once you have passed Part 1.
- You must pass the OSCE within two years of the date you passed the Part 1 exam.
- You cannot have more than four attempts at the OSCE.

VALIDITY PERIOD
Though you must pass the OSCE within two years of passing Part 1 of the PLAB exam, there is no limit on the time within which you must apply for registration after you pass the OSCE. Your registration and visa are applicable for a certain number of years. So some of you may want to delay your registration process for personal reasons.

ATTEMPTS AT OSCE
You may have four attempts at the OSCE, which must be within two years of passing the Part 1 exam. If you do not pass at the fourth attempt, you must retake the IELTS and Part 1 of the PLAB test. There are no exceptions to this rule.

PASS RATE
There is no set pass rate for the OSCE. A few candidates believe that some centres have better pass rate than other centres. This is not true.

OSCE TEST CENTRES
You can take the OSCE only in the United Kingdom. The centres are London, Leeds, Edinburgh and Liverpool.

Once your form has been processed, you will be sent a letter offering you a place in the OSCE and a map showing you where your centre is located. You may or may not get a centre of your choice. If there are no places available, you will receive communication about other OSCE dates.

OSCE DATES
The OSCE is run approximately 10 times in a year, approximately every six weeks. The closing date for each OSCE is just over two weeks before

the OSCE takes place. However, remember, this does not mean that you will definitely get a place if you apply before the closing date. The GMC advises you to apply for the OSCE at least four months in advance.

ARRIVAL AT THE CENTRE
In the letter offering you a place, you will be given a time for arrival at the centre. You may be tested in the morning or in the afternoon.

Some candidates will be asked to arrive at the centre in the morning but will not be tested until the afternoon. This is to ensure that no candidate feels disadvantaged because he or she thinks that candidates taking the exam in the afternoon have prior awareness of the stations. If you will be tested in the afternoon, the letter offering you a place will evidently state this fact. As a consolation, you will get a sandwich lunch.

DURATION OF THE OSCE
The OSCE will last one hour and thirty-six minutes. In practice it may take up to two hours. If you are taking the test in the afternoon, you will have to be at the centre for more than three hours.

PROOF OF IDENTITY
You must take proof of your identity to the OSCE together with the letter from the General Medical Council offering you a test place. These will be checked before the OSCE.

The identification document must bear your photograph and the following are acceptable forms of identification:
- Passport
- UK Immigration and Nationality department identification document
- Your Home office travel document
- Your UK Driving license.

DURING OSCE
You will be provided with all the materials you need for the OSCE. You may not use or refer to any other materials.

The prohibited and unacceptable practices are:
- Copying, stealing, appropriation or use of the work of another person.
- Permitting or assisting another to copy or use one's own work.
- Using or attempting to use dishonest method to gain advantage in any part of the OSCE process.
- Removal from the OSCE centre, any papers, answer sheets or other OSCE materials.
- Writing in or attaching to any papers, or giving orally, any message or appeal to the examiner.

SCORING
The OSCE will be marked in the UK by computer technology.

You will be given your grade for each station. However, the overall result of the OSCE will be either PASS or FAIL. This overall result will be your PLAB test result.

The GMC will send you the results by post two weeks after the date of the OSCE. The results will also be posted on the GMC's website.

PASS IN OSCE
If you pass, you will be eligible to apply for limited registration. You will be sent forms for and details about applying for limited registration.

Before you are granted limited registration:
- Your primary qualifications must be checked.
- You must have been selected for appropriate employment.
- You must satisfy the GMC that you are of good character.

FAIL IN OSCE
You will be sent forms enabling you to re-apply, unless you have failed at your fourth attempt.

APPEAL AGAINST RESULTS
You may not appeal against the mark you received for the OSCE. The examiners decision

is final. However, candidates wishing to verify any mark or marks, by means of a clerical check, shall apply to the head of the PLAB test section.

FORMAT OF THE OSCE

The OSCE takes the form of 14 clinical scenarios or stations as well as two test stations, or one rest station and a pilot station. There will, therefore, be a total of 16 stations.

Each station requires you to undertake a particular task. Some tasks may involve talking to, or examining patients; some may involve demonstrating a procedure on an anatomical model. You will be required to perform all tasks. Each station lasts five minutes.

You will be told the number of the station that you should begin in when you enter the examination room. This will be your first station booth.

Once inside the OSCE room, stand outside your first station booth. You will find an instruction sheet at the entrance of the booth. You will have one minute to read the instructions. Do not enter the booth until the bell rings for the start of the station.

The instructions will give basic information about the patient such as name, age and major symptoms. You should read these instructions carefully to ensure that you follow them exactly. An example might be, 'Mr. Jones has been referred to you in the rheumatology clinic because he has joint pains. Please take a short history to establish supportive evidence for a differential diagnosis.'

At the end of 60 seconds, a bell will ring. You may then enter the station.

Inside the booth, there will be an examiner. In some stations, in addition, there may be an observer and/or a simulated patient. There will also be an additional set of candidate instructions inside the station for you to refer to, if you wish to do so.

When you enter the room, the examiner will greet you and check your name and candidate number as shown on your badge, which will be given to you at the candidate briefing.

The examiner will also check that you understand the instructions. Once you have started, do not speak to the examiner unless the candidate instructions ask you to do so. An actor, who has been provided with a detailed script beforehand, is playing the patient. The examiner has a checklist of points to consider when marking a marksheet that is pre-printed for each individual candidate.

When there is a manikin at the station, address any comments or explanations to the examiner and not to the manikin.

When there is a simulated patient, the candidate instructions for that station will tell you whether you should address to the examiner or to the patient.

The tasks at some stations, in particular those tasks requiring practical skills, may take less than five minutes to complete. A bell will ring after four and a half minutes to warn you that there are only 30 seconds remaining. If you finish early, you must remain in the station until the five-minute bell rings and do not speak to the examiner or to the patient during this time.

The stations are numbered clearly. There will be one minute between stations.

Your first station may be a rest station, in which case, there will be no one present at the booth. The rest stations will be clearly labelled.

Each station has a number of objectives like communication, past history, diagnosis, which you do not see, but they are set out on the examiner's marksheet.

The examiners shall award grades as follows:
- A = excellent = 5 marks
- B = good = 4 marks
- C = adequate = 3 marks
- D = fail = 2 marks
- E = severe fail = 1 mark

For the purpose of calculation, the grades will be converted to marks. The objective is weighed with the total weighing for each station adding up to 100%. An overall grade is calculated for each station. You must obtain a 'C' or above in 10 or more stations to pass the exam. You should not get an 'E' in more than one station.

Each objective is worth a certain percentage of the total marks for the station. The examiner does not know this percentage. Multiplying the marks given for each objective by the percentage allocated, and then adding up the results give the overall marks. The results are then converted to grades.

OSCE SYLLABUS

The main skills tested are:
1. Communication skills
2. History taking
3. Clinical examination
4. Practical skills
5. Emergency management.

Communication Skills

Communication skills are tested through the observations of interaction between the candidate and another person, usually a simulated patient or the examiner. You are expected to know the major legal and ethical principles set out in duties of a doctor.

Examination of communication skills that may be tested are:
• Explaining diagnosis, investigation and treatment
• Involving the patient in decision making
• Checking understanding
• Communicating with relatives
• Communicating with health care professionals
• Breaking bad news
• Seeking informed consent for an invasive procedure or a post-mortem
• Dealing with anxious or angry patients or relatives

• Giving instructions on discharge
• Giving advise on lifestyle, health promotion or risk factors.

History Taking

You should be competent in taking a history from any of the patients and reaching at an appropriate diagnosis, if required.

The following are examples of symptoms of presenting patients:
• Diarrhoea
• Wheezing
• Vaginal bleeding
• Palpitations
• Abdominal pain
• Headache
• Anxiety
• Weight loss
• Joint pains
• Ear pain
• Difficulty in swallowing
• Episodes of loss of consciousness.

Clinical Examination

a. You will be assessed on your ability to conduct a clinical examination of a standardised patient.
b. You are expected to be competent to carry out any basic physical examination. Examples are examination of the chest, heart, breast, hand, hip, knee and shoulder. You must be able to perform a rectal or bimanual vaginal examination. You must also be able to use the appropriate equipment in carrying out the examination of, for example, the ear or the eye.
c. The candidate's ability to maintain effective records may be tested through the writing up of findings from a physical examination. The marking will focus on completeness, legibility and clarity.
d. Examination of the mental state is treated as a form of clinical examination for this test.
e. You will also be marked on your ability to treat

a patient you are examining with respect for their privacy and dignity and attention to their discomfort.

Practical Skills

The practical skills may include:

- Taking blood pressure
- Venepuncture
- Inserting a cannula into a peripheral vein
- Giving intravenous injections
- Mixing and injecting drugs into an intravenous bag
- Giving intramuscular and subcutaneous injections

- Suturing
- Interpreting an ECG, X-ray, or the results of other investigations
- Basic respiratory function tests
- Bladder catheterisation
- Taking a cervical smear
- Safe disposal of sharps.

Emergency Management

Examples include dealing with post-operative collapse, acute chest pain, trauma assessment, administering oxygen therapy safely and basic adult and paediatric CPR.

18 Applying for the PLAB Part 2 Exam

◆ Completing the application form, where to send them, and information on cancellation procedures is included.

Completing the Application Form

The following notes are intended to help you complete your application form.

Name

You should use the name you gave to the General Medical Council when you made your first enquiry.

If this name differs from:

- The name on your IELTS certificate;
- The name on the proof of identity you intend to use at the Examination;
- The name shown on your diploma or other evidence of qualification;

You will be required to provide *original* documentary evidence that the names on the different documents refer to you. This could be your marriage certificate or a declaration from the IELTS awarding body that both the names refer to the same person.

Date on which you would like to take the Examination

An up-to-date list can also be found at the GMC website: www.gmc-uk.org. Please choose your preferred centres and dates from the list.

Enclosures

Fees: The fee of £ 430 must be paid in advance in sterling. Personal callers to the General Medical Council's office in London may pay fees in cash. Otherwise, fees paid in the United Kingdom must be in the form of a cheque, money order or postal order payable to 'General Medical Council'. Fees sent from other countries, or paid in other countries, must be by sterling bank draft or money order. These must be made payable to 'General Medical Council'. Please remember, where appropriate, to consider bank charges when paying the fee.

Do not enclose evidence of your primary qualification at this stage

The General Medical Council will check this when you apply for limited registration.

Declaration

Please check the form carefully to ensure that the information is correct, and sign and date it. Then return it with the appropriate enclosures to the address at the end of the form.

Send the completed application form to:

PLAB Test Section (Candidate Services)
General Medical Council
178 Great Portland Street
London
W1W 5JE
United Kingdom

Notification of a place

Once your form has been processed, you will be

sent a letter offering you a place in the Examination and a map showing you where the Examination centre is located.

If there are no places available, they will write to you about other Examination dates.

Cancellation by candidate

If you want to cancel your place, please give the office, which offered you the place, as much notice as possible. You must return the letter offering you an Examination place. If you cancel early, they may be able to offer your place to another candidate waiting to take the Examination. You may not pass the letter offering you a place to anyone else.

If you cancel your place, you will be charged a fee. This will normally be deducted from the fee you paid to enter the Examination. The amount charged depends on the amount of notice you give.

Cancellation charges

The current cancellation charges are as follows:

UK centres:

Period of notice	Cancellation charge
Four months or more	£70
Between 21 days and four months	£100
Less than 21 days	£145

If you do not want to re-book a place, the office will refund the balance of your fee.

Postponement, cancellation or invalidation of Examinations

If exceptional circumstances cause the office to postpone or cancel an Examination, or to declare the results of an Examination to be invalid, you will be entitled to a full refund of the Examination entry fee. The General Medical Council will not be liable for any other costs.

19 Courses and Sponsorship Schemes for PLAB Part 2 Exam

> ◆ There are a plethora of courses and sponsorship schemes available for the Part 2 exam and you will go bananas deciding which one of them to take up. I have provided here the positive and negative aspects of each of them to help you make a decision.

PLABWISE

They are in all probability, the only company providing courses for PLAB Part 2 in Manchester—a city that is away from the havens for plabbers such as East Ham in London. Nevertheless, Manchester is a good choice for plabbers in terms of cost of living and the comparative ease of procuring clinical attachments. The PLABWISE provides a comprehensive service to facilitate your preparation for the PLAB examinations right up to securing your first job in the UK. You can choose to take advantage of all their services or select from amongst them (CV embellishing, Arranging Clinical Attachments, Interview preparation) according to your needs.

PLAB Part 2 Course

Location   : Manchester
Duration   : 5 days
Cost   : £ 225
Pay if you pass : Yes, £ 75 upfront; £ 175 after
                   you pass and get a job = £ 250

The PLABWISE Part 2 course is an intensive 5-day course with thorough revision of all aspects of the OSCE. The sessions include lectures, demonstrations, videos, manikin practice and physical examinations practice. All the tutors are doctors in the NHS who are experienced with the

PLAB system. These courses are held approx. 7 to 10 days before each examination.

Manikins Only

Location   : Manchester
Duration   : 1 day
Cost   : £ 45

It is intended for those who are confident with their core subject knowledge and communication skills, but wish to augment their practical skills. It provides hands-on experience on manikins similar to those used by the GMC. This course is held a week before each OSCE.

Sponsorship Scheme

Location   : Manchester
Duration   : 3 weeks
Cost   : £ 470
Pay if you pass : Yes; £ 95 upfront +
                   £ 400 after you pass and get a
                   job = £ 495

Inclusions...

- Accommodation for 3 weeks
- Food for 3 weeks (3 meals)
- Enrollment on PLAB Part 2 course
- Sponsorship letter for visa purposes detailing the provisions that have been made for your stay in the UK.
- Pick and drop facility from Manchester airport/train or coach station.

Format of the Sponsorship Scheme

Arrival in the UK : 3-4 days before the course

Duration of the course : 5 days

Final revision : 7-10 days

Relaxing period : 1 or 2 days after the exam.

Contacting Plabwise

Postal Address

50 Brandon Avenue
Heald Green
Cheadle
SK8 3SQ
United Kingdom

Tel

0011-8456-442-883
(Mon-Fri 9:00 am - 5:00 pm UK time)

Email

info@plabwise.co.uk

Emergency Contact

0011-771-590-7919

FISCHTEST LTD

This course is more apt. More apt for candidates doing clinical attachments because it is usually held on weekends and therefore does not demand a leave from the attachment for 5 to 7 days. It is probably one of the most professional (and expensive) of all the courses offered. All the course instructors are practicing doctors and most of them have sat and passed the OSCE. The only disadvantage is that the courses are not held as often as the OSCE exams.

Location : London

Duration : 2 days

Course Fee : £300.00 (includes course handbook, sandwich lunch and refreshments)

Pay if you pass : Yes, £ 80 upfront and £ 300 after getting a job.

The Course Covers

- Counselling and history taking, physical examination skills, including per rectal and bimanual examination, simulated on realistic polymer models very similar to those used in the OSCE.

- Basic techniques of suturing. Each participant will suture at least two types of cuts commonly encountered in the OSCE (Linear and Z-Cuts). A *Suture Training Simulator CD-ROM* aid provided.

- Taking blood using the Vacutainer system, and ordinary syringe and needle.

- Male and Female catheterisation .

- Intravenous cannulation using Venflons.

- Peak Flow measuring.

- Basic Life Support (CPR) on an advanced Cparlene Model with light indicators to show correct technique.

- Fundoscopy using the Eye Retinopathy Trainer. This shows various pathological conditions.

Sample Time Table

Day One

09.00 : Registration, coffee and Handing out of Free Book

09.15 : The OSCE technique

10.00 : Counselling and History Taking

11.00 : System Examination, including thyroid, breast and nerves

13.00 : SANDWICH LUNCH

13.45 : Blood Pressure, Peak Flow measurement

14.00 : Cervical Smear, Prostate exam, Bi-manual exam.

14.30 : Venepuncture, IV cannulation

15.15 : TEA

15.45 : More Simulator exercises - CPR, Suturing, Otoscopy

17.00 : Discussion and close

Day Two

09.00 : Coffee

09.10 : Counselling and History Taking

11.00 : Examination of Joints: Knee, Hip. Shoulder, etc

12.00 : Male and Female Catheterisation

12.30 : SANDWICH LUNCH

13.30 : Simulation exercises (Revision)

17.00 : Discussion and close

Manikins Only

The dummy sessions are supervised day-long practice sessions on all dummies. No formal teaching is done during dummy sessions as all formal teaching takes place only on the PLAB II course.

Candidates can Practice

Bimanual examination, Cervical smear, Suturing, Blood pressure measurement, Peak flow, measurement, Prostate examination, Otoscopy, Taking blood using the Vacutainer system and ordinary syringe and needle, Male and Female catheterisation, Intravenous Cannulation using Venflons, Peak Flow measuring, Basic Life Support (CPR) on an advanced Cparlene Model with light indicators to show correct technique, Fundoscopy using the Eye Retinopathy Trainer

Cost : £ 50

Contacting Fischtest

Postal Address

Fischtest Ltd
7 Miller House
Westgreen Road
London
N15 3DR
United Kingdom

Tel

0011 870 429 4739.

PLABMASTER

Debatably, one of the oldest and most popular companies providing coaching for PLAB 2 along with sponsorship schemes. They also show off other services such as visa facilitation, single airfares (which any travel company can provide) and so on. There has been a lot of speculation in recent times about the standard of coaching provided by PLABMASTER. Many people who have attended the course feel that they do not get the attention they deserve. Conversely, there are others who strongly recommend it. They have recently introduced PLABMASTERONLINE for online coaching for the OSCE.

PLABMASTERONLINE for the OSCE will have information about the exam, the course contents, examples of past questions, and actual teaching with voice files about counselling, pictures and action-pictures of various manikins and career guidance as well. It was programmed to launch in March 2003, but had not started till May 2003.

PLAB Part 2 Course

Location : London, East Ham
Duration : 1 week
Course Fee : £ 270 includes one extra dummy session.
Pay if you pass : Yes, £ 80 upfront, £ 190 after you pass and get a job.

Sponsorship Scheme

Location : London
Duration : 3½ weeks
Cost : £ 100 upfront and £ 450 when you pass and get a job = £ 550

Includes...

- Lodging for 24 days
- Boarding
- Coaching.

Their sponsorship scheme does not, anymore, include a pick up facility from Heathrow or Gatwick airport.

Additional accommodation is available for £ 50 per week.

Contacting PLABMASTER

In India : Y.B.E.S.,
4, "Neelkamal", Near "Daya Kshama Shanti",
Bhaskar Colony, S.V. Road, Naupada,
Thane (W) - 400 602, INDIA

In UK : 1st Floor, 2A Burges Road, EastHam,
London E6 2BH, United Kingdom

Email : info@ybes.org

VISHWA MEDICALS

Universally known as the 'Cardiff Course' or Dr. Mane's course, it is an intensive 2-day course held in Cardiff in Wales. The course is conducted for over ten hours on both days with just a 30-minute break for lunch. The course has got a good repute and is pretty cheap compared to the other courses if you decide to pay the payment in full. However, since it is held in Cardiff, you must also think about the travel and accommodation expenses involved, which could easily shoot up your total expenditure.

Apart from offering the "Hands On" Training on all models, they also provide the Video recording and playback on big screen for each candidate to analyse their individual performance. **Mock Simulated Exam circuits** help you to get a feel of the real exam. You are given a feedback of your OSCE scores in the circuit, giving an objective assessment of your preparation.

PLAB Part 2 Course
Location : Wales, Cardiff

Duration : 2 days
Cost : £ 195, or Rs.4000 in India and £ 150 in UK.
Pay if you pass : No

Accommodation, if required during the course is provided for about £ 15 to £ 20 per day.

STAY and STUDY Facility
Location : Cardiff, Wales
Duration : 2½ weeks
Cost : £ 345, or Rs.4000 in India and £ 300 on arrival in UK.

Includes...
• Accommodation
• Coaching
• Computer and printer access for 24 hours
• Internet access for 24 hours
• Facilities like washing machine, microwave, fridge/freezer and all basic kitchen utensils.

This scheme does not include food.

PLAB Part 2 Course in INDIA

This is a fresh introduction from the Vishwa Medicals group.

The Course Covers
• Mock circuit
• Video recording, replay and personal feedback
• Tips to improve communication skills
• Models for practice
• Videos of past candidates to learn from
• List of past exam OSCEs that you should know
• Books to read
• CV preparation and Career guidance
• Guidance on clinical attachment
• Guidance on travel to the UK and Visa matters.

Course Fee : INR 3000/- includes free stay for 3 nights and daytime food.

CONTACTING VISHWA MEDICALS
In India : 1st floor, Laxmi-Sohum

building, Near Smita Soc., Shastrinagar, Dombivli (W), Dist-Thane, Pin-421202

In UK : 1, Peppercorn Close, Turner Rise, Colchester, CO4 5WS, United Kingdom

PLABTUTOR

This one is the 'New kid on the block' but is fast mounting in reputation as one of the most sought after course for the PLAB 2 aspirants.

The course runs over 7 days, in the evenings from Monday to Friday and the whole day on Saturday and Sunday. It is an intensive course and consists of speciality-based two-hour sessions. Interactive workshops include resuscitation skills, communication skills and individual practical sessions. Comprehensive study material and course information is provided to all students at no extra cost. Refreshments are provided everyday and lunch is provided on Saturday. All those who attend the course irrespective of the sponsorship scheme receive a sponsorship letter for visa purposes.

PLAB Part 2 Course

Location : East Ham, London
Duration : 5 full days and 2 half days
Course Fee : £ 210
Pay if you pass : Yes, £ 100 upfront and £150 after you pass = £ 250

Accommodation can be prearranged for the duration of the course for £ 50-65 exclusive of food.

Sponsorship Scheme

Up to 10 well deserving and needy students can avail of the sponsorship scheme per course.

Location : East Ham, London
Duration : 4 weeks
Cost : £ 100 upfront + £ 575 when you pass and get a job = £ 575 (£ 100 returned for expenses in UK)

Includes...

- Sponsorship letter provided to all who join the course
- Course fee
- Course notes
- Accommodation for 4 weeks prior to the exam
- £ 100 for your living expenses while you are in the UK.

Please note that for the PLABTUTOR and the PLABMASTER sponsorship schemes, the sponsorship letter will reach you only 3 weeks ahead of the course. This might holdup your visa application process.

Contacting PLABTUTOR

London, UK
1, Wades Grove, Winchmore Hill, London N21 1BH
Phone and Fax: 0044 208 8820376
Bangalore, India
87/46/2, 13th Cross, 8th Main, Wilson Gardens, Bangalore- 7
Phone: 0091 80 2127807
Email:contactus@plabtutor.com

EASY EXAM LTD

Popularly known as the Fahmida's course, it seems she started this in an effort to help her friends, and ever since, it has grown in popularity to be one that provides individual attention at its best.

Apart from providing the course, if you register as a member for £ 70, you get access to the library. It includes materials to read, group study place, manikins on weekends, photocopying and computer facility. All materials for the PLAB, IELTS, MRCS, MRCP, etc., are available. This facility is given for a period of one month before exam.

PLAB Part 2 Course

Location : East Ham, London
Duration : 5 days
Cost : £ 150
Pay if you pass : No

Manikins Only Course

Duration   : 1 day
Cost   : £ 60

Contacting EASY EXAM LTD

Email: fahmida@easyexamltd.com

BIRMINGHAM PLAB COURSE

They provide courses that run on Saturdays for a period of ten weeks. It is useful for those who arrive in the UK more than three months before their exam to do a clinical attachment or for any other purpose. Candidates are allowed unlimited access to the manikins.

Location   : Birmingham
Duration   : 10 days
Cost   : £ 150
Pay if you pass : No

Contact

Email: birminghamplabcourse@yahoo.co.uk

PLABDOCTORS

They have a modern clinical skills lab, which has been extremely beneficial for the doctors to pass the OSCE Part in PLAB 2, with unlimited hands-on training, especially before each exam. They also provide reasonably cheap accommodation.

Location   : London
Duration   : 5 days
Cost   : £ 240
Pay if you pass : £ 100 upfront and £ 170 after you pass and get a job = £ 270

Sponsorship Scheme

Location   : London
Duration   : 4 weeks
Cost   : £ 100 upfront and £ 500 when you pass and get a job = £ 600

Includes...
• Accommodation and food for 4 weeks
• Course fees

• Access to clinical skills lab
• Unlimited manikin practice
• Computer and internet facilities

Contacting PLABDOCTORS

Email: mmcdoctors@hotmail.com

NHS RECRUITS

This recently launched company provides packages that include PLAB-2 courses and arrangements for clinical attachments. The first part of the course will be during the first weekend of you arriving in the UK. During this you shall be given a brief introduction on PLAB 2 and booklet with practical hints on most clinical studies.

The second part of the course is the practical part. It consists of five days. We will go over clinical scenarios in small groups. Hands-on experience with dummies (same or similar to exam situation). An exam on last day is optional.

Location   : London
Duration   : 1 + 5 days
Cost   : £ 310
Pay if you pass : Yes, £ 100 upfront and £ 210 when you pass and get a job = £ 310

For the package deal, you have to pay £ 500 and it includes the course and arrangement for clinical attachment for 3 weeks. This too can be divided into the 'pay if you pass' scheme. You have to pay £ 100 upfront and £ 400 when you get a job.

Contacting NHS RECRUITS

Website: www.nhsrecruits.com

FASTTRACKMEDICS COURSE

This is an intensive 2-day course designed to prepare candidates for all aspects of the exam including:
• History taking from British patients (played by professional as in the real exam).

- Scenarios are taught in an interactive way using actors, teachers and doctors. All scenarios are based on those found in the exam.
- Procedures on patients/actors or manikins as in the exam.
- Tutor based training in the use of the manikins found in the GMC exam including repeated demonstrations of correct technique. (See Manikin list). Plenty of time is set aside for each candidate to practice on each manikin.
- Also provided are course file and guide to starting your NHS portfolio and CV preparation (needed for interviews).

- Lunch and refreshments include, catering for Halal and vegetarian diets.

Location	: Northwick Park Hospital, London
Duration	: 2 days
Cost	: £ 325
Pay if you pass	: No

Contacting FASTTRACKMEDICS
By phone: 07984 764810 or 0208 9227493
By e-mail: *fasttrackmedics@yahoo.com*

Table 19.1: Comparison of PLAB Part 2 courses

Course	Days	Cost	Pay if you pass	Remarks
PLABWISE	5 days	£ 225	£ 75 + £ 175	Other valuable services, 12 hrs/day
PLABMASTER	7 days	£ 270	£ 80 + £ 190	Reviews not very good
PLABTUTOR	7 days	£ 210	£ 100 + £ 150	Well organized
FAHMIDA'S	5 days	£ 150	No	Individual attention
BIRMINGHAM	10 days	£ 125	No	Run only on Saturdays for 3 months
VISHWA	2 days	£ 195	No	Very intensive…10 hrs/day !
FISCHTEST	2 days	£ 300	£ 80 + £ 300	Most professional of the lot!
PLABDOCTOR	5 days	£ 240	£ 100 + £ 170	—

Table 19.2: Comparison of sponsorship schemes

Provider	Duration	Cost	Remarks
PLABWISE	3 weeks	£ 95 + £ 400	Airport transfers, Early Sponsorship letter, Other facilities
PLABMASTER	3½ weeks	£ 100 + £ 450	No Airport transfers, Late sponsorship letter, No other facilities
PLABTUTOR	4 weeks	£ 100 + £ 575 (- £ 100)	Late sponsorship letters
PLABDOCTOR	4 weeks	£ 100 + £ 500	Access to Clinical Skills Laboratory.

20 Preparation Material for the PLAB Part 2 Exam

> ◆ There is not much preparation you can get from books for the OSCE. It is more about your clinical knowledge acquired and retained. Included here is a review of the OSCE books available, other recommended reading and useful websites.

THE COMPLETE PLAB—OBJECTIVE STRUCTURED CLINICAL EXAMINATIONS

Author	: M.A.Mir, S.Madhusudan, Freeman
Publisher	: Churchill Livingstone
No. of pages	: 487
Cost	: £ 23
Edition	: 2003
Order	: www.amazon.co.uk
Content	: ✱ ✱ ✱ ✱ ✱
Accuracy	: ✱ ✱ ✱ ✱ ✱
Presentation	: ✱ ✱ ✱ ✱
Price	: ✱ ✱

100 OBJECTIVE STRUCTURED CLINICAL EXAMINATIONS

Author	: Una Coales
Publisher	: Royal Society of Medicine Press
No. of pages	: 256
Cost	: £ 20
Edition	: 2001
Order	: www.amazon.co.uk
Content	: ✱ ✱ ✱ ✱
Accuracy	: ✱ ✱ ✱ ✱ ✱
Presentation	: ✱ ✱ ✱
Cost	: ✱ ✱

PLAB PART 2—A PRACTICAL APPROACH FOR SUCCESS AT THE OSCE

Author	: Jyothi Kulkarni, G.Ram Mohan
Publisher	: Paras Publishers
No. of pages	: 257
Price	: INR 150
Order	: Any medical bookshop in India, PARAS MEDICAL PUBLISHERS
Content	: ✱ ✱ ✱
Accuracy	: ✱ ✱ ✱
Presentation	: ✱ ✱ ✱
Price	: ✱ ✱ ✱ ✱ ✱

PLAB 2 COURSE MANUAL

Author	: Sanjay Patwardhan, Manasi
Publisher	: Jaypee Brothers
No. of pages	: 88
Cost	: INR 100
Order	: Any medical bookshop in India, JAYPEE BROTHERS
Content	: ✱ ✱
Accuracy	: ✱ ✱
Presentation	: ✱ ✱
Price	: ✱ ✱ ✱ ✱

PLAB PART 2 MADE EASY—OSCE WITH DISCUSSION

Author	: Jonathan Treml, E.Mukherjee
Publisher	: Pastest
No. of pages	: 280
Cost	: £ 14.95 + postage
Order	: www.amazon.co.uk
Content	: ✴ ✴ ✴
Accuracy	: ✴ ✴ ✴ ✴ ✴
Presentation	: ✴ ✴ ✴ ✴
Price	: ✴ ✴

PLAB 2 CLINICAL TEACHING VIDEOS

Author	: Asrar Rashid
Publisher	: Medicbyte
Edition	: 2002
Cost	: £ 145
Order	: www.amazon.co.uk
	www.medicbyte.com
Content	: ✴ ✴ ✴ ✴
Accuracy	: ✴ ✴ ✴ ✴
Presentation	: ✴ ✴ ✴
Price	: ✴

LONDON HANDBOOK FOR PLAB PART 2

Author	: Hemanth Kaukuntla
Publisher	: Paras Medical Publishers
Cost	: INR 266
Order	: Any medical bookshop

OTHER RECOMMENDED READING

1. Oxford Handbook of Clinical Medicine
2. Oxford Handbook of Clinical Specialities
3. Oxford Handbook of Acute Medicine
4. Clinical Examination—MacLeod's
5. Chest X-ray made easy
6. Abdominal X-ray made easy
7. ECG made easy—John Hampton
8. Clinical Medicine—Kumar and Clark
9. House Surgeons Survival Guide
10. A Hands-on Guide for House Officers
11. Seven Sisters Notes for PLAB Part 2

RECOMMENDED WEBSITES

1. www.mcqs.com
2. www.eurekamedica.com
3. www.i-medicine.net

> ◆ *This chapter will give you an insight into the type of OSCE's you will encounter.*

1. A patient complains of diarrhoea. Take history and give differential diagnosis.
2. HRT advice—A 49-year-old lady complains of ten months of amenorrhoea, mood swings. She is feeling low and tired and having hot flushes and sweating. She is complaining of vaginal dryness and dyspareunia. She is working as a shopkeeper and not mobile. Her mother who is 78 -year-old is suffering from brittle bones. Talk to her whether HRT is needed or not and explain.
3. An 18-year-old known epileptic lady has come to you. She is going to another town for higher studies. She wants to know about alcohol and recreational drugs and about contraception. Talk to her about her condition and answer her queries.
4. Basic life support—You are working in a ward. Suddenly, you hear a noise of a fall from an adjacent cubicle. On entering the cubicle, you find a man (manikin) lying on the floor. You are only present there. You need to assess the condition quickly and need to do what you are supposed to do in such a condition. (Perform basic life support) (Resuscitation stations have repeated).
5. A mother of a 5-year-old has come and tells you that her daughter is not doing well and always seems to be lethargic since a cough and cold a week before. Take history from the mother and come to a diagnosis and explain what you are going to do.
6. A 60-year-old man has peripheral vascular disease affecting his lower limbs. Examine him and give your diagnosis.
7. A 17-year-old girl has come with weight loss, apathy and depression. Talk to her very politely, take history and give diagnosis.
8. A 19-year-old lady has come to you with pain in the right lower abdomen and bleeding per vagina. Take relevant history and give your diagnosis.
9. Do cranial nerves examination.
10. A blood sample has to be drawn and relevant things to be done (model).
11. A man has come with a cut over his forearm. Assume that local anaesthesia has been given. You need to perform two stitches. Do it accordingly (model).
12. A middle-aged lady has come with pain in right upper abdomen radiating towards the back. Take history and perform an abdominal examination.
13. A 64-year-old lady was suffering from endometrial carcinoma. A total abdominal hysterectomy and bilateral salpingo-oopherectomy was done 7 days back. She was well after the operation. Yesterday she suddenly died following a suspected pulmonary embolism. You were present during the resusci-

tation. Take an initial verbal consent for autopsy from her next of kin in a very sympathetic way.

14. A 25-year-old lady is feeling dizzy particularly after standing from a sitting position. You need to measure her blood pressure.

15. A 50-year-old gentleman is complaining that his right great toe became painful and was swollen six months back. Three months back his left knee was affected. Take a relevant history to arrive at a diagnosis.

16. A lady is there on the phone. Her 18-month-old daughter is having diarrhoea. She is also having diarrhoea. Her daughter had another attack of diarrhoea six months back. Take history from the mother and give her relevant advice, as she is very anxious.

17. A 35-year-old alcoholic lady is complaining of loss of sensation over her lower limbs. Perform a neurological examination of her lower limbs for sensory system and reflexes and explaining to the examiner at every stage what you are going to do.

18. A 60-year-old diabetic lady does not follow doctor's advice regarding her diet or her medications. She is a non-insulin dependent diabetic since last 15 years. She is now complaining increasing visual difficulty. Perform a fundoscopic examination on her and discuss your diagnosis with the examiner (manikin supplied).

19. A 35-year-old lady is suffering from panic attacks for the last three months. You are a psychiatric SHO. Take a relevant psychiatric history in a very sympathetic way and advise her accordingly.

20. A 60-year-old gentleman (manikin) is having increasing difficulty with passing his urine. Since last 12 hours, he has not passed adequate urine. You are required to pass a per-urethral catheter.

21. You are working in a ward. Suddenly, you hear a noise of a fall from an adjacent cubicle. On entering the cubicle, you find a man (manikin) lying on the floor. You are only present there. You need to assess the condition quickly and need to do what you are supposed to do in such a condition. (Perform basic life support).

22. In this OSCE station you need to perform a bimanual vaginal examination on an anatomical model assuming it to be a real patient. Describe your findings to the examiner. (Speculum examination or smear not required).

23. A 25-year-old lady is having pain over the right upper abdomen. Confirm the history from her and perform an abdominal examination to arrive at a diagnosis. Do not give more stress on the history.

24. A 35-year-old lady has been diagnosed of having an ovarian cyst on the right side. On ultrasonography, the cyst is 8.5 cm in diameter. A decision to perform right ovarian cystectomy has been made. Explain the condition to the patient and take her informed consent. She is expected to remain five days in the hospital after the operation and the Surgeon concerned will be using a bikini incision and sub-cuticular wound closure using a fine prolene as suture material. A 6-week restricted activity is normally advised after such a procedure. You are the SHO in the department of gynaecology.

25. Perform a cardiovascular system examination and describe whether the patient is in heart failure or not.

26. Examination of diabetic feet.

27. Counselling for tubal sterilisation.

28. Take a cervical smear from an anatomical model. Fix it properly and do the necessary for sending it to the laboratory.

29. Take history from the mother of a 5-year-

old child who is suffering from breathing difficulty.

30. Perform a mini mental state score on an elderly demented person.

31. Venous cannulation for intermittent drug use (on a model).

32. A 50-year-old gentleman is suffering from non-Hodgkin's lymphoma for the last five years. He had been taking co-proxamol and co-codamol for his pain relief. However, his pain is no longer under control with the above medications. Your Consultant has decided to start him on morphine sulphate sustained release preparation 40 mg once daily. Explain the treatment to the patient.

33. A 25-year-old lady is complaining of severe headache over the occipital region since last four hours. Take relevant history to arrive at a diagnosis and explain to her regarding the exact nature of the problem.

34. A young man is having pneumonia. Talk to him regarding the condition and give him relevant advice.

35. A 28-year-old lady is complaining of pain over the left knee joint following an injury during a skiing holiday and presenting to you three days after the injury. You are the Orthopaedic SHO in the clinic. Perform a knee examination on her and give your diagnosis.

36. Hand Examination—Examine and describe the features and give differential diagnosis.

37. You are working in a ward. Suddenly you hear a noise of a fall from an adjacent cubicle. On entering the cubicle, you find a man (manikin) lying on the floor. You are only present there. You need to assess the condition quickly and need to do what you are supposed to do in such a condition. (Perform basic life support) (Resuscitation stations have been frequently repeated).

38. Prostate Examination—Perform a digital rectal examination on an anatomical model.

A 60-year-old man comes with retention of urine. Talk to the examiner as patient. At the end present the findings.

39. Rectal Bleeding—A 47-year-old man complaining of bleeding per rectum. Elicit history and discuss the differential diagnosis.

40. Trauma Management—History of fall from a ladder. Airway and breathing is normal. The patient cannot move his right knee joint. Do a secondary survey and arrive at a diagnosis and outline the management.

41. Cardio-vascular system examination and describe whether the patient is in heart failure or not.

42. Drug Advice—A patient was taking minocycline for acne. Yesterday she has read an article about the drug and its side effects. You have not read the article. She is worried now. Counsel her.

43. Chest Examination—History of chronic obstructive airway disease. Do a chest examination and give your findings.

44. Coma—A patient was found unconscious on the road, brought to A and E by ambulance, airway and breathing normal, blood glucose normal. After entering the station, assess the patient's level of consciousness. Examiner will provide you the GCS Chart.

45. Post Natal Depression—A 27-year-old lady delivered a baby 4 weeks before. She is now feeling low and her appetite has gone down. You are a Psychiatric SHO, take history and explain management.

46. Venepuncture—A 60-year-old lady found to be anaemic, draw blood sample for full blood count. Talk to the examiner assuming him to be the patient.

47. Discharge Instruction Post Myocardial Infarction—A patient with uncomplicated myocardial infarction is going to be discharged and got his drugs from the pharmacy. Explain about the drugs and nothing else.

(The drugs were GTN spray, atenolol and aspirin tablet).

48. Large volume spacer—A child admitted with acute breathlessness was treated and discharged. Explain to the parents how to fit and use the spacer device and drugs.

49. A 51-year-old lady has come with complaint of cough and breathlessness. Examine her respiratory system and give your diagnosis.

50. An old man is suffering from end stage metastatic prostatic carcinoma. His daughter has come. Explain her regarding the condition and tell her about terminal care.

51. Pain right upper abdomen—history and examination.

52. Vaginal examination on a model.

53. Measure B P—A 25-year-old lady is feeling dizzy particularly after standing from a sitting position. You need to measure her blood pressure.

54. Breast examination on an anatomical model.

55. ECG—anterior MI (T—wave inversion, Q wave) and CXR showing acute LVF. Management of both. Contraindications for the use of streptokinase.

56. A patient with whiplash injury. X-rays are normal. He is still in pain. The patient is feeling low. Talk to the patient.

57. A patient had right hemicolectomy done six hours back. He suddenly collapses. Temperature, BP and pulse chart given. Call your registrar over the phone and explain.

58. Examine hip joint of a patient.

59. An 18-year-old patient recently diagnosed with epilepsy. She is on carbamazepine. Counsel her.

60. A patient anxious about a hernia operation. Take informed consent.

61. Manikin—Examine the fundus, talking through the procedure to the examiner.

62. This patient complains of dizziness. Measure her blood pressure.

63. The mother has brought her child to the A and E. You have examined the child and diagnosed as having respiratory tract infection. She is worried that her child may be suffering from meningitis. Counsel her.

64. Manikin—You are in the ward. Suddenly, you hear a patient collapsing to the floor. Perform CPR.

65. This 56-year-old woman is suffering from non-Hodgkin's lymphoma. She has had radiotherapy and chemotherapy. She has taken paracetamol and ibuprofen tablets, which she says is not relieving her pain now. The consultant has decided that you start on sustained release morphine. Counsel her.

66. Manikin—This patient sustained injury to his forearm. Deep tendon/other soft tissue injury is ruled out. Local anaesthesia has been given. Suture the wound with two sutures.

67. Take history from a 40-year-old with c/o chest pain since yesterday, unilateral, left sided.

68. This 25-year-old woman was admitted with c/o pain, lower abdominal pain. You are suspecting ectopic pregnancy. The pregnancy tests and ultrasound are planned for tomorrow morning. But the patient wants to leave the hospital today. Talk to her.

69. This patient comes with c/o breathlessness and tightness of chest. Examine the respiratory system and teach him to use peak flow meter.

70. This 25-year-old patient came with c/o pain right hip. Examine his hip.

71. This patient came to undergo surgery for ingrowing toenail. Pre-operative investigation shows increased mean corpuscular volume. He is a chronic alcoholic. Take history about alcohol intake.

22 PLAB Part 2—OSCE Revision Aid

HISTORY TAKING

The purpose of history taking at the OSCE stations in the PLAB exam is to assess whether candidates, can take an effective history from the patient and make a competent initial assessment. Most postgraduate doctors know the fundamentals of history taking and believe that they can cope up with these encounters. However, the exam setting, the time limit, and the presence of the examiner possibly with an observer; all add to the stress of having to take a history. Knowledge of what you are likely to encounter and some practice, however, will make you confident in your ability to obtain all the relevant facets of a history and draw the appropriate conclusions.

GENERAL CONSIDERATIONS

Introductory Information
- Introduce, shake hands.
- Name, What age are you now [name clues: ethnicity or age-specific disease].
- Where from [if relevant].

Presenting Complaint
- What is the problem lately. Alternatively: What is the problem that brought you to hospital [record in patient's own words].

History of Presenting Complaint

SOCRATES
- **S**ite: where, local/diffuse, "Show me where it is worst."
- **O**nset: rapid/gradual, pattern, worse/ better, what did when symptom began.
- **C**haracter: vertigo/lightheaded, pain: sharp/ dull/ stab/ burn/cramp/crushing.
- **R**adiation [usually just if pain].
- **A**lleviating factors, "What do you do after it comes on?"
- **T**ime course: when last felt well, chronic: why came now.
- **E**xacerbating factors, "What are you doing when it comes on?."
- **S**everity: scale of 1 to 10.
- Associated symptoms.
- Impact of symptoms on life: "Does it interrupt your life."
- "Were you referred here by your GP, or did you come in through casualty?"

Past Medical, Surgical History
- Past illnesses, operations.
- Childhood illness, obs/gyn.
- Tests and treatment prescribed for these.
- Drugs remaining relevant: corticosteroids, OCP, anti-HTN, chemotherapy, radiotherapy.
- Checklist of disease's:
  MJ THREADS:
  MI
  Jaundice
  TB
  HTN ["Anyone told you, you have high BP?"]
  Rheumatic fever
  Epilepsy
  Asthma

Diabetes
Stroke
- Problems with the anaesthetic in surgery.

Gynaecological History
- Time of menarche, if periods regular, menopause.
- Possibility of pregnancy number of children, number of miscarriages.
- Length of cycles, length of period, first day of your last period.

Family History
- The current complaint in parents/siblings: health, cause of death, age of onset, age of death [e.g., heart disease, bowel CA, breast CA].
- Health of parents/ siblings/ children: "Are your parents still alive?" "How is the health of your..."
- Hereditary disease suspected: do a family tree.

Social, Personal History
- Birthplace, residence.
- Race and migration [if relevant].
- Present occupation [and what do they do there], level of education.
- Any others at workplace with same complaint.
- Social habits [if relevant].
- *Smoking:* "Ever smoked, how many per day, for how long, type [cigarette, pipe, chew]."
- *Alcohol:* Do you drink? If yes: type, how much, how often?
- *Travel:* Where, immunisation/prophylactic status when went [if relevant].
- Marital status [and quality], health of spouse/ children, sex activity [discretely, if relevant].
- Other household members, pets [if infectious/ allergies], social support, whether the patient can manage at home: "Who's there with you at home?".
- Diet, physical activity.

- *Community care:* Home help, meals on wheels.

Drug History
- Prescriptions currently on [don't trust their written doses, do your own when re-prescribe].
- Over-the-counters.
- OCP.
- Supplements, HRT.
- Alternative medications.
- Recreational drugs.
  Allergies: Drugs [and what was reaction], dyes. The patient often will confuse side effect with a reaction.

INDIVIDUAL HISTORY TAKING

1. Abdominal Pain in a Woman

DD's

UTI, STD, PID, appendicitis, ectopic pregnancy, acid peptic disease, pancreatitis, renal and gallstones.

Good morning Miss Tracey I am Dr. John, Senior House Officer in the Department of Obstetrics and Gynaecology. I would like to ask you a few questions regarding your abdominal pain, is that all right with you?
- When did the pain start?
- Could you point out with one finger exactly where the pain is?
- What type of pain do you have?
- Is the pain radiating anywhere?
- What makes the pain better and what makes it worse? Is the pain getting better now?
- Is there any variation in the intensity of pain during the day?
- Do you have any nausea, vomiting and abdominal distention?
- What is the colour of the vomit? Is there any relation to food?
- Does it wake you up at night (severity)?

- How is your appetite? Have you lost weight?
- Are you opening your bowels regularly?
- Are your stools formed? Is it hard to flush? What is the colour of your stool? Is there any relation to exercise?
- Do you feel breathless or sweat excessively?
- When was your last period? Are you on any contraceptives? Could you be pregnant?
- Do you have burning micturition, h/o urinary tract infection or vaginal discharge? Does the vaginal discharge foul smell? What is the colour of the discharge? Have you had a similar episode in the past?
- Do you have family history of bowel disease or carcinoma?
- Do you smoke or consume alcohol? Are you on any medications?
- Do you have history of acid peptic disease, angina, appendicectomy, STD, PID, IUCD, ectopics?

2. Alcoholism

A series of questions called CAGE screening tool can help determine if a patient has a problem with alcohol:

1. Have you ever felt you should cut down on your drinking?
2. Have people annoyed you by criticising your drinking?
3. Have you ever felt bad or guilty about your drinking?
4. Have you ever had a drink first thing in the morning to steady your nerves or to get over a hangover? (Eye-opener).

A positive answer to any of these questions signals an increased risk for alcohol-related problems.

- When did you start drinking?
- How much do you drink?
- Have you ever tried to cut down drinking?
- Has anybody criticised on your drinking habit?

- Have you ever felt bad or guilty about drinking?
- Have you ever had a drink first thing in the morning?
- Who has referred you here?
- Do you have any mood changes?
- Have you got any phobias? Do you feel anxious about small things?
- How is your memory?
- Have you noticed any personality disturbances in you?
- Have you ever tried to end your life?
- Have you ever tried to stop drinking?
- Do you have any vomiting of blood, abdominal distension?
- Do you have loss of your pubic hair, or has your testis atrophied? Do you have abdominal pain, pruritis?
- Do you have any marital and sexual problems? Have you got any family problems?
- Have you got a job?
- Do you have any financial problems?
- Do you drive while you are drunk?
- Are you involved in crime and homelessness?
- Do you have health problems like difficulty to fall asleep, agitation, hypertension, DM, acid peptic disease or jaundice?
- Have you had any hospital admissions in the recent past?
- Have you had fits, falls and blackouts?
- Are you on any medication or are you involved in drug abuse?

3. Anxiety

- Do you get tensed or agitated very often?
- Have you got trembling; feeling of impending doom?
- Do you have difficulty falling asleep or poor concentration?
- Do you have history of collapse?
- Do you hyperventilate when you are anxious?
- Do you have chest pains, ringing in the ears, tingling and numbness of hands and feet?

- Do you have abdominal pain?
- How are your bladder and bowel habits?
- Are your menstrual periods regular?
- Have you had spasms or posturing of your hands?
- Do you have headaches, sweating, palpitations or nausea?
- How is your appetite? Do you have the feeling of something stuck in your throat or lump in the throat?
- Do you have excessive concern about self and bodily functions?
- Do you get repetitive thoughts or do activities like thumb sucking, nail biting, bed wetting?
- Are you terrified about certain situations or objects?
- Are you under stress for any reason? Have you had any bad experience recently?
- Are you married? Any marital problems?
- Are you happy with your job?

4. Epilepsy

- When do you get such attacks?
- How often do they occur? For how long do they last?
- Do they occur during any particular time of the day?
- Is there a warning? e.g., an aura preceding the attack.
- What are the exact circumstances in which they occur?
- Do you go pale or flush during an attack?
- Is it related to movement?
- What happens during an attack? Do you get injured or become incontinent?
- What is your pulse during the attack?
- Was the patient confused or sleepy after the attack?
- How much does the patient remember of the episode?
- Were there any other accompanying symptoms?

- Can the patient prevent the attack?
- Do you have any headache, photophobia, weakness of limbs, blurring of vision?
- Do you smoke or consume alcohol?
- Is the patient on any medication for BP? Is he a diabetic?
- Does he have recurrent episodes of hypoglycemia?
- Do you have HTN or heart disease? Do you have h/o neck stiffness, head injury, fits or migraine? Is there a family h/o heart disease?

5. Depression

- Since how long are you feeling this way?
- How is your appetite?
- Have you lost weight?
- Do you have early morning waking and difficulty in falling asleep?
- Do you experience frequent mood variations?
- Is there anything that makes your mood better?
- How is your thought process?
- Have you noticed any change in your sexual activity?
- How is your ability to concentrate?
- Do you get feelings of worthlessness, guilt and self-blame?
- Do you get thoughts of death and suicide? Have you attempted suicide?
- Do you smoke or consume alcohol?
- Do you take recreational drugs?
- How is your job scene?
- Do you have any problems at home? Have you experienced a major blow recently?

6. Chest Pain

DD's

Acute myocardial infarction, angina, pericarditis, myocarditis, aortic dissection, PE, pleurisy, pneumothorax, oesophagitis + spasm, acid peptic disease, cholecystitis and pancreatitis, shingles, nerve root lesion and chest wall pathology.

- When did the pain start?

- For how long have you been having this pain?
- If episodic, how long does it last?
- Could you point out the exact site of the pain?
- How is the pain, pricking, squeezing, burning?
- Is this the first time?
- Does the pain go anywhere else—to the jaw, arm or to the back?
- Do you have associated features like nausea, vomiting, sweating and breathlessness?
- Do you have any cough with expectoration?
- Are you running a temperature?
- Do you have any history of regurgitation, heartburn?
- Any history of trauma to the chest?
- What makes the pain come on? (Anxiety, emotion and palpitations). What makes it go? (Stopping exercise).
- Any diurnal variations?
- Any relation of the pain to food?
- Do you smoke or consume alcohol?
- Do you have h/o DM, HTN, acid peptic disease, stroke? Any family h/o heart disease?

7. Diarrhoea

DD's

Inflammatory bowel disease, celiac disease, parasitic infestations like amoebiasis and tropical sprue, malabsorption syndromes, gastroenteritis, carcinoma colon.

- When did it start?
- Was it sudden or has it been there for some time?
- Have you had similar episodes previously?
- How many times per day or week do you normally open your bowels? How many times per day do you pass stools now?
- Do you have pain while passing motions?
- What is the colour of the stool?
- Have you noticed blood or slime?
- Are the stools hard to flush? Are the stools fully formed or watery in consistency?
- How much do you pass in the sense do you pass more stools as compared to your normal stool quantity?
- Do you have abdominal pain?
- What aggravates or relieves your symptoms?
- Have you noticed any relation to foods like bread, cakes, oats etc.?
- Have you lost weight?
- Are you running temperature?
- Have you consumed from outside recently?
- Have you changed your diet off late?
- Have you travelled outside from your home-town recently?
- Are you on any medications? Do you take laxatives/purgatives?
- Have you had constipation before?
- Do you smoke or consume alcohol?
- Do you have family history of bowel problems?
- Are you a diabetic? Have you had bowel diseases, bowel surgeries or any other illnesses?

8. Headache

DD's

Refer revision aid for PLAB Part 1.
- When did the headache start?
- How did it start? Was it sudden?
- Is there anything you were doing like straining when it started?
- Where is the headache?
- Have you had similar episodes in the past?
- Do you suffer from migraine?
- Do you have any preceding symptoms?
- Is the headache getting better or worse?
- Is there any diurnal variation?
- Is the pain episodic, lasting for weeks and then absent for months?
- Do you have vomiting, nausea which are more in the morning?
- Do you have fever, cough or cold?
- Do you have a stiff neck?
- Do you have history of visual flashes or blurring of vision?

- Have you got a sore neck? Have you noticed rashes on your body?
- Did you suffer from ear infections in the recent past?
- Do you have a sinus problem or toothache?
- Any history of trauma?
- Any history of recent infections like meningitis?
- What is your job? Where do you work?
- Are you under a lot of stress?
- Are you on any medication? Do you smoke or consume alcohol?
- Do you have a family history of headaches?

9. Ectopic Pregnancy
- When did the bleeding start?
- How much have you bled or how many pads have you changed?
- Is the blood dark red or bright red?
- Have you passed clots or bits of tissue?
- Where is the tummy pain?
- For how long have you been having this pain?
- Did the pain precede the bleeding or vice-versa?
- Does the pain go anywhere else?
- When was your last period? Do you have any history of post-coital bleeding?
- Were your periods regular?
- Are you sexually active?
- Do you have an IUCD in place? Are you on any other contraceptive?
- Are you on any medication?
- Have you got a sexually transmitted disease?
- Do you have children?
- Do you have past h/o similar complaints?
- Have you undergone any abdominal surgery?
- Are you a diabetic or hypertensive? Do you have any other medical problems?

10a. Infertility—Female
- When was your last period?
- Are they regular? Do you have any pain during menses?

- Do you have any idea about the fertile period in your cycle?
- Do you use any type of contraception?
- Have you ever been pregnant?
- Have you suffered from pelvic inflammatory disease?
- Do you have history of ectopic and tubal pregnancy?
- Are you a diabetic?
- Do you have a history of TB or contact with TB?
- Do you have any problems with your thyroid?
- Do you have any visual field defects, headache, milk secretion?
- Have you undergone any abdominal or pelvic surgeries?
- Are you on any medication?
- Do you smoke or consume alcohol?

10b. Infertility—Male
- Have you fathered a child before?
- What is your occupation?
- Have you suffered from mumps as a child?
- Have you had infection of the waterworks?
- Are you a diabetic?
- Have you had a sexually transmitted disease?
- Have you been operated for any abdominal problems?
- Are you on any medication?
- Do you smoke or consume alcohol?

11. Suspected Meningitis
- Introduce yourself and calm the mother.
- When did the fever start?
- Is the child sick? If yes, how many times has he vomited?
- Have you noticed any rash?
- Does he have any head banging or pulling of hair?
- Was the glass test performed? If so what is the result?
- Is the child refusing food? Is he very irritable?
- Does he cry excessively?

- Is the child active and responding to commands or drowsy?
- Is there a past history of similar episodes?
- Has the child been immunised to date?
- Is there any health problem in the siblings and other members of the family?
- Does anyone in his school suffer from meningitis?

12. Palpitations

DD's

Heart disease, Thyroid, drugs, alcohol, obesity, anxiety.

- When did the palpitation start?
- Are they fast or slow?
- Can you tell the exact circumstances of their occurrence?
- Are they regular? Do you know the rate?
- Have you got any associated features like vomiting, sweating, chest pain, dyspnoea, dizziness, and collapse?
- Are you a very anxious personality?
- Have you lost weight?
- How are your bowel habits?
- Do you get tremors or panic attacks?
- What makes the palpitations worse and what makes them go?
- Are you on drugs?
- Do you consume alcohol or smoke?
- Do you have any medical problem like MI, DM and thyroid disease?

13. Rectal Bleeding

DD's

Diverticulitis, colorectal carcinoma, hemorrhoids, polyps, trauma, fissure *in ano*, angiodysplasia, arteriovenous malformation, radiation proctitis.

- Since when have you been passing blood per rectum?
- Is this the first episode?
- Is it frank blood or blood mixed in the stool? Are you passing any slime?

- Is the blood in the beginning or end of passing stool? Is the stool coated with blood?
- How many times do you open your bowel?
- Do you feel any thing coming down while passing bowels?
- Do you have to strain to pass your motion (Tenesmus)?
- Do you have pain while passing motions?
- Do you have fever?
- Do you have any skin rashes.
- Is there any breathlessness, fatigue?
- Do you have abdominal pain?
- Do you feel better after opening the bowel?
- How is your appetite? Have you lost weight?
- Do you have problems with your joints?
- Are you on any medication?
- Do you have history of IBD, Ca and bleeding disorders?
- Do you smoke or consume alcohol?
- Does any one in your family have similar complaints?

14. Post-Coital Bleeding

- When did the bleeding start?
- How much have you bled?
- Is it only after sex? Is the intercourse painful?
- When was your last period? Are the periods regular?
- How many days do you bleed?
- When was your first period?
- When did you start having sex?
- Are you in a steady relationship?
- How many children have you got?
- Are they from the same partner?
- Do you get your cervical smears done regularly? When was the last smear test done?
- Any other discharges? What is the consistency? Does it smell?
- Have you had any problems with your waterworks? Does it burn or pain while you pass water?
- Have you lost weight?

- Do you have any history of bleeding disorder?
- Did any one in the family suffered from similar complaint?
- Are you on any medications?
- Do you smoke or consume alcohol?
- Do you have any medical problems?
- Are you a diabetic or hypertensive?

15. Post-Menopausal Bleeding

- How old are you?
- When did the bleed start? For how long have you been bleeding?
- Have you noticed bleeding after sex?
- Did you pass clots or have you noticed only spotting?
- Have you got any abdominal pain?
- Is there any discharge from your front passage? What is the colour and consistency of the discharge?
- Have you lost weight?
- How old were you when you got your first period?
- When did you attain menopause?
- When did you have the last cervical smear?
- Do you have h/o hot flushes, night sweats and dry vagina?
- How many children have you got?
- Do you smoke or consume alcohol?
- Are you on any other drugs or HRT?
- Have you had any other gynaecological problems or operations?
- Do you suffer from any medical problem?
- Is there a family history of genital cancer?

16. Amenorrhoea

DD's

Primary amenorrhoea, anorexia nervosa, hypo-thalamic-pituitary-ovarian failure, polycystic ovary syndrome, ovarian failure, Asherman's syndrome, post-pill amenorrhoea, tumours and necrosis, Sheehan's syndrome.

- What is your age? Have you ever had periods?

- Do you have any sisters? When did she start her periods?
- When did you mother have her first period?
- Have you developed axillary hair? When did you notice them?
- Have your breasts developed?
- Do you get lower tummy pain?
- Is there any chance, that you could be pregnant? Do you use any contraceptives?
- Are you emotionally stressed for any reason?
- Are you preparing for any exam?
- Have you lost weight?
- Do you have any medical problem?
- Do you have past h/o D and C?
- Do you have any thyroid enlargement, any tremors, diarrhoea, constipation, weight gain or loss, intolerance to cold or heat?

17. Post-Natal Depression

- How is your thought process?
- Do you have frequent mood changes?
- How is your appetite?
- Do you look forward to happy moments with your baby?
- Is there any change in your sleep patterns?
- How is your ability to concentrate?
- Since when have you been feeling low?
- Is the pregnancy planned? Did you have any complications during antenatal period?
- How did the labour go? Did you have any complication?
- For how long have you been staying in the hospital?
- How is the baby doing? Are you breast-feeding?
- Is there anyone to share the household work? Is your partner caring and helpful?
- Are you feeling worthless or guilty?
- Do you have suicidal thoughts? Have you ever attempted one?
- Have you ever tried to harm the baby?
- Do you have a job?

- Do you smoke or consume alcohol?
- Are you on any medication?

18. Stridor

DD's

Croup, epiglottitis, foreign body inhalation, tracheo malacia.

Tumours (papilloma or haemangioma)
- When did it start?
- Did it start off suddenly or has it been of a gradual onset?
- Did this happen while you where eating?
- Did you choke any foreign body?
- Have you been having this problem since your birth?
- Are you able to swallow your saliva or does it drool?
- Do you go blue during the attacks?
- Do you feel breathless?
- Do you have fever?
- Do you have cough or cold? Barking cough?
- Is it worse at night?
- Have you been immunised against HIB?

19. Vomiting

DD's

Gastroenteritis, acid peptic disease, pancreatitis, ICSOL, gallstones, pregnancy.
- How long have you been sick?
- How many times do you vomit in a day?
- When do you vomit? Is the vomiting worse in the mornings?
- Is the vomiting effortless?
- Does the vomiting occur in relation to meals?
- How much do you vomit? Is the vomit copious and watery?
- What is the colour of the vomit? Is the vomit blood or bile (green) stained? Is there any food in the vomit?
- Do you have fever?
- Have you lost weight?

- Do you bring up acid?
- Is there an associated abdominal pain?
- Do you get an unpleasant feeling before you vomit or does it just happen?
- Do you feel better after vomiting?
- Have you travelled recently?
- Does any other member of the family have similar complaints?
- Are you on any medication (morphine, digoxin)?
- Could you be pregnant?
- Do you consume alcohol?
- Do you have any medical problem like acid peptic disease, pancreatitis, ICSOL, gallstones or angina?

20. Child with Diabetes
- How old is he?
- Is he lethargic and drowsy?
- Is he having temperature and any coughs and colds?
- How much does he drink?
- How often does he go for a wee?
- Does he wake up at night for a drink?
- How is his appetite? Has he lost weight?
- Does he pass loose motions?
- Does it sting during wee?
- Has he had any problems with his waterworks? Does he complain of pain or burning sensation while passing water?
- Has he had similar illness in the past?
- Has he suffered from head injury or meningitis?
- Has he been immunised to date?
- Is there a family history of diabetes?

21. Pain in the Great Toe
- How long has the pain been there? (Duration)
- Is it there all the time or does it come and go? (Periodicity).
- Can you tell me exactly where the pain is? (Site).
- Does it spread? (Radiation)

- Do you have pain in other joints?
- Do you feel any heat over the toe? (Septic arthritis).
- Any skin rash? (SLE)
- Any redness of eye or pain on passing water? (Reiter's syndrome)
- Have you had a similar pain before?
- Ask about predisposing factors to gout: have you had any injury or surgery recently?
- Do you have any disease, blood disease?
- Any recent illness?
- Are you on any medication? Aspirin?
- Do you eat a lot of red meat? Are you on any diet?
- Do you drink at all? How much of alcohol?
- Has anyone else in your family had similar condition?
- Do you have any tummy pain?
- Any kind of problem?
- Is it painful when you touch it, any swelling, and any redness?

22. Numbness in the Hand

- When did that happen?
- How long did it last?
- Have you had similar conditions in the past?
- Have you had any weakness in the arm or leg?
- Have you had any change or loss of vision?
- Have you had any giddiness or dizziness? Is there any difficulty with hearing?
- Have you had any difficulty with speaking?
- Do you have any headache?
- Have you had any loss of consciousness?
- Have you had any trauma to the head?
- Do you have any pain in the neck, joint, or heart problem?
- Do you have DM, hypertension?
- Do you smoke? How many cigarettes a day?
- What about your diet? Do you eat a lot of fatty meals or salt?
- Has anyone else in your family had similar condition?

- Does anyone in your family has hypertension, DM, CVA, early death, or hyperlipidaemia?
- Are you on any medication? Did you use contraceptive pills?

23. Weight Loss

- When did you notice that you are losing weight?
- What was your weight before? And what is it now?
- Through how much time you lost this amount of weight?
- Do you have any fever, any feeling of tiredness, cough, shortness of breath, chest pain, and infection?
- Do you feel thirsty and pass water more than usual? (DM)
- Have you noticed any recent intolerance to heat, sweating, and tremor? (Thyrotoxicosis)?
- How many times do you open your bowel? And do you have diarrhoea? Did you notice that the waste couldn't be flushed away easily? (Steatorrhoea).
- Do you have any stress at home, at school? (Stress).
- How is your appetite? Do you take any special diet?
- Do you think that you are thin, have usual weight or overweight? (Model, Ballet dancer).
- Do you ever induce vomiting or use medication to decrease weight?
- Do you exercise to lose weight?
- What about your periods? Are they regular?
- How do you feel in yourself?
- Do you have any mood changes during the day?
- What about your sleep? What about your concentration?
- What about your memory?
- Do you still enjoy things you used to like them before?

- Do you think that life is worth living nowadays?
- Do you have any disease?
- Do you take any medication?
- Do you have any disease in the family?

COUNSELLING

Unfortunately, communication skills are not part of the medical curriculum and are not taught as a subject in many colleges. Doctors learned communication by a process of osmosis as they went along on ward rounds, or sitting in as students in the outpatient clinics. This inevitably left many gaps in the communication skills of younger clinicians. The older ones tended to learn from their own and others' mistakes. As a result of an increasing emphasis on communication and counselling, there will be at least three stations in the OSCE where the spotlight will be on communication skills.

The basic components of counselling follow the mneumonic **GATHER**

Greet the patient and introduce yourself

Ask the patient his/her reasons for the procedure, e.g., sterlisation

Tell the patient about the alternative options

Help him/her decide

Explain the procedure

Return for follow-up—be available for further questioning.

1. Counselling a Mother who has a Child with Cleft-Palate

Good morning Mrs. Tracey I am Dr. Rahul, Senior House Officer in the Department of Paediatrics. Congratulations on the birth of your baby boy. I have come to talk to you about the defect that you see in his upper lip. This is called a cleft lip. The defect also extends to the roof of his mouth. And this is called a cleft palate. This happens due to the failure of fusion of the two parts of lip and the palate in the middle. I understand that you are anxious to know what will happen to him. I would like to reassure you that this defect although common, is not a life-threatening condition.

In the near future he will need a surgery to repair the defect. The operation is performed by plastic surgeons. It is possible to close the defect and leave behind only a very small scar. The lip is repaired at three months and the palate at one year.

At this second, however, it is important to concentrate on his feeding. If you are breast-feeding, you might need some help from our breastfeeding nurse. If you are planning to bottle feed, he will need a special teat so that the defect of his palate will be covered. This prevents milk from going into his nose.

Other than that you need not take any other special precautions. I will also refer you to the CLAPA team, i.e., cleft lip and palate association. One of the nurses from this team will talk to you again about feeding techniques.

That's all for now Mrs. Tracey, Thank you.

2. Counselling a Mother who has a delivered a Baby with Down's Syndrome

Hello Mrs. Tracey! I am Dr. XYZ, Senior House Officer in the Department of Paediatrics. Congratulations on the birth of your beautiful boy. I would like to have a little chat to you about him. You might have noted that he looks somewhat different to other babies. I have examined him carefully and I am sorry to tell you that I believe he has a condition known as Down's syndrome. Have you heard about this at all?

Down's syndrome is a chromosomal disorder. Now, children with Down's syndrome can have a variety of features. The most obvious ones are the upward slanting eyes. They have a large tongue and can be rather floppy. This might lead to feeding problems in the early life.

Occasionally, these children can have heart defects and malformations in their guts. This does not seem to be the case with your son, as I have listened to his heart and examined his tummy.

I don't want to paint a very gloomy picture. Children with Down's syndrome are very pleasant and lovable. They enjoy music very much.

It is important to do a blood test to look at the chromosomes to confirm this. We will also do an ultrasound for his abdomen.

It must be a lot for you to take in, in one session. I will be happy to clarify any queries that you may have.

Thank you, Mrs. Tracey.

3. Counselling an Epilepsy Patient who is being Discharged

Introduction, then you may begin by saying: "You are going to have a wonderful time in the next few weeks. Where are you going? With whom are you going? Before you go, I would like to say a few words about what you should avoid while being on holiday.'

Advice About Medication

First make sure that you take enough medication with you. You are going to a very sunny place and you are on carbamazepine treatment. Remember that this medication makes you more sensitive to sunlight. Therefore, you can easily get sunburn. To avoid this, don't stay in the sun between 11:00 am and 3 pm; keep yourself covered, especially during the hottest time of the day. Don't wear clothes that you can see through if you hold them up to the light, they let UV light through. Try to wear a hat (especially if light coloured hair). Always use high-factor sun-protection cream. Apply regularly, especially if you are swimming.

General Advice

Let other people with you know that you have epilepsy, so that they can help if necessary.

It is a good idea to wear Medic-Alert chain or bracelet, which is a very useful way of letting other people know that you have epilepsy, so that they can help, should this be necessary.

Sports

You can play tennis, basketball, go jogging, running, swimming and what is important about swimming, that you shouldn't do it alone. Always go with a strong swimmer who can help you in case an attack occurs. Also, avoid excessive exercise and allow yourself enough time to rest.

Sports that could be dangerous are those where people cannot reach you easily, should a seizure happen, such as horse riding, parachuting, hang-gliding, para gliding; or those involving water such as scuba diving.

Sleep, TV, and Disco

Sleep is also very important, less sleeping hours would trigger an attack, this is most likely to happen after getting up early following late nights. A regular pattern of sleep should reduce this risk.

The flashing light of disco, and flicking light of TV can trigger an attack. Try to limit the period of time you spend in disco and try to stay away from flashing light. When watching TV, stay at least eight feet away from screen and three feet away when playing computer games.

At Home

a. *Living room:* Stay away from fire, and if possible choose a soft carpet. Fit safety glass in windows and doors.

b. *In kitchen:* Don't cook on your own. In general, microwaves are safer than cookers, but if you use a cooker, then use the back burners and turn the sauce pan handle towards the back of the cooker to make them less likely to knock over. Carry the plates to the pan and not vice versa.

In bedroom: Choose a wide-low level bed.

d. *In bath room:* Let people, living with you, know that you will have a shower or bath, and don't lock the door. In general, showers are safer than baths. But if you use bath, don't have the water too hot and turn off the tap before you get in, and it is better to keep the water shallow.

e. *At work:* Avoid works that involve operating machinery or going up to high open spaces.

f. *Driving:* You must not drive by law until you are one year fit free, with or without medication and you need to inform the driving and vehicle licensing authority.

4. Counselling the Mother of a Child who has had Febrile Convulsions

I know that was a very fear-provoking experience for you. You may even have thought that your child was dead or dying. Many parents think that when they first see a febrile convulsion. However, febrile convulsions are not as serious as they look. It is an attack brought on by fever in a child usually aged between 6 months and 4 or 5 years. A convulsion is an attack in which the person becomes unconscious and usually stiff, with jerking of the arms and legs. It is caused by a hurricane of electrical activity of the brain. The words convulsions, fit and seizure mean the same thing.

I will now advise you on some precautions to be taken:

If your child is having fever, you can take the temperature by placing the bulb of the thermometer under his armpit for three minutes with his arm held against his side. Keep him cool. Don't overclothe him or over heat the room. Give plenty of fluids to drink. Give children paracetamol medicine to get his temperature down.

When your child is fitting, you should lay him flat on his side, with his head at the same level or slightly lower than his body. Note the time and wait for the fit to stop. It is not necessary to do anything else. We will give a medicine to insert into your child's bottom. This is called rectal diazepam. If the fit carries for more than five minutes, give rectal diazepam. This should stop the fit in 10 minutes. If it doesn't, bring him up to the hospital or dial 999 if necessary. In any event let your doctor know what had happened.

5. Counselling the Mother of a Child who suffered from Birth Asphyxia

Hello Mrs. Smith I am Dr. XYZ, Senior House Officer in the Department of Paediatrics. I would like to have a little chat with you regarding your son. As you know, we have to admit him to the special care baby unit yesterday.

Unfortunately, he went through a tough time when he was born. He was very distressed because of the cord prolapse and his brain was starved of oxygen for a while. Due to this he was floppy when he came out and needed help with his breathing. As you can see now, he is on a ventilator, a machine that breathes for him.

Unfortunately, he also started to fit yesterday and he is on medication to control his fits. We have done a scan of his brain, which shows some swelling. We are hoping that this will go down in the next few days.

We need to monitor his progress carefully over the next few weeks.

We will also be doing more blood tests and head scans. We will let you know any results immediately.

In the meantime, try not to worry too much, as these are early days. I know it is hard. We will encourage you to spend as much time with him as possible, here on the baby unit.

Before discharging your baby, we will notify the physiotherapist, health visitor, social worker and GP. We will arrange regular appointments for follow-up of your son.

Do you have any questions? Thank you, Mrs. Smith.

6. Counselling the Mother of a Child who is suffering from Leukaemia

Hello Mrs. Tracey. How are you doing?

I would like to speak to you about your son's condition. He has been suffering from multiple bruises, bodyaches and recurrent infections. We have done a few blood tests, which suggest that he has a condition called acute leukaemia. This means that his bone marrow is producing a lot of abnormal white cells. As a result, there is a deficiency of the other cells, which is leading to him developing frequent infections and bleeding manifestations.

I am sorry to say that this is a form of cancer. Nevertheless, we would first have to confirm the diagnosis by doing a bone marrow test. Subsequent to that, we will start him on chemotherapy to suppress the cancer. There are some side effects from the drugs like hair loss, vomiting, bleeding and diarrhoea. We hope his condition responds to chemotherapy. If not, he might need a bone marrow transplant.

I know that this is a lot of information to digest at the moment.

We will explain things on a daily basis. If you have any doubts do not hesitate to ask. Thank you.

7. Counselling the Mother of a Baby suffering from Nappy Rash

Hello Mrs. Tracey, I am Dr. Rahul, Senior House Officer in the Department of Paediatrics.

You brought your son Robert to the hospital because he has a sore bottom. I have examined him. It appears to me that he has a common condition called ammoniacal dermatitis.

It is quite common in small children. It is due to irritation of the skin from the urine in the nappy. However, it is a reasonably easy condition to treat. I will, however, need your help in the treatment.

You will have to change his nappy regularly. You can apply an emollient cream or a nappy cream to prevent irritation to other areas.

Also, avoid any tight fitting clothes. If possible give your baby some time off from the nappies if you can. If you are using reusable nappies, you have to wash them thoroughly after use.

This condition should soon go away. However, if it is no better in a few days time, you should come back to see me again.

If you have any queries, you can ask me now.

Thank you Mrs. Tracey, I shall leave now. Take care.

8. Counselling a Victim of Needle-Stick Injury

Hello Mrs. Tracey. I am Dr. Rahul, Senior House Officer in this A and E Department.

I can see you have brought your little boy Thomas. I understand he pricked himself with a needle. I need to ask you a few questions.

- Do you know whom the needle belongs to?
- Do you have any idea where did he found it?
- When did the injury happen?
- Have you cleaned the wound?
- When did he last have his tetanus immunisation?

There are a few things we need to do. We will dispose of the needle for you. Thomas needs a blood test to check his hepatitis status. We will then give him the first shot of the vaccine. He will need two further boosters at 1st month and 2nd month, which he should get from your GP. He will also need an additional blood test after the vaccination to see if the vaccine is working. Regarding the risk of AIDS, I can assure you that the risk is very small.

I hope I have cleared all your doubts. I will write to your GP about what needs to be done. It is important that Thomas receives the full course of the immunisation.

I will give you an information leaflet as well. If you have any doubts later, please don't hesitate to contact us.

Thank you Mrs. Tracey.

9. Counselling for Sterilisation—Male

Introduction, then you may say: "As far as I know, you asked about sterilisation that is what we call vasectomy.

Vasectomy is the procedure by which tubes that carry sperms from your testicles to the penis are cut and blocked. This operation is usually done under local anaesthesia. That is the type of anaesthesia that numbs the (sac) scrotal area. So you will be awake during the procedure, but you will not feel pain. The doctor will make a small cut in the skin of the scrotum, which is the sac of the testicle to reach the tubes, then will remove a small piece of each tube and close the ends.

The cuts will be very small and you may not need any stitch, but if needed, dissolvable stitches will be used. The operation takes 10 to 15 minutes and you will be able to leave the hospital shortly afterward. But you should not drive yourself home; you should rest for the remainder of the day. The stitches used are dissolvable and will disappear within a week. After the operation, the scrotum may feel bruised, swollen and painful. You can help that by wearing tight-fitting underpants to support your scrotum day and night for one week. Avoid heavy exercise for at least a week.

Some men may get bleeding or infections. If this happens, you should contact your doctor. You can have sex after the operation as soon as it is comfortable; however, you have to use another method of contraception until sperms disappear from your seminal fluid, and this may take up to 2 to 3 months. We have to have two clear semen tests, so that you can rely on vasectomy for contraception. Your testicle will continue to produce male hormone as before, your sex drive, ability to have erection and climax will not be affected. The appearance and amount of semen should be the same as before. There is a suggestion about link between vasectomy and cancer of testicle and prostate, but it is not yet proven.

You should consider vasectomy as a permanent method of contraception. Reversal is complicated and may not work. Failure rate is 1/1000-2000 and reversal rate is 50 per cent. You should not attempt vasectomy if you are not sure that you don't want more children and you should discuss it carefully with your partner as well as the possibility of the use of available method of contraception.

It doesn't protect against STD.

10. Counselling for Sterilisation—Female

Introduction, then you may say: "As far as I know, you want to do permanent sterilisation. I would like to ask you a few questions, and discuss the condition with you."

- How old are you?
- Do you have children? How many?
- Do you have a partner? Does he know about your decision?
- Does he agree?
- Why do you want to be sterilised?
- Do you know about contraception methods available, such as OCP, coils, condoms, diaphragm and cups?

Female sterilisation is a procedure by which the fallopian tubes—the tubes between the womb and ovaries—are cut, sealed or blocked. This stops eggs moving down them to meet sperms. The operation can be done in several ways; the most common method is by the use of laparoscopy. This is usually done with the use of General Anaesthesia, where you will be put to sleep; a doctor will make two tiny cuts, one just below your navel and the other just above the bikini line in the lower part of your tummy. They will then insert a laparoscope which is a thin telescope-like instrument with magnifying lenses to look at your reproductive organs.

The second way is by what we call it mini-laparotomy, usually done under General Anaesthesia, the doctor will make a small cut in your tummy, just below the bikini line to reach the fallopian tubes.

The third way is to reach the reproductive organs through the vagina. The fallopian tubes are then blocked either by tying (ligation), or by removal of a small piece, and then sealed by heat, or by applying clips or rings.

The period you need to stay in the hospital depends on the type of anaesthesia and operation. It is usually around couple of days. After operation, if you have General Anaesthesia you may feel unwell for a few days and you may have some bleeding and pain, which are slight. You must consider sterilisation as the permanent method of contraception.

However, there is an operation to reverse sterilisation, but it is complicated and may not work. The failure rate of female fertilisation is 1 to 3 per 1000. Pregnancy rate after reversal is around 50 per cent with high-risk of ectopic pregnancy.

The advantage is that it does not interfere with sex; your womb and ovaries will remain in place. Ovaries will still release an egg every month. Your sex drive and enjoyment will not be affected. Actually, they may improve, as fear of pregnancy is no more an issue.

Occasionally some women find their periods to be heavier, but it is usually because of their age and stopping contraceptive pills. You can start sex as soon as comfortable. You must continue contraception until the time of operation and if you use an intrauterine contraceptive device (ICUD), it should be left till the next period. You should contact your doctor if you think that you are pregnant, or if you missed a period and, especially, if it's accompanied with tummy pain.

11. Counselling for Abortion

Hello Mrs. Tracey, I understand that you want to terminate your pregnancy.
- How old are you?
- Are you sure that you are pregnant?

- Why do you want a termination? I don't mean to be intrusive, but have you considered the pros and cons of this?
- You have to live with the decision for the rest of your life.
- Have you discussed with your partner?
- Have you considered the other alternatives like adoption of the baby?

I will have to examine you and do a screen to confirm that you are pregnant. I will need to do some blood tests, too.
- When was your last cervical smear?
- Do you have any vaginal discharge?
- Are your menstrual cycle's regular?
- When were your last periods?
- Are you on any contraception?
- Is this a planned or unplanned pregnancy?
- Have you had any terminations of pregnancy before this one?
- Are you having any medical problems?
- Are you on any medication?
- Do you smoke or consume alcohol?

Mrs. Smith as you are more than 9 weeks' pregnant, the TOP is done under General Anaesthesia. The cervix is dilated and the womb is evacuated.

When you wake up, it may be sore and bleed. If there are no problems, you can go home the same day.

Thank you Mrs. Tracey that would be all.

12. Counselling the Mother of a Child with Diabetes Mellitus

Good Morning Mrs. Tracey. The results of Robert's investigations have arrived and I am afraid he is suffering from diabetes mellitus. I would like to tell you something about this disease:

Due to the lack of insulin, which is produced by the pancreas, the blood sugar always remains high. The child may pass a lot of urine and he may be dehydrated. There is an increased risk of infection and boils.

It can't be cured but can be kept under control by insulin injections. The cause of this is not known. The good news is he can grow as a normal child with insulin. It is important that he takes insulin regularly.

He should not skip meals or exercise excessively at one go. It is advisable to always carry sugary drinks or chocolate. He will go into hypoglycaemia if he skips a meal. Hypoglycaemia presents as irritability, sweating, drowsiness, light-headedness and abdominal pain. It is important to recognise these symptoms. If he is ill, he should still take insulin regularly with sugary drinks.

Regular monitoring of his blood glucose will be required. If it remains persistently high, he could have problems with his waterworks, his eyes and could also affect his brain.

Our diabetic nurse will have a word with you regarding his diet. He will have regular follow, ups. His GP will be informed. If you have any doubts, please don't hesitate to ask.

Thank you, Mrs. Tracey.

13. Counselling a Patient with Inguinal Hernia

Introduction, and then you may say: "I am going to have a word with you about your hernia and possibility of surgical treatment. And to take your consent about the operation."

Do you know what a hernia is?

In anyone there are weak areas in the lower part of the front of the tummy. The coverings of the tummy contents together with some of these contents, such as part of the gut, may push through these weak areas into the upper part of the thigh, groin area or sometimes down the scrotum that is the sac of the testicles.

The predisposing factors that can lead to hernia are: lifting heavy objects, straining as in constipation, being overweight, and chronic cough.

As the gut and coverings pass through these weak areas, it might happen that the inside of the gut get blocked, and in this case we need to do emergency operation with higher possibility of complications than if we do planned operation.

In the operation we return the contents of the tummy, as gut and covering, back into the proper position and the weak area is repaired either by the use of synthetic mesh or darning by nylon or reposition of the muscles.

About anaesthesia, well, you will have either general anaesthesia, where you will be put to sleep and then wake up after the operation. Or spinal anaesthesia where you will be given injection into the backbone and you will feel numb from waist below.

You will wake up from general anaesthesia in the recovery area and once you wake up, you will be taken back to ward. You will probably feel sleepy for a couple of hours, you may feel sick, get headache or sore throat, this will pass but be sure to inform the nursing or medical staff should this become worse.

As any operation, this may have complications like:
1. Wound infection.
2. Bleeding and collection of blood in the area.
3. Recurrence of hernia.
4. Pain, sensation of pins and needles in the area of operation.
5. Infertility. (Very rare< %1) and as you are in good hands, we will find the structures related to fertility and put them away from the work field.
6. General: urine retention, chest infection, clots in the leg and lung.

You will remain in the hospital for 1 to 2 days after operation, if dissolvable suture are used, then they will dissolve by themselves if not removed within seven days.
1. You have to rest for one week.
2. Back to work within two weeks (desk work), after thre months (manual work).

3. Drive within 1 to 2 weeks or when comfortable.
4. Sex: as soon as it is comfortable.
5. Diet: a lot of vegetables and fruits.
6. Smoking: stop it, if possible.

Is everything clear to you? Do you have any questions to ask me? This is the consent for operation. Would you mind reading and signing it please?

14. Counselling for Hormone Replacement Therapy (HRT)

Introduction, then you may begin by saying: "I have heard that you are here to discuss the HRT. You know every woman goes through the menopause. This occurs when a woman's ovaries produce no more the female sex hormones, which are oestrogen and progesterone."

Oestrogen has an effect on every cell in the body, whether it is in the skin, bone, blood vessels, womb and vagina. So when the level of oestrogen in the body falls, women get features of hot flushes, night sweats, mood changes, forgetfulness, sleep disturbances, and loss of concentration. In addition, lack of oestrogen causes a type of protein, called collagen, to be gradually lost from the skin, so the skin becomes thinner, drier, and easily bruised. Also, the vagina becomes thinner, less flexible, drier leading to painful sexual intercourse, and less resistant to infections. But the most important effect of oestrogen lack is on the bones causing what we call osteoporosis, which means that the bones loose mass, so they become weak, brittle, and much more likely to break, causing a number of minor injuries such as a fall.

Another important effect is on the heart, where before menopause women rarely get heart diseases, while after menopause, the possibility of getting heart attack increases. And within 10 years, they catch up with the heart attack incidence in men.

Fortunately, there is an effective way of dealing with the problem that is the use of HRT, which consists of these lacking hormones, oestrogen and progesterone.

There are many ways of taking the HRT; the first is tablets, which are taken by mouth every day, the second is patches that stick to the skin and should be changed twice weekly. Another way is implants that are inserted under the skin under local anaesthesia and their effect lasts for 3 to 6 months. The fourth way is the gel, which is applied to the skin daily. But you should not bath after application for one hour. If vaginal dryness is the main problem, we could give you cream or pessary to place inside the vagina.

With the HRT, hot flushes usually disappear within a few weeks. It also helps dryness of vagina, improves mood, and sleep disturbances. And the most important effect of the HRT is that it can dramatically decrease the risk of osteoporosis, hence fractures. And substantially decreases the risk of heart attacks.

There are a very few reasons why a woman cannot take the HRT, such as in liver disease, cancer of the womb, or cancer of the breast, and in case of abnormal bleeding from vagina that has no obvious cause. Like any other medication, the HRT has some side effects, most of them are minor and often disappear if you stop the treatment. Some women feel sick, that is with tablets. Some may put on weight, some may get breast pain and mood changes before periods, which will re-appear with the HRT. Some may get skin irritation with the usage of patches.

With the use of oestrogen hormone, there is a slight increased risk of womb cancer and to decrease that risk, we add progesterone, which has protective effect on the womb. Therefore, in women who have had their womb removed, this combination of drug is not necessary. The most common reason people are worried about in the HRT, is breast cancer, however if you use the

HRT for five years, is the risk, still minimal. But once you get beyond that, e.g., 10 to 15 years, the then the risk tends to increase bit more and we usually teach women how to do self-examination of the breast. Also, we tell them to report, immediately, any vaginal bleeding if happens. One more thing is that the HRT is not a contraception method and the woman should continue to use her usual contraception method for one year after the last menstrual period.

15. Counselling before Inserting IUCD

Hello Mrs. Tracy. I would like to give you some advice before I insert this intrauterine contraceptive device (IUCD).

- How old are you?
- Have you completed your family?
- How many children do you have?
- Were the deliveries normal?
- When was your last period?
- Do you have regular periods?
- Do you have any history of ectopic pregnancy or fibroids?
- When was your last cervical smear?
- Have you been treated for any genital infection?
- Do you have any history of heart disease, diabetes or Wilson's disease? Are you on any medication?

An IUCD is a small plastic and copper device with two soft threads on the ends. It prevents the egg from settling in the womb. The IUCD doesn't interfere with sex. It needs to be changed once in 3 to 5 years.

The periods you have henceforth may be heavier or painful. There is a tiny chance of infection. In the first 20 days your womb may expel the IUCD out. There is also a rare chance of perforation. If you do become pregnant, there is the risk of an ectopic pregnancy. The IUCD does not protect against the STD. You don't have to really worry about all these problems.

We will see you again immediately after the next period and then once every six months. You should regularly feel for the thread. Come immediately to the hospital if the thread is missing, if you have excessive bleeding, pain and fever.

That's all I guess. Thank you Mrs. Tracy.

16. Counselling For TURP

Hello Mr. Shyam, I am Dr. Sharma, Senior House Officer in the Department of Surgery.

I understand that you have a problem when passing urine. Your stream is not very good. You have also said that you need to go very often to the toilet. We have examined you and found that your prostate is enlarged. As it is a benign enlargement, we would like you to undergo an operation called TURP, transurethral resection of the prostate.

This means that we will insert a small camera through your urethra and with it we can remove all the abnormal tissue. The procedure will be done under general anaesthesia. The Anaesthetist will come and have a word with you.

There are a few risks associated with this operation and I should be informing you about them. There is a miniature chance that you may become infertile after the operation. You might notice a little blood in your urine for the first two weeks.

After the operation, you should not drive for two weeks. You need to avoid sex for two weeks.

Your ejaculate may be decreased and this is due to backward flow into the bladder. This can make the urine look cloudy. You might have to go to the toilet more frequently, but this should settle in a few weeks time.

Do you have any questions? Thank you Mr. Shyam.

17. Counselling an HIV Patient

Good morning Mr. Shyam, I am Dr. Mohammed Ali, Senior House Officer in the Department of

Medicine. The result of your blood test came today morning.

I am afraid to say that the blood test confirmed that you are having the HIV virus which cause AIDS. I can understand that this is a very awful news for you. I would like to ask you a few questions to put things in perspective.

- Do you have any history of blood transfusion?
- Do you use any recreational drugs?
- Do you practice safe sex?
- What are your sexual preferences?

Mr. Shyam, having the virus doesn't mean that you are having AIDS. We really don't know how the disease progresses. Some people can be free of symptoms for a long time. However, it is important that you use medication to prevent further deterioration in your condition.

The symptoms you might experience could be bodyaches, lethargy, swelling of your glands, headache, weight loss, skin infection, diarrhoea, etc. You will also require regular follow-up with us.

Mr. Shyam you should practice safe sex. You shouldn't donate blood or share needles and razors. This is an entirely confidential matter, but I feel you should tell your GP and your partner about it.

That's it Mr. Shyam. Hope you will take my advice sincerely!

18. Counselling a Patient after Cervical Smear

Hello Mrs. Smith, I am Dr. XYZ, Senior House Officer in the Department of Obstetrics and Gynaecology. We have got the results of your smear test back. I am afraid we have detected some abnormal cells. Let me put in plain words what it means.

Some of the cells from the cervix have shown some changes. This could be due to an infection. So we will check and treat if there is any infection. It is necessary to repeat the cervical smear and

then we will decide the further course of action. I would like to reassure you that this is not cancer.
or

Some of the cells from the cervix have undergone changes. So we would like to do another test called colposcopy. Here we have a direct look at the cervix with a microscope. At the same time a biopsy can be taken. We will let you know about the biopsy as soon as the report is back. I would like to reassure you that this is not cancer. But it might develop into cancer if left alone untreated. The treatment of abnormal cells is quite a minor one and if the treatment is done early enough, it almost always leads to a complete cure. But you need to have a smear test every year to check that everything is still fine.

If not all the cells are removed, I am afraid we would do further tests to know the extent of the disease. You might have to have a hysterectomy then. I am sorry about the bad news. I am going to arrange, for you to have a biopsy.

If you have further doubts, don't hesitate to ask. Thank you.

19. Counselling a Patient with Crohn's Disease

Good morning Mr. Tom, I am Dr. Danny, Senior House Officer in the Department of Medicine; I would like to talk to you about your condition.

In view of your symptoms, we had to do some investigations. I am afraid we have diagnosed a condition called Crohn's disease. It is also called inflammatory bowel disease.

I am going to explain it to you. This means that the lining of the bowel is inflamed and that is why you are experiencing these symptoms. The cause for the inflammation is not known. Unfortunately, there is no cure for this condition, but we can definitely offer you treatment to relieve your symptoms.

We are going to start you on some medication. One of them is prednisolone, which will keep the inflammation under control. The other medicines are called sulphasalazine and azathioprine. We will also give you a course of antibiotics called metronidazole, to get rid of any gut infection.

In addition to these drugs, you need to be careful with your diet. The dietician will talk to you as well.

We will monitor your progress regularly by clinic appointments and blood tests. In some chronic and resistant cases, we sometimes advice surgery.

Surgery

This would involve removing the diseased end of the bowel and performing what is known as an ileostomy. This is when the healthy part of the bowel is brought to the outside through a hole in the abdominal wall. This is called a stoma. You will be opening your bowels through the stoma into a bag attached to it. This stoma stays permanently. I can imagine that it sounds horrible, but we have quite a few patients who have a stoma. The stoma nurse will talk to you about it in detail.

There won't be any smell and you can carry on your daily activities normally. I will give you some leaflets about stoma care that you can go through.

That's all, Thank you.

20. Counselling the Relatives of a Patient with Alzheimer's Disease

It is sad to know that your brother is suffering from Alzheimer's disease. This disease is usually progressive with mental function getting steadily worse. Some problems, such as aggression, may improve over time. The rate of change and the length of life vary greatly.

You will need to listen carefully to what advice I will be giving you now.

You should lock up any rooms in the house that are not in use, he will not notice this restriction.

Lock up any drawers, which contain important

papers or easily spoiled items. This will prevent the patient storing inappropriate things in them.

Remove locks for the lavatory, so that the patient cannot get locked in.

His normal sexual relationship will probably stop.

You should psychologically prepare yourself for the day when your brother will no longer recognise you.

21. Counselling Regarding OC Pills

Introduction, I have heard that you are here to discuss about the oral contraceptive pill (OCP). There are two main types of OCP.

1. Combination Oral Contraceptives (COC)

The first type is the combination oral contraceptives (COC): where the tablet contains two hormones, oestrogen and progesterone. This type stops the woman from releasing an egg each month.

Advantages: A very reliable method of contraception with less than 1/100 will get pregnant in a year. It does not interrupt sex, often decreases bleeding, period pain and premenstrual tension. It also protects against cancer of womb and ovaries.

Disadvantages: The most important disadvantages are the risk of vascular diseases as clot in the leg, heart attack, and stroke. That is why it should not be given to women at risk of these diseases. Women with cardiac diseases, liver diseases, some cases of migraine, gross obesity and immobility also abnormal vaginal bleeding. It should be stopped in a smoker at the age of 30 years and should not be used by breastfeeding mothers.

How to take the pills: They should be taken daily for 21 days, and then stopped then for seven days. Taking pills should starts on the first day of cycle (the first day when blood is seen), on the day of termination of pregnancy (TOP), three weeks postpartum (if the mother is not breastfeeding the baby), and two weeks after major surgery (if the patient is immobilised). If the pills are forgotten for more than 12 hours, you should keep taking the pills as usual thereafter, but you should use another type of contraception for seven days. This is also applied in case of diarrhoea where you should use another type of contraception on the day of diarrhoea and for another seven days thereafter. It is also applied in case of taking of drugs known to interfere in the action of combination oral contraceptive pills (COP) like anticonvulsants, and antibiotics.

If you start taking (OCP) you have to come for follow-up every six months to check your BP, and do breast exam (if >35 yrs).

The OCP should be stopped in case of severe headache, severe chest pain, and tummy pain.

2. Progesterone-Only Pills (POP)
The second type is POP (progesterone-only pills): This type contains only the progesterone hormone which causes changes making it difficult for sperm to enter the womb or for womb to accept a fertilised egg, and in some women it prevents the release of eggs.

Advantages: It is a reliable method, with careful use; the failure rate is 1/100 per year. It does not interrupt sex. It is useful for women who smoke and those who cannot take the COP for any cause. Also, it can be taken in breast-feeding mothers.

Disadvantages: It has some side effects like headache, acne, putting on weight. The periods may be irregular with some bleeding in between. And it is less reliable than the (COP).

How to take the pills: The same as the COP, and should be taken at the same time of everyday. If you miss by three hours, you should use another type of contraception for a week and also if you get diarrhoea, use another type of contraception for the period of diarrhoea and for one week thereafter.

Any woman on the OCP should have every six months check of: BP, breast exam, cervical smear.

That's all I have to say about the OC pills to you.

22. Counselling for Colposcopy
Introduction, then you may start as follows: "Now we have had the results of your cervical smear test back and it showed some changes in the lower part of your womb, that is the neck of your womb."

Now we need to do further exam called colposcopy, which is a simple exam that allows the doctor to have a closer look at the changes on the neck of your womb. You will lie comfortably on bed, and the doctor will gently insert a speculum into your vagina just as when you had your cervical smear done. After that the doctor will look by a colposcope that is a specially adapted type of microscope. It is just a large magnifying glass with a light source attached to it. It neigher touches you nor gets inside you. The doctor will then dab liquids onto the neck of your womb, which helps the area with changes to appear white and if any such area appears, then the doctor will take a sample of tissue (which is just a size of pin head). The exam takes about 15 minutes; it should not be painful, may be a bit uncomfortable. You may feel a slight stinging during the tissue sample taking.

After colposcopy, if you have had a biopsy, you may have a light blood stained discharge for a few days, this is nothing to worry about and should clear by itself and it is better to avoid sexual intercourse for five days to allow site to heal.

You will get the results back of your biopsy after one or two weeks, they will tell you about that. If the result showed any condition that needs treatment, the doctor will tell you about the treatment, which is simple, and virtually

100 per cent effective. The treatment is usually carried out with the use of colposcopy and the procedure is similar to your initial exam. There are several ways of treatment, either to apply heat or freeze the area or apply laser. All treatment types aim at destroying the cells with changes. After treatment you may have blood stained discharge for 2 to 4 weeks. During this period, and during your menses you will need to use sanitary towels rather than tampons and it is better to avoid heavy exercise and sexual intercourse to allow the area to heal.

The treatment will have little or no effect on your further fertility, nor on risk of having miscarriages. After treatment you will have a follow-up visit after six months during which you will have a cervical smear and colposcopy exam and if everything is satisfactory-you will have a follow-up smears every year for the following 4 to 5 years.

You are welcome to arrange for a friend or relative to come with you for colposcopy. You may need to bring a sanitary towel with you just in case some discharge appears.

Intercourse does not make the condition worse, enjoy sex as usual but use effective contraception, it is important not to get pregnant until the condition is dealt with. This is because hormones during pregnancy make treatment more difficult. You cannot pass changes or abnormal cells to your partner.

Abnormal smear does not mean cancer, it is very common 1/12, it is just a warning sign and the treatment is simple and virtually 100 per cent effective.

Colposcopy is performed in lithotomy position and liquid used is 5 per cent acetic acid.

23. Counselling for Laparoscopy

Introduction, then you may start by saying: "Now, we have had a good look at your tests that we run. And according to the results of the tests, the examination, and what you complained of, there is a high possibility that you have what we call ectopic pregnancy that is a pregnancy outside your womb. This can be in the tubes between your womb and ovaries as in most cases, or at the ovary or inside the tummy, which is very rare."

And since the pregnancy is not in the usual place, it cannot continue to term. In addition, it may bleed suddenly or even cause damage to the tube, which could cause you some harm.

To avoid these problems, we have first to be sure that you have ectopic pregnancy and the best way to do this is by laparoscope. That is the procedure by which we insert a tube with lenses within a small incision in your tummy, after we put you into sleep. So we could look at your womb and tubes. And to treat the condition, there are two ways. Either by laparoscopy, where we could either, inject a medication called methotrexate or remove the pregnancy by incision. The second way to deal with this condition is by operation to remove the pregnancy. And in either ways of treatment we will try to conserve the tube, but if it is damaged by this condition, then the only way to deal with it, is to remove the tube.

Is everything clear or do you want me to repeat anything for you?

Are there any questions that you would like to ask me?

You will remain for 2 to 3 days in the hospital.

You can return to work after six weeks (sick leave).

24. Counselling for Sexually Transmitted Diseases (STD)

Introduction, then you may say: "I have heard that you are here to discuss about STD. They are infections that can pass from one person to another during sexual contact; anyone can get an STD from an infected partner if no protection has been taken. There are several types of STD:

Some are Common

Genital warts, genital herpes, *Chlamydia*, none specific urethritis, gonococal infection.

Less Common

Trichomonas vaginalis, syphilis (the pox), HIV (the virus that causes AIDS), hepatitis B and C, infestations like scabies, and pubic lice (crabs).

Method of Spread

STDs usually spread when an infected blood, semen, or vaginal fluid comes into contact with another person during sex, but some infections can be transmitted by blood or sharing needles such as AIDS or hepatitis. Some of them like none-specific urethritis, gonorrhoea, hepatitis and HIV spread by penetrative sex, some as *Trichomonas vaginalis* by vaginal sex, some as warts, herpes, and syphilis by body contact.

Safe Sex

This can be achieved by preventing the infected persons' blood, semen, or vaginal fluid from getting inside their partner's body. This can be done by use of male or female condom, which can even protect from AIDS. When using condom, be sure if you want to use a lubricant to use water-based ones as KY jelly or boots lubricant jelly. And do not use oil-based lubricants such as Vaseline. For anal sex use stronger condom as Durex, and plenty of water-based lubricant.

- *How do I know if I have an STD?*

There are some features to look for:

1. Unusual thick, cloudy or smelling discharge from vagina.
2. Discharge from penis.
3. Itchy, rash, sores, blisters, or pain in genital area.
4. Pain or burning sensation when passing water.
5. Passing water more than usual with little quantity.
6. Pain during sex.

But remember that an STD can have no feature at all, or features that may not appear for months. Some features may disappear and you may still have the disease, and this could lead to many problems if untreated.

The patient may ask: Where can I go for help?

You can go to Genitourinary Medicine Clinics; they offer free check-up and treatment of an STD. All information is kept strictly confidential; you can go to any clinic anywhere in the country. You will complete a registration form and they will give you a number to retain your anonymity.

A full sexual health check includes:

1. Examination of your genitals and sometimes the lower part of your body, mouth, and skin.
2. Taking swabs, which is a type of cotton bud used to take sample from any secretion or discharge from genitalia.
3. Urine sample for examination.
4. Blood test for syphilis

You also may be offered:

1. HIV test with your consent.
2. Cervical smear in women.
3. Blood test for hepatitis B and C.

It better not to have sex until it is all clear. When you have an STD, it is important to tell your sexual partner so he/she can have a sexual health check-up, too.

25. Counselling a Post-MI Patient for Lifestyle and Medications

Introduction, and then you may say: "You remember that you came a few days ago with sudden chest pain, you are coming along very nicely and you are ready to go home tomorrow. I think it would be a good idea if we have a little chat before going home."

The tests showed that you had heart attack, which is a condition where one of the vessels which supply blood to the heart becomes blocked by a clot. That area is damaged and is replaced by a scar. This process takes from days to weeks and it is better not to put a great strain on the heart at this time. Within 2 to 3 months at most, the hearts of many patients are functioning just about, as well as they were before the attack.

Apart from medication which I'll talk to you about later, there are some points about a little change in your lifestyle:

1. *Diet:* It would be a good idea if you consider reducing your weight and avoid saturated fat, especially high-fat diary products such as butter, fatty meat, palm, coconut oil. You can eat more fresh fruit and vegetables, chicken (without skin), fish, skimmed, and semiskimmed milk, grill, don't fry.

2. *Exercise:* You can start exercise gently and increase it with time. Try to avoid walking in cold winds and climbing up steep hills. About sports you can take up with golf, cycling, swimming, beside walking; but avoid sports with vigorous exercise as squash and weightlifting.

3. *Smoking:* You should give up smoking as it increases risk of recurrent attacks.

4. *Alcohol:* One or two glasses of wine or ½-1 pint of beer/ one measure of spirit don't affect the heart but more than this may give harm to the heart.

5. *Sexual intercourse:* It increases the work of the heart and in some people causes chest pain or shortness of breath. But in majority of cases, sexual activity can be resumed as soon as you are able to take other forms of moderate exercise as walking up stairs without symptoms. The glyceryl trinitrate (GTN) tablet before intercourse, can help but you should give up immediately if you get chest pain.

6. *Driving:* You can start after four weeks and it is better if you try short runs in the neighbourhood accompanied by a friend. Inform your driving license authority.

7. *Work:* You can go back to work in 4 to 12 weeks depending on the type of work.

8. *Stress:* It would be a good idea if you take up relaxation therapy and avoid stressful condition as much as you can.

9. *Travel:* Avoid air travel for at least six weeks.

Take the beta-blocker bottle and show it to the patient: This is propranolol. It prevents chest pain. You should take one tablet every six hours for the first 2 days, and 2 tablets twice a day afterwards. Swallow the tablet with a glass of water. It is a long-term treatment (usually for 2 to 3 years). Please do not stop taking this medication suddenly. Because this may cause the pain to worsen and will affect your condition. This medication sometimes causes side effects in some people. If you get any of the following symptoms, tell your doctor immediately: headache, sleepiness, bad dreams, dizziness, light headedness, shortness of breath, wheeze, slow pulse, skin rash, dry eye, tiredness, cold hands and feet.

Show the patient the bottle of Aspirin: This is Aspirin, you should take it once a day with a glass of water, sometimes causes irritation of stomach, and to prevent this it should be taken after meal (on full stomach). This is a long-term treatment. This drug prevents blockage of the blood vessels of the heart, which may result in another heart attack. The side effects are mainly stomach irritation, it might cause tummy pain, blackish discolouration of stool, shortness of breath and wheeze. If you notice any of these features, or if you notice any bleeding, contact your doctor immediately.

Show the patient the bottle of glyceryl trinitrate (GTN): This is GTN, you should take it if you have chest pain, or you can take it before exercise, it will increase your exercise limit. Put one tablet under your tongue and wait till it dissolves in your mouth. Don't swallow it. The possible side effects include headache, flushing, dizziness, especially when you get up suddenly (postural hypotension). These side effects are usually short term. If you notice any of these, consult your doctor. I would like to assure you that it is not habit forming or addictive,and it has a very short expiry date.

26. Counselling for Peak Flow Meter Usage

Peak flow meter is the instrument used to monitor the progress or response to treatment. PEFR is the maximal speed in L/min which a patient can blow air out of his lung. It changes with sex, age, height, and time of the day (lowest in the morning in asthmatics).

Introduction, then you may say: "Now I would like to examine your lung function. You should stand up in order to breathe more easily. This instrument is called Peak flow meter; you should put your mouth here around mouthpiece. And catch the instrument from the side to allow the marker to slide freely. Then blow or breathe out into it sharply. This will cause the marker to fly up and show me the result which we call PEFR. Please breathe out into it as hard as you can."

(After the patient breathes). Thank you, one more time please.

(After breathing for second time). Thank you and for the last time.

(After breathing for the third time) Thank you.

We take the result and plot it on the chart. There are two types of charts, one for men and another for women. Each has the horizontal axis showing height, and left vertical showing PEFR. The graph in the middle shows the age.

Remind the patient of important clues:
1. You must hold it horizontally.
2. You must take a deep breath.
3. There are charts for two weeks, and one month.
4. Ask the patient to repeat the reading in the

morning and evening for two weeks at home.

27. Counselling in Stillbirth

Introduction, then you may say: "How do you feel in yourself now? I understand that it is not easy to come to terms with."

Do you want to see your baby, hold or take a photograph with him? You can even take a lock of hair or palm print, if you want.

You can name him, and for funeral you can make it a private one if you want, or the hospital can arrange a funeral for him.

I want to take a blood sample from you, also to take a swab from vagina, blood from the baby and send it for examination that would help us to know the cause of what has happened.

It would be so useful for us to know the cause of what has happened and to arrange for future pregnancy if we can send him to post-mortem examination, that is an operation-like examination. This may help avoiding such condition in the future.

If she refuses, then ask her for permission to take a type of X-ray (MRI) and a sample of tissue for examination.

I'm going to give you a medication to decrease breast milk secretion. You need to use it, one tablet today, then two tablets daily for two weeks and we will give you an appointment to discuss future plans when the results of these tests come back.

We will give you a certificate of stillbirth that you need to take it to the registrar of birth and death within 42 days.

I will give you the address of the local branch of bereavement counselling which might be useful for you.

It is preferable not to get pregnant in the next six months to one year.

EXAMINATION

Most of you would have had to do clinical examination at different stages through medical school and all of you will have had to pass them in the final year. The purpose is to test your ability to carry out a physical examination of a system or a sub-system. There are a few differences, however, between this exam and your final exam. At each patient, you will have the same task, the same time limit, the same patient, the same examiner and the same marksheet. This makes it a much fairer teat than the traditional format. The other difference is that you will mostly see a 'patient', who is usually an actor who has been trained to display the same signs to each candidate.

1. EXAMINATION OF THE RESPIRATORY SYSTEM

Environment
- *Table:* inhalers, cigarettes.
- Ventilator, O_2 mask, nasal tube.
- Sputum cup.
- Pneumatic boots (PE risk).

General Appearance
- Ask the patient to sit over edge of bed, if well enough.
- Colours.
- Cyanotic.
- Pink (emphysema, CO_2 toxicity).
- White (anaemia).
- Jaundiced (lung CA metastatic to liver).
- Dyspnoea, wheeze, difficulties.
- Breathing rate [normal: 14 breaths/min].
- Using accessory muscles of respiration.
- Oedema.
- Cough type.
- Thyroxicosis (goitre impinging on trachea).

Nose, Sinuses
- Deviated septum (nasal obstruction).
- Nasal polyps (asthma).
- Swollen turbinates (allergies).
- Palpate sinuses for tenderness (sinusitis).

Cough, Sputum
- Productive cough (typical pneumonia, bronchiectasis, chronic bronchitis).
- Dry cough (ACEi, asthma, atypical pneumonia, bronchial CA).
- Bovine cough [lacks initial hard sound] (paralysed vocal cords).
- *Sputum:* colour, amount, consistency, blood, purulence.
- Red jelly sputum (*Klebsiella*).
- Rusty sputum (*Strep pneumonia*).

Trachea
- Doctor's middle finger on sternal notch.
- Keeping middle finger on notch, put index on one side, then ring on other side.
- Assess deviation (enlarged thyroid, intrathoracic disease).
- If deviated, focus ensuing chest exam to upper lobe problem.

Chest

Chest: Inspection
- Ask the patient to undress to waist.
- Chest shape.
- Barrel chest (emphysema).
- Pigeon chest aka pectus carinatum (rickets).
- Funnel chest aka pecus excavatum (congenital defect).
- Harrison's sulcus [depression above costal margin] (rickets, childhood asthma).
- Asymmetry during respiration.
- *Spine curvature:* kyphosis, scoliosis, lordosis, kyphoscliosis (polio, Marfan's).
- Chest drains.
- Scars.
- Radiotherapy marks.
- Veins (SVC obstruction).
- Local swellings. If on breast, See *Breast Examination.*

Chest: Palpation
- Ask the patient if any part tender: examine that last.
- Ribs (fracture).

Chest: Palpation: Expansion
- The patient leans forward, crossing arms to get scapula out of the way for palpation, percussion, auscultation of back.
- The patient lets his breath all the way out.
- Doctor places palms on the patient's back, thumbs together.
- The patient breathes all the way in.
- Doctor records how far thumbs have spread, and whether one thumb moved less than the other.
- Usual expansion is 4 cm.
- Alternatively: use a measuring tape.

Chest Palpation: Vocal Fremitus
Vocal fremitus (consolidation):
- Ulnar edge of doctor's pronated, flattened hand slips into upper intercostal space.
- The patient says "99."
- Doctor's hand moves to opposite side, and repeat down intercostal spaces.
- Listening for a change in sensation (consolidation).

Chest: Percussion
- Percuss by comparing left to right each time as move from top to bottom of lung.
- Supraclavicular region.
- Back.
- Tidal percussion (diaphragm paralysis).
DDx:
- *Dull:* solid (liver, consolidated lung).
- *Stony dull [very dull]:* fluid (pleural effusion).
- *Hyper-resonant:* hollow (pneumothrorax, bowel).

Chest: Auscultation
- Have the patient cross arms. Ask to "breath in

and out, through your mouth, on your own time."
- Breath sounds.
- Adventitious sounds.

Chest: Auscultation: Resonance
- The patient says "99" each time the doctor listens to each part of chest
- Clearly heard aegophony speech [bleating goat] means consolidation.
- Muffled is normal.
If aegophony, assess "whispering pectoriloquy":
- The patient whispers "1, 2, 3, 4."
- See if you can hear the whisper clearly with stethoscope (extreme consolidation).

Nails
- Nicotine stains.
- CLUBBING (Lung disease: hypoxia, lung cancer, bronchiectasis, CF).
- Emphysema, chronic bronchitis **don't** cause clubbing.
- Leuconychia (hypoalbuminism 2° to cirrhosis).
- Muehrke's lines (hypoalbuminism 2° to cirrhosis).

Hands
- Peripheral cyanosis.
- *CO_2 flapping tremor (CO_2 retention):*
  - The patient does a policeman "stop" position with both hands.
  - Unlike liver flap, both hands go down at once.
- HPO (lung CA).
- Erythema (CO_2).
- Tremor (asthma inhaler).
- Veins (CO_2).
- *Muscle wasting of hands:* Inspect, then ask the patient to adduct/abduct against doctor's resistance (brachial plexus palsy 2° to lung CA).

- Pallor of palmar creases (anaemia 2° to blood loss).
- *Pulse:* rate (asthma has tachycardia), rhythm, character, pulses paradoxus (severe asthma).

Arms
- Blood pressure, if relevant.

Eyes
- *Horner's syndrome* (lung CA in apex):
  - Ptosis.
  - *Miosis:* partially constricted, but reacts normally to light.
  - *Anhydrosis:* Doctor's back of finger over each eyebrow to compare sweating.
- [tear that doesn't drop] (CO_2 retention).
- *Eye fundus:* papilloedema
- *Conjunctiva:* pale (anaemia).

Mouth, Voice
- *Lips blue:* (peripheral cyanosis).
- Pursed lips breathing (emphysema, not chronic bronchitis).
- *Teeth:* Nicotine stains.
- *Teeth:* Broken, rotten (pneumonia or lung abscess).
- *Tonsils:* Tonsils inflamed (upper RTI).
- *Pharynx:* Reddened (upper RTI).
- *Tongue:* Leucoplakia (smoking, spirits, sepsis, syphilis, sore).
- Under tongue (central cyanosis).
- *Voice:* Hoarseness (recurrent laryngeal nerve).
- *Voice:* Stridor (upper airway obstruction).

Neck
- Expose the patient's chest and neck, covering women's breasts with loose material.
- Hypertrophied accessory muscles of inspiration.
- Obese neck with receding chin (obstructive sleep apnoea).

- Signs of tracheostomy, other surgeries.
- Goitre (trachea impingement).
- Lymph nodes.

JVP
- Landmark is sternal notch to heads of SCM to earlobe.
- Anything > 3 cm is significant.

Anterior Chest
- Palpate apex beat for presence, deviation.
- Pemberton's sign (SVC obstruction):
  - The patient raises arms over head.
  - The patient develops facial plethora, non-pulsatile JVP elevation and inspiratory stridor.

Heart
- The patient at 45°.
- Have a quick listen to heart.

Abdomen
- Abdominal breathing: more than normal.
- Palpate liver if RHF.

Legs
- Peripheral cyanosis.
- Ankle swelling (DVT, so PE risk).

2. EXAMINATION OF CARDIOVASCULAR SYSTEM

Environment
- ECG leads, machine.
- Support hosiery.

General Appearance

- *Colours*
  - Cyanotic.
  - Pallor (anaemia).
  - Jaundiced.
  - Hyperpigmented (hemochromatosis cardiomyopathy, Addisonian hypotension).

- Weight loss.
- Glaring breathing problems.
- *Syndromes:* Down's, Marfan's, Turner's.
- Leg hanging over edge of bed: peripheral vascular dz.

Nails
- Ask the patient to sit at 45°.
- Clubbing, stage 1 to 5 (cyanotic heart disease, IE).
- Splinter haemorrhages (IE).

Hands
- Peripheral cyanosis.
- Arachnodactyly (Marfan's).
- Pallor of palmar creases (anaemia 2° to blood loss, malabsorption).
- Osler's nodes [0.5 to 1 cm red-brown painful subcutaneous papules on fingertips, palmar eminences] (IE).
- Janeway's lesions [rare, painless flat erythematous macules on thenar and hypothenar eminences] (IE).
- *Wrist:* Tendon xanthoma [yellow deposit over extensors] (type II hyperlipidemia).
- Heat (thyrotoxicosis).
- Tremor (thyrotoxicosis).
- *Pulse:* Rate, rhythm, character, radiofemoral delay, radioradial inequality. Say "character, volume better assessed at the carotid". (See APPENDIX for PULSE)
- *If suspect AR, assess 'water hammer pulse':*

Arms
- Take blood pressure.
- IV drug injection scars (IE).
- Optionally raise arm to see if less circulation.

Face

- *Facies*
  - Apprehension, pain (angina, MI, PE, etc).
  - Cushing's (HTN).

- Acromegaly (CHF, HTN).
- Paget's (high-output failure).
- Malar flush [thin face, purple cheeks] (mitral stenosis).
- Earlobes (cyanosis).

Eyes
- Xanthelasma [yellow plaque periobital deposits] (hypercholestolaemia, DM).
- Lid oedema (myxoedema, SVC syndrome, nephrotic syndrome, etc).
- Exophthalmos, lid retraction (thyrotoxicosis).
- Corneal arcus (severe hypercholesterolemia).
- Blue sclera (Marfan's, Ehlers-Danlos's [AR, ASD, MVP]).
- Subluxated lenses (superior: Marfan's, inferior: homocystenuria).
- Argyll Robertson pupil (syphilis).
- *Ophthalmoscope fundi:*
  - Roth's spots [small red haemorrhage with pale centre, due to vasculitis] (endocarditis).
  - Hypertensive changes.

Mouth
- *Lips:* Central cyanosis.
- *Tongue underside:* Central cyanosis.
- Tongue enlargement (amyloidosis).
- High-arch palate (Marfan's).
- *Breathing:* Dyspnoea + wheezing (asthma, COPD, asthma, LV failure).
- *Breathing:* Cheyne-Stokes breathing (stroke, CHF, sedation, uremia).

Neck
- Tell the patient to remove shirt now or during chest exam. Cover women's breasts with loose material.
- Using accessory muscles of respiration (pulmonary oedema, asthma, fulminant pneumonia, COPD).
- *Carotid:* Inspect for carotid pulsations.
- *Carotid:* Compress one carotid at a time [fingers behind neck, thumb at or below cricoid

cartilage level. Optionally use just L thumb to assess R carotid—some teachers disapprove but carotid pulse outweighs thumb].

Assess:
- Amplitude.
- Contour of pulse.
- Variations in amplitude.
- *Carotid: auscultate bruit:*
  - Use bell of stethoscope.
  - Tell the patient to hold his breath while the doctor listens.

JVP
- The patient must be at 45°. The patient's head tilted upwards and facing slightly away from the doctor.
- Use the internal jugular, not external jugular. External jugular is lateral to SCM and easier to see. Internal jugular is medial/behind the clavicular head of SCM.
- Shine a torch [light] on internal jugular vein at an oblique angle.
- Extend torch out horizontally from the highest point of JVP pulsations, use ruler to measure vertical height from sternal notch to torch.
- Height > 3 cm above sternal angle is pathologic (raised ventricular filling pressure or volume overload often from RHF).
- In normal person, usually can't see the JVP when the point is at 45°, but can see when the patient is at 90°.
- *Optionally:* auscultate heart or feel carotid pulse to help identify JVP by its complex waveform.
- Test for Kussmaul's and hepatojugular reflux if required—See APPENDIX.

Chest: Inspection
- Scars, including mitral valvotomy laterally on L breast.
- Deformities.
- Visible pulsations.
- Apex beat.

Chest

Chest: Palpation
- Ask the patient if any part is tender, examine that last.
- Pacemaker boxes.
- Apex—see APPENDIX for abnormalities of apex.

Normal landmark
- Palpate sternal angle [angle of Louie], which is 2nd rib.
- Space below is 2nd intercostal space.
- Count down to 5th intercostal.
- 1 cm medial to midclavicular line.

Palpating deviation
- The doctor makes a claw.
- Put middle finger in 5th intercostal space on lateral ribcage.
- Place rest of the hands' fingers in spaces above and below.
- Move claw around medially, finding the apex beat.
- *Parasternal impulse:*
  - Heel of the doctor's hand to L of sternum.
  - If RV, LA dilated, heel will lift on systole.
- *Thrills and heaves:*
  - The doctor's hand horizontal under L pectoral, then vertical up medial side R pectoral, then horizontal across centre of ribcage, below sternal notch.
- *Diastolic thrill:* doesn't coincide with apex beat.
- *Systolic thrill:* coincides with apex beat.
- Pulmonary component of S2.

Chest: Auscultation
- Heart sounds, 1st, 2nd split.
- Murmurs.
- Time according to carotid pulse (atrial fibrillation: not all apex beats become pulses).
- Dynamic auscultation.

- If systolic murmur, do Valsava manoeuvre (hypertrophic cardiomyopathy).
- If mitral stenosis, hear thrill by rolling the patient onto the patient's L side [brings apex closer to chest wall].
- *Heart sounds:*
  Auscultation sites
  - **A**ortic: 2nd right intercostal space.
  - **P**ulmonary: 2nd left intercostal space.
  - **T**ricuspid: 4th intercostal space, at lower left sternal border.
  - **M**itral: 5th left intercostal space, 1 cm medial to midclavicular line.
  Auscultation order
  - Mitral: bell.
  - Mitral diaphragm.
  - Tricuspid.
  - Aortic.
  - Pulmonary.
  - See APPENDIX for heart sounds and their abnormalities.

Back
- The patient leans forward.
- Inspect for deformities (ankylosing spondylitis, with AR).
- Percuss back (exclude an RVF pleural effusion).
- Palpate sacral oedema.

Abdomen
- *Liver:* Find, examine edge.
- *Liver:* Pulsatile liver (tricuspid regurgitation).
- Splenomegaly (endocarditis).
- AAA.

Legs
- *Inspect:* oedema.
- *Inspect:* peripheral vascular dz.
- May also see marks of the patient squeezing thigh to increase perfusion.
- Femoral pulse.
- Varicose veins.
- Ulcers.

Feet
- Rest of peripheral pulses.
- Achilles tendon xanthomata.
- Same signs as *Hands* and *Fingernails*.

3. EXAMINATION OF THE NERVOUS SYSTEM

Environment
- *Bed:* One side rail raised (hemiplegia).
- *Bed:* The patient's bad eye side placed against wall so they can't be surprised (stroke).
- *Bed:* Soft mattress to avoid pressure sores (mobility difficulty).
- *Bed:* V-shaped posture pillows since the patients are unable to support self.
- *Tables:* all medications, etc. within reach of non-side railed arm (hemiplegia).
- *Room:* hoist, wheelchair, walker (paralysis).
- *Room:* NG tube (palsy of throat CN's).
- *Room:* ventilator, life support machines.

General Appearance
- Age of the patient (Parkinson's usually 45+, etc).
- Chorea (Huntington's, rheumatic fever, drugs, etc).
- Ethnicity (Scandinavian: multiple sclerosis).
- Ballismus, dystonia (usually drugs), noticeable tremor.
- *Posture:* leaning to one side (hemiplegia).
- *Posture:* stooped forward (Parkinson's).
- Only using one hand on tray (hemiplegia).

Handedness, Speech
- Ask to shake hand, ask if R or L-handed.
- Ask name, present location, how long in hospital.
- See APPENDIX for speech disorders.

Head
- Asymmetry, unilateral facial drooping (stroke).

- Ptosis.
- Serpentine stare (Parkinson's).
- Licking of lips.
- Scars of previous operations.
- Trauma, injury, abnormalities.
- Mental retardation syndrome facies: Down's, etc.
- *Eyes:* exophthalamos (thyroxicosis), Kayser-Fleisher rings (Wilson's).

Neck, Neck Stiffness

- *Neck:* thymectomy scar (MG).
- *Neck:* thyroidectomy scar (thyrotoxicosis).
- Beware of performing manipulation on a cervical spine injury patient.
- Hand under occiput, flex neck to chin and see for resistance.
- *Resistance causes:* raised ICP, cervical fusion or spondylosis, Parkinson's, meningitis.
- If suspect meningitis (fever, photophobia) do Kernig's sign.

Cranial Nerves

- See *later*

Upper Limbs

Upper Limbs: Inspect

- The patient sits over side of bed facing you.
- For rest of examination, comparing L side to R side.
- Asymmetry.
- *Deformities:* wrist drop, waiter's tip, claw hand.
- Muscle wasting, fasciculations. Include shoulder girdle.
- *Tremor:*
  - Intention (cerebellar).
  - Resting with pill-rolling (Parkinson's).
  - Action tremor (**BAT: B**enign essential tremor syndrome, **A**nxiety, **T**hyrotoxicosis).

- Feel hand for heat (thyrotoxicosis), grip.
- *Pronator drift:* The patient's eyes closed, arms extended, with palms up. Tap patient's arms briskly downward (arm drifting into pronation: UMNL, cerebellar, post. column loss).
- Pseudoathetosis from proprioceptive loss.
- Muscle bulk, tenderness.

Upper Limbs: Tone

- Ask patient if any tenderness in any joints, so won't hurt them when manipulating them for tone.
- Grasp under elbow and wrist, and rotate the 2 joints to assess resistance:
  - If Parkinson's, cogwheel rigidity in wrist [combination of tremor and increased tone].
  - If Parkinson's, lead pipe resistance when flexing forearm.
- If ulnar nerve indicated, Froment's sign:
  - Give the patient a piece of paper for each hand.
  - Ask the patient to grasp papers by moving straightened thumb to radial side of index finger.
  - Affected thumb is forced to flex at interphalangeal joint to grip paper.
  - If median nerve indicated, pen touching test:
    - The patient's hand supine.
    - The doctor hold's pen above thumb
    - Ask the patient to lift thumb to touch it.
    - Affected thumb can't touch pen.

Upper Limbs: Power

- Assess shoulder, elbow, wrist, fingers:
  - Assess by ability to push against doctor's hand.
  - Assess across a single joint at a time [e.g.: doctor's hand on bicep, not forearm, to assess shoulder power].
- If MG suspected:
  - The patient holds arms above head.
  - An MG patient will lose power after contractions.

- 0: No movement
  1: Twitch
  2: Movement, but not against gravity
  3: Movement against gravity, but not resistance
  4: Movement against resistance, but not entirely normal
  5: Normal

Upper Limbs: Reflexes

- Supinator/Brachioradialis (C5-6).
- Biceps (C5-6).
- Triceps (C7-8).
- Fingers (C7-T1).

Upper Limbs: Coordination

- The patient's finger touches the doctor's fingers, then to the patient's nose.
- Dysdiadochokinesia:
  - The patient's palm on dorsum of their opposite hand.
  - The patient's flips their hand quickly so the two hand dorsums touch.
  - Repeat quickly.

Upper Limbs: Sensory

- Dorsal columns (vibration):
  - Place on sternum [the last area lost] so the patient knows how the buzzing feels.
  - The patient's eyes shut and 128 Hz fork on distal interphalangeal joint: ask if felt.
  - If can feel, ask the patient to say when it stops, then later stop it.
  - If deficient, assess dermatomes at wrist, elbow, shoulder, both anterior and posterior.
- Dorsal columns (proprioception):
  - Grasp the patient's distal phalanx, move up and down to show what to do.
  - Tell the patient to close eyes and repeat this, saying whether it's up or down.
- *Spinothalamic (pain, forget temperature):*
  - Sterile toothpick or broken wood tongue depressor on forehead or anterior chest.
  - The patient closes eyes, tells if sharp or dull.

- Stick each dermatome looking for cord, dermatome, peripheral nerve, stocking glove.
- *Light touch:* Cotton wool. Dab skin lightly, don't stroke.
- If lesion, feel for thickened nerves:
  - Ulnar at elbow
  - Median at wrist
  - Radial at wrist
  - Axilla.

Lower Limbs

Lower Limbs: Inspect

- Asymmetry.
- Muscle wasting, fasciculation's, tremor.
- Muscle bulk: quads, anterior tibials.
- Foot bruising, infections from peripheral neuropathy.

Lower Limbs: Tone

- Orthopods may roll legs for a quick preliminary inspection of tone.
- Tone of knees, ankles.
- Test clonus by pushing lower end of quads sharply down towards knee (sustained contractions: UMNL).

Lower Limbs: Power

- *Power:* hips, knees, ankles. "Lift leg, don't let me push it down." "Push leg down, don't let me push it up."

Lower Limbs: Reflexes

- Knee (L3-4).
- Ankles (S1-2).
- Plantar (L5, S1-2).
- Ankle clonus test:
  - Place the patient's knee bent, thigh externally rotated.
  - The doctor lifts The patient's heel in The doctor's cupped hand.
  - The doctor quickly dorsiflexes The patient's ankle and holds it flexed for 3 seconds.
  - Clonus if sustained movement afterwards.

Lower Limbs: Coordination

- Heel-shin test:
  - The patient kicks a heel out, then touches that heel to other shin.
  - Repeat in a smooth motion loop.
  - Alternatively: heel sliding up and down on opposite shin.
- Toe-touching test.
- Tapping of feet.

Lower Limbs: Gait

- Walk a few feet, then walk back.
- *Notice signature gaits:*
  - Trendelenburg gait (proximal myopathy).
  - Shuffling gait (Parkinson's).
  - High-stepping gait (foot drop).
  - Hemiplegic gait [swinging one leg in lateral arc] (usually stroke).
- Walk heel to toe (hard: midline cerebellar).
- Walk on heels (hard: L4-5 foot drop).
- Squat or sit then stand up (proximal myotrophy).
- Romberg sign positive if unsteadiness is worse when eyes closed.

Lower Limbs: Sensory

- Sensory pin prick, vibration, proprioception, light touch. Same as was for *Upper Limbs*.
- If peripheral sensory loss, try to establish sensory level.
- Examine sensation in saddle region.
- Test anal reflex (S2-4).
- See APPENDIX for dermatomal references.

Spine

- Back: deformity, scars, neurofibromas.
- Palpate for tenderness over vertebral bodies.
- Straight leg raising test:
  - The patient tries to lift straight leg.
  - Full lifting will be prevented if slipped disc.

Carotid Bruit

- Auscultate for bruits (atherosclerotic disease).

Aspiration

- Paralysed pt may have aspirated fluid.
- Feeding assistance devices, such as PEG (dysphagia, usually 2° to neurological damage, like stroke).

4. EXAMINATION OF CRANIAL NERVES (CN)

Setup

- The patient sitting over edge of bed.

Cranial Nerves (CN)

CN I: Olfactory

- Usually not tested.
- Rash, deformity of nose.
- Test each nostril with essence bottles of coffee, vanilla, peppermint.

CN II: Optic

- With the patient wearing glasses, test each eye separately on eye chart/card using an eye cover.
- Examine visual fields by confrontation by wiggling fingers 1 foot from the patient's ears, asking which they see move.
- Keep examiner's head level with the patient's head.
- If poor visual acuity, map fields using fingers and a quadrant-covering card.
- Look into fundi.

CN III, IV, VI: Oculomotor, Trochlear, Abducens

- Look at pupils: shape, relative size, ptosis.
- Shine light in from the side to gauge pupil's light reaction.
- *Assess*
  - Assess both direct and consensual responses.
  - Assess afferent pupillary defect by moving light in arc from pupil to pupil. Optionally: as do arc test, have the patient place a flat

hand extending vertically from his face, between his eyes, to act as a blinder, so light can only go into one eye at a time.

- "Follow finger with eyes without moving head": test the 6 cardinal points in an H pattern.
  - Look for failure of movement, nystagmus [pause to check it during upward/ lateral gaze].
- Convergence by moving finger towards bridge of the patient's nose.
- Test accommodation by the patient looking into distance, then a hat pin 30 cm from nose.
- If an MG suspected: the patient gazes upward at The doctor's finger to show worsening ptosis.

CN V: Trigeminal

- Corneal reflex: The patient looks up and away.
  - Touch cotton wool to other side.
  - Look for blink in both eyes, ask if can sense it.
  - Repeat other side [tests V sensory, VII motor].
- Facial sensation: Sterile sharp item on forehead, cheek, jaw.
  - Repeat with dull object. Ask to report sharp or dull.
  - If abnormal, then temperature (heated/ water-cooled tuning fork), light touch (cotton).
- *Motor:* The patient opens mouth, clenches teeth (pterygoids).
  - Palpate temporal, masseter muscles as they clench.
  - Test jaw jerk (pseudobulbar palsy).

CN VII: Facial

- Inspect facial droop or asymmetry.
- If indicated, look at external auditory canals, eardrums.

CN IX, X: Glossopharyngeal, Vagus

- *Voice:* hoarse or nasal.

- The patient swallows, coughs (bovine cough: recurrent laryngeal).
- Examine palate for uvular displacement. (unilateral lesion: uvula drawn to normal side).
- The patient says "Ah": symmetrical soft palate movement.
- Gag reflex [sensory IX, motor X]:
  - Stimulate back of throat each side.
  - Normal to gag each time.

CN XI: Accessory

- From behind, examine for trapezius atrophy, asymmetry.
- The patient shrugs shoulders (trapezius).
- The patient turns head against resistance: watch, palpate SCM on opposite side.

CN XII: Hypoglossal

- Listen to articulation.
- Inspect tongue in mouth for wasting, fasciculation's.
- Protrude tongue: unilateral deviates to affected side.

5. DEEP TENDON REFLEXES

General Considerations
- Always compare one side to the other.
- Let hammer fall by gravity in most cases.
- Don't keep hammering a patient, if can't elicit it.

Upper Limb Reflexes

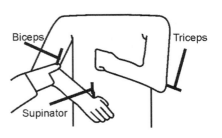

Fig. 22.1: Upper limb reflexes

Supinator/Brachioradialis (C5-6)
- The patient's elbow at 90°, relaxed.
- Hand pronated and resting on pelvis.
- Hammer falls on distal end of radius.

Biceps (C5-6)
- The patient's elbow still at 90°, relaxed.
- The doctor's finger over biceps tendon.
- Hammer falls on doctor's finger.

Triceps (C7-8)
- The patient's arm crossed over, onto chest.
- Hammer swings into triceps tendon.

Fingers (C7-T1)
- The patient's hand palm up, fingers very slightly flexed.
- The doctor's finger pads overlie The patient's finger pads.
- Hammer taps doctor's fingers.

Knees (L3-4)
- If supine, the doctor lifts both knees with 1 arm, flexing legs slightly.
- Hammer falls on patellar tendon.

Lower Limb Reflexes

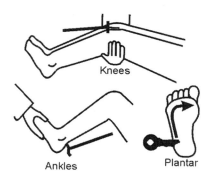

Fig. 22.2: Lower limb reflexes

Ankles (S1-2)
- Need ankle and knee joints both now at 90°

angle, abducted and externally rotated. Two options of doing this:
- The patient's lateral side of heel lies overtop opposite shin. Tell pt: "Place your heel on your opposite shin."
- Tap Achilles tendon.

Plantar (L5, S1-2)
- Tell the patient about what to do.
- Use key to stroke from heel, up lateral sole, then medially across to ball of foot.
- See if big toe goes up (UMNL) instead of its normal down.
- Alternatively: try with a fingernail first, before the key, so less pain to the patient.

Increasing a Reflex
If can't elicit a reflex, can increase its visibility via any of three methods:
1. Clenching teeth.
2. Jendrassik's manoeuvre:
   - The patient clasps hands together tightly.
   - The patient releases hands just before tap hammer.
3. Gripping an object.

Obviously, teeth clenching is the only appropriate one while testing upper limbs.

6. MINI MENTAL STATE EXAMINATION
Points are in square brackets. Maximum score is 30.

Orientation
- Knowledge of time [1 each]:
  - Date
  - Day
  - Season
  - Year
  - Month

- Knowledge of location [1 each]:
  - Country
  - State/Province
  - Town
  - Hospital
  - Ward

Registration
- The doctor says three objects.
- The patient repeats them [1 each correct].
- Note number of trials needed.

Attention and Calculation
- Count backwards from 100 by 7's [1 each for 1st 5 correct].
- Alternatively: spell WORLD backwards [1 each correct].

Recall
- The patient recalls the names of items in Registration [1 each correct].

Language
- The patient names two shown objects [2].
- Pt repeats statement: "No ifs, ands or buts" [1]
- The patient follows command [1 for each step]:
  - Take paper in right hand.
  - Fold in half.
  - Put it on table.
- The patient reads the phrase "CLOSE YOUR EYES" and can do it [1].
- The patient reads the phrase "WRITE A SENTENCE" and can do it [1].
- Copy this design (See Figure 22.3) [1 if all angles present and figures intersect].

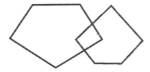

Fig. 22.3

7. EXAMINATION OF THE ABDOMEN

Environment
- NG tube.
- Feeding tube.
- Cans of special food.

General Appearance
- Colours:
  - Anaemic (iron malabsorption, haemorrhage, CA).
  - Jaundiced (liver disease).
  - Hyperpigmented (hemochromatosis).
- Hydration and nutrition.
- Weight loss vs. gain, wasting.
- Shocked.
- Postural hypotension.

Inspection

Abdomen: Inspection
- The patient is supine, abdomen visible from nipples to pubic symphysis.
- Scars.
- Stoma from surgery, trauma.
- PEG (dysphagia, usually 2° to neurological damage, like stroke).
- Distension (**f**at, **fo**etus, **fa**eces, **f**latus, **f**luid, **f**ull-sized tumours).
- Local swellings (enlarged organs, hernia).
- Pulsations (AAA).
- Peristalsis visible (thin person, intestinal obstruction).
- *Skin:*
  - Herpes zoster (abdominal pain).
  - Grey-Turner's sign [discoloured skin] (acute pancreatitis).
- *Striae:*
  - Regular striae (ascitis, pregnancy, weight loss).
  - Purple, wide striae (Cushing's).
- *Dilated veins location:*
  - Anterior leg (IVC block).

- Caput medusae (portal HTN)
- Costal margin (normal).
- Dilated vein flow direction. Test by occluding with fingers:
  - Flows superior (IVC block).
  - Flows inferior (SVC block).
  - Navel radiation (portal HTN).
- *Umbilicus:*
  - Sister Joseph nodule (metastatic tumour).
  - Cullen's "black eye" (acute pancreatitis, extensive hemoperitoneum).
- *Groin:* brown freckles (Peutz-Jeghers).
- Squat to the patient's stomach level, and watch for asymmetrical movement during breathing (mass, large liver).

Palpation

Palpate General Abdominal

- Warm hands.
- Ask the patient if any part tender: examine that last.
- Abdominal muscles relaxed, the patient bends knees if necessary.
- Light palpation.
- Deep palpation.
- Note rigidity, rebound tenderness, involuntary guarding (peritonitis).
- Record mass characteristics.
- Distinguish abdominal wall mass from intra-abdominal mass:
  - The patient folds arms and sits halfway up.
  - Wall mass if size is same, tenderness same or greater.

Palpate Liver

- Find edge:
  - The doctor's R hand held still at base of RLQ, parallel to costal margin.
  - Ask the patient to breathe slowly.
  - During each inspiration, see if liver edge strikes radial edge of index finger.

- During each expiration, The doctor's hand moves superiorly 2 cm.
- Palpate liver surface, edge:
  - Hard vs. soft.
  - Regular vs. irregular.
  - Tender vs. not.
  - Pulsatile (tricuspid incompetence) vs. not.
- Find top border by percussing down R midclavicular line [normal: 5th rib in midclavicular line].
- Calculate span [normal span: 12.5 cm].

Palpate Gallbladder

- The doctor's fingers placed perpendicular to R costal margin near midline, then moved medial to lateral to palpate.
- *Do Murphy's sign:* Cessation of inspiration upon palpation.
  - Murphy's point: costal margin in midclavicular line.
  - Courvoisier's law: **S**tones= **s**tays **s**mall since **s**carred.

Palpate Spleen

- Bimanual technique:
  - The doctor's L hand posterolaterally, below The patient's L ribs, compressing on rib cage.
  - The doctor's R hand below The patient's umbilicus, parallel to L costal margin.
  - Advance R hand superiorly to L costal margin.
  - 1.5x-2x enlarged spleen is palpable.
  - If miss spleen, roll the patient's towards the doctor (so the patient lies on the patient's R side) and repeat palpation.
- *Alternatively:* palpate like liver edge with just R hand, starting from RLQ diagonally over to LUQ.
- *Alternatively:* combine the two methods: start to palpate from RLQ like liver edge with just R hand, but then as get closer, reach with L

hand around to The patient's L ribcage and pull, while continuing advancing with R hand.
- Assess spleen characteristics [these also help differentiate from kidney]:
  - Size
  - Shape, notch vs. no notch.
  - Percussion dullness vs. not.
  - Moves on respiration vs. not.

Palpate Kidneys
- The doctor's L heel of hand slipped under The patient's R loin, L fingers under R back.
- R hand held over RUQ.
- The doctor flexes L MCPs in renal angle.
- The doctor R hand feels strike as kidneys float anteriorly.
- Repeat for the other side.

Auscultation

Auscultate Stomach
- Perform on empty stomach.
- Stethoscope on epigastrium.
- Then shake both iliac crests.
- While shaking, listen to splash from retained fluid.
- Audible splash called "succussion splash" (ulcer or gastric CA).

Palpate Pancreas
- Palpate for a round, fixed, swelling above umbilicus that doesn't move with inspiration (pseudocyst, acute pancreatitis, CA in thin patients).

Palpate Aorta
- Palpate in midline, superior to umbilicus.
- The doctor's two fingers on outer margins of aorta, watch if fingers diverge (AAA).
- Normally felt in thin the patient

Palpate Bowel
- Sigmoid usually palpable in severe constipation.

- Whether indents (feces) or doesn't indent (masses).
- Sometimes can feel CA, megarectum.

Palpate Bladder
- Ask patient when last urinated, and whether was complete emptying..
- Usually palpable if full, usually not palpable if empty.
- Look for palpable, empty bladder (swelling).

Palpate Testes
- Atrophy (liver disease).

Abdomen

Abdomen: Percussion
- Liver border for loss of dullness (necrosis, perforated bowel).
- Spleen for splenomegaly.
- Kidneys.
- Bladder for enlarged bladder, pelvic mass.
- Percuss masses.

Abdomen Percussion: Ascites
- *Shifting dullness:*
  - The doctor's percussing finger placed vertically, so the doctor's finger pointing toward The patient's legs.
  - Starting at midline, percuss laterally to dullness on L flank, and mark site of dullness with non-permanent marker.
  - Roll patient towards doctor's, so the patient now lying on R side.
  - Patient stays lying on R side for 30 min, then repercuss while still lying on R side.
  - Ascites present if the dullness has moved medially (i.e. the point of dullness is now resonant).
  - *Optionally*: percuss laterally on both R and L flanks, and mark both before rolling the patient so can assess them both moving.
- Dipping:
  - Flex MCP joint fast to displace fluid and palpate a mass.

- Fluid thrill:
  - The doctor puts hands on each of the patient's flanks.
  - If patient is obese, the patient places lateral edge of hand vertically on midline at umbilicus.
  - The doctor flicks hand on right flank, by quickly flexing MCPs.
  - Ascites if the doctor feels resulting thrill on left flank.

Abdomen: Auscultation

- Below umbilicus to assess bowel sounds for:
  - Rushing sound called "borborygmi" (diarrhoea).
  - No sound for three minutes (ileus, paralysis).
  - "Tinkling" sound (obstructed bowel).
- Above umbilicus for:
  - AAA bruit.
  - Venus hum [blood flowing in caput medusae] (portal HTN).
- R and L above umbilicus for renal artery stenosis.
- Over liver for:
  - Friction rub [grating during breathing] (peritonitis, Fitz-Hugh-Curtis, others).
  - Bruit (CA, alcoholic hepatitis).
- Over spleen for splenic rub (splenic infarct).

Groin, Hernias, Rectal

- Palpate lymph nodes.
- Check for Hernias
- Do a PR if required.

Nails

- CLUBBING (UC or Crohn's, Biliary cirrhosis, GI malabsorption).
- Koilonychia (iron deficiency 2° to GI bleeding).
- Leuconychia (hypoalbuminism 2° to cirrhosis).
- Muehrke's lines (hypoalbuminism 2° to cirrhosis).

- Blue lunulae (Wilson's).
- Nicotine stains (some GI CA's).

Hands

- Asterixis (PSE 2° to alcoholism):
  - The patient stretches out hands in policeman's stop position, fingers spread out.
  - Coarse flapping tremor, "liver flap", is seen.
- Pallor of palmar creases (anaemia 2° to blood loss, malabsorption).
- Palmar erythema (cirrhosis).
- Dupuytren's contracture [fibrosis, contracture of palm's fascia, usually contracting ring finger] (alcoholism, manual labour).
- Palmar xanthomata [yellow deposists on palm of hand] (Type III hyperlipidemia).
- Tendon xanthomata [yellow deposits on dorsum of hand, arm] (Type II hyperlipidemia).

Arms

- Scratch marks (itch from jaundice).
- Spider naevi (alcoholism).
- Bruising (clotting factors 2° to liver damage).
- Tuboeruptive xanthomata [yellow deposits on elbows, knees] (Type III hyperlipidemia).

Eyes

- Cornea rings (Wilson's).
- *Sclera:* jaundice.
- Iritis: IBD.
- Xanthelasma [yellow plaque periorbital deposits] (elevated cholesterol).

Mouth

- Temporalis muscle wasting.
- *Lips*
  - Telangiectasia (Osler-Weber-Rendu)
  - Brown freckles (Peutz-Jeghers).
- *Breath*
  - Fetor hepaticus (alcoholism).
  - Ethanol.

- *Mouth*
  - Ulcers (Crohn's, coeliac disease).
  - *White Candida* patches (spread down throat).
  - Cracks at mouth edges (iron deficiency anaemia).

- *Teeth*
  - Cavities (acid 2° to vomiting).
  - Nicotine stains.

- *Gums*
  - Hypertrophy.
  - Bleeding.
  - Gingivitis.

- *Tongue*
  - Leucoplakia (smoke, spirits, sepsis, syphilis, sore teeth).
  - Atrophic glossitis [withered tongue] (deficiencies, Plummer-Vinson).
  - Macroglossia (B_{12} deficiency).

Neck, Chest, Back
- Cervical nodes:
  - Supraclavicular nodes for Virchow's node (lung CA, GI malignancy).
- Gynaecomastia (chronic liver disease).
- Hair loss (chronic liver disease).
- Back: neurofibromas.

Legs
- Oedema.
- Bruising.
- Tuboeruptive xanthomata [yellow deposits on elbows, knees] (Type III hyperlipidemia).
- Toenails and foot showing same symptoms as *Fingernails* and *Hands*.

8. EXAMINATION OF THE HAND

Environment, General Appearance
- Check for any rheumatoid features

- For hand examination, place sitting The patient's hands on pillow, palms down.

Nails
- Vasculitic changes [2 cm black lesions, due to local infarction] (RA).
- Splinter haemorrhages (SLE, RA).
- Periungual telangiectases (SLE, scleroderma).
- Pin-sized pitting (psoriatic arthritis).
- Hyperkeratosis [thickening] (psoriatic arthritis).
- Onycholysis [nail separates from distal nail bed] (psoriatic arthritis).
- Discolouration (psoriatic arthritis).
- Ridges (psoriatic arthritis).
- Anaemia.
- Nail folds with magnifying glass: dilated capillary loops (scleroderma).

Fingers
- Move from DIP to MCP, as examine.
- Redness (inflammation).
- Sausage-shaped digits (psoriatic arthritis, sometimes ankylosing spondylitis or Reiter's).
- Nicotine stains (NSAID s/e increased risks).
- Arthritis mutilans [fingers shortened] (advanced destruction).
- Tophi (gout).
- Swan neck deformity (RA).
- Boutonniere's deformity (RA).
- Z deformity of thumb (RA).
- Bouchard nodes [PIP] (OA)
- Heberden's nodes [DIP, 1st MCP] (OA).
- Finger ulnar deviation [MCP] (RA).
- Ulnar nerve deformity (nerve entrapment).
- Contraction deformity of fingers (scleroderma).
- Calcinosis [palpable calcium nodes] (scleroderma).
- Telangiectasia (scleroderma).

Dorsum, Wrist
- Scars.

- Rashes, erythema.
- Skin tightening (scleroderma).
- Muscle wasting on dorsum of hand.
- Ulnar deviation.

Palm
- Scars from operations.
- Erythema.
- Wasting.
- Anaemia.

Forearm
- Subcutaneous nodules at elbow (RA).

Wrist Dorsum: Palpate, Move
- Ask the patient about tender areas.
- The patient's hand is placed palm down.
- Both thumbs of the examiner are placed on the dorsum of the wrist in the midline, fingers under wrists.
- Palpate for synovitis, effusions.
- Palpate ulnar styloid tenderness (RA).
- Dorsiflexion [normal: 75°].
- Palmarflexion [normal: 75°].
- Abduction [normal: 75°].
- Adduction [normal: 75°].

Fingers: Palpate, Move
- Palpate with two thumbs as with *Wrist*
- Nodules (RA).
- Tenderness.
- Warmth.
- Swelling.
- Volar subluxation test:
  - The patient holds hand like showing off an engagement ring.
  - The doctor grips a proximal phalanx between the doctor's thumb and forefinger.
  - The doctor moves an MCP joint back and forth.
  - Normal joints will have little movement.

Palmar Side: Palpate, Move
- *Tinel's sign (carpal tunnel):*

- The doctor taps on the patient's flexor retinaculum.
- *Positive test:* paresthesia over median nerve distribution.
- *Palmar tendon crepitus (tenosynovitis):*
  - The doctor's fingertip pads on the patient's palm.
  - The patient flexes and extends MCPs.
  - Listen for crepitus during motion.
  - Palpate for thickened tendons, nodules.
- *Trigger finger (RA):*
  - Similar to above but flexion is prevented at a point.
  - The patient increases force until it snaps, and continues flexing inward.

Function Tests
- *Grip strength:*
  - The patient's squeezes examiner's fingers.
- *Opposition test:*
  - The patient holds thumb to little finger.
  - Does the patient have difficulty then in moving them apart?
- *Paper grip:*
  - The patient holds piece of paper between thumb and index fingertip pads.
  - While holding, can the patient then open other fingers.
- *Daily activity test:*
  - Writing name with a pen.
  - Grasping a utensil.
- *Wrist flexion test (carpal tunnel):*
  - The patient flexes both wrists for 30 seconds
  - Parasthesia arises in affected hand.

9. BREAST EXAMINATION

General Examination
- *Liver:* For secondary deposits, lungs and bones for metastasis.
- Rectal and vaginal examinations are also necessary to detect Krukenberg's tumour of the ovary.

Setup
- The patient removes upper body clothing, in gown, sitting up.
- Briefly describe examination to the patient
- The patient removes gown.
- The patient relaxes arms by side.

Inspection

Inspect: Whole Breasts
This is carried out in four positions:
- With the arms by the side of the body,
- With the arms raised above the head,
- With the hands on the hips pressing and relaxing
- Bending forward so that the breasts fall away from the body.
  - Symmetry.
  - Swelling.
  - Visible masses.

Inspect: Skin
- Dimpling.
- Peau d'orange (CA).
- Skin retraction.
- Veins: bilateral vs. unilateral (CA).

Inspect: Nipples
- Nipple position, inversion, retraction (fibrosis, CA, normal).
- Red, bleeding (Paget's disease of nipple).
- Discharge.

Inspect: Manoeuvres
- *The patient raises arms above head. Look for:*
  - Change in a mass's relative position.
  - Nipple or skin tethering.
- Examine axillae while the patient's arms are raised.
- *The patient pushes hands down on hips. Look for:*
  - Dimpling.
  - Fixation.

- Large breasts: The patient leans forward, hands on knees.

Palpate: Nodes
- Axillary nodes.
- Supraclavicular nodes.
- See *Hemolymphoid Examination*.
- If exam normal so far, tell the patient

Palpate: Quadrants
- The patient lies down.
- The patient places hands behind head.
- Ask if any part tender before palpate (inflammatory).
- If sores visible, wear gloves.
- Use fingerpads of middle 3 fingers.
- Press breast against chest wall by rolling fingers in small, circular motions.
- Press lightly for superficial layers, medium pressure for middle layer, firmer pressure for deepest layers.
- Start at sternoclavicular junction.
- Move in overlapping vertical strips, until all 4 breast quadrants are covered.

Palpate: Nipples
- Palpate around areola.
- Palpate depression under nipple.
- Gently press nipple between thumb, index finger, noting discharge.

Axillary Tails
- The patient places arms above head.
- Palpate tail between fingers and thumb.

10. EXAMINATION OF LEVEL OF CONSCIOUSNESS
- Press knuckles over sternum to cause pain and assess consciousness.
- Note stage:
  - *Drowsiness:* normal sleepiness, can we roused to wakefulness.
  - *Stupor:* unconsciousness, can be aroused with effort, purposeful pain responses.

- *Light coma:* unconscious with reduced semi-purposeful response.
- *Deep:* no response, no reflex.

Glasgow's Coma Scale

Table 22.1: Glasgow's coma scale

Eye opening	Verbal response	Motor response
4: Spontaneous	5: Oriented	6: Obeys command
3: To command	4: Confused conversation	5: Localises pain
2: To pain	3: Inappropriate words	4: Withdraws from pain
1: None	2: Incomprehensible	3: Abnormal flexion to pain
	1: None	2: Extension response
		1: None

11. EXAMINATION OF THE BACK

Introduction, then you may start: "I am going to examine your back, please get undressed to your underwear, and stand up so that your back is in front of me."

Inspection

With the patient standing, observe from behind for scoliosis, and from the side checking that there is normal lordosis.

Palpation

Palpate with fingers for tenderness on spinous processes and paraspinal muscles. Then perform light percussion with the fist to elicit bone tenderness.

Movement

Ask the patient to extend backward, bend forward with leg straight, then on each side trying to touch side of knee. Then ask the patient to sit on couch and rotate to right and left with fixed hips.

Tests

i. *Straight leg raising test (SLR):* The patient is lying supine. With knee flexed. Check passive hip flexion. With knee extended, raise leg on unaffected side by lifting the heel with right hand while preventing knee flexion with left hand. Repeat this on the affected side asking the patient to report any pain or paraesthesia. (Normal straight leg raising test are 90°). When this limit is reached, now gently dorsiflex the ankle if the patient feels pain, Bragaard test is positive.

ii. *Bow string sign:* Perform SLR test at the limit, flex the knee, reducing tension on the sciatic roots and hamstrings. Now further flex the hip to 90°. Gently extend the knee until pain is once again reproduced (Lasegue's sign). Apply firm pressure with thumb first over the hamstring nearest the examiner, then in the middle of the popliteal fossa and finally over the other hamstring tendon. Ask the patient which manoeuvre exacerbates the pain. The test is positive if the second manoeuvre is painful and if the resultant pain radiates from the knee to the back.

iii. *Sitting test:* Ask the patient to sit up from the lying position, ostensibly to inspect the back. Only in the absence of sciatic nerve irritation will the patient be able to sit up straight with legs flat on the bed.

iv. *Flip test:* Ask the patient to sit with hips and knees flexed to 90° on the edge of the couch and test the knee reflexes. Then extend the knee, ostensibly to examine the ankle jerk. When there is genuine root irritation, the patient will flip backwards to relieve the tension. The malingerer, distracted by attention to the ankle jerk test, may permit full extension of the knee, which is the equivalent of full 90° SLR.

v. *Femoral stretch test:* Ask the patient to lie prone, or on the unaffected side if there is a painful flexion deformity of hip. Flex the knee slowly asking the patient to report onset of pain. If this fails to produce pain, gently extend the hip with the knee still flexed. The accompanying neurological deficit is in femoral roots compression: numbness on anteromedial aspect of the thigh and weakness of knee jerk.

Examine sacroiliac joint with the patient in prone position, apply firm pressure over the sacrum.

Femoral nerve: L2, L3, L4

Sciatic nerve: L4, L5, S1, S2, S3

Useful language: I'm going to tap your back (percussion)

For prone position: Lie on your front, or tummy.

12. EXAMINATION OF THE KNEE

Introduction, then you may say: " I'm going to examine your knee, please undress your bottom half to your underwear, and stand up for me (Slip your trousers and leave your underwear/don't worry about it)."

Inspection

With the patient erect, then supine for limb alignment, bony contour, erythema, swelling, muscle wasting, and any genu valgus or varus.
Measures: Muscle girth at 10 cm above patella (both sides).

Palpation

With knee extended palpate soft tissue, collateral ligaments for tenderness and temperature with dorsum of your hand. With knee flexed palpate along the joint line anterior and posterior for tenderness.

Movement

With the patient supine, put your left hand on the knee to detect crepitation; ask the patient to fully flex knee and then to extend it. With the patient in prone position, thigh supported on the couch and legs projecting from couch. Observe the level of heels (test minor limitation of extension).

Tests

1. *Massage test:* (for effusion) With the knee extended, massage any fluid in the anterior compartment of thigh into suprapatellar pouch. Then firmly stroke the lateral side of the joint with the palm of your hand. Observe any fluid impulse on medial side of the joint.

2. *Patellar tap:* (for effusion) With the knee extended, empty suprapatellar pouch with pressure from the palm of your left hand. And with index of right hand, press patella firmly against femur.

3. *Patellar apprehension test:* (stability of patella) With the knee extended, apply pressure with your both thumbs on medial border of patella, and maintain pressure while slowly flexing the knee passively to 30°.

4. *Anterior and posterior draw test:* (cruciate ligament test) Flex the knee and sit on the patient's foot. Grasp upper tibia with your both hands and try to draw it forward (anterior cruciate ligament). Try to push it backward (posterior cruciate ligament).

5. *Lachman test:* (isolated cruciate ligament tear with intact collateral ligament) Flex the knee to 20°, push the lower part of thigh in one direction and pull tibia in the other direction, then reverse directions.

6. *Collateral ligament test:* With the knee fully extended, hold the patient's ankle between your elbow and side with both hands on upper tibia and attempt to abduct and adduct femur on tibia with knee straight.

7. *Pivot shift test:* (rotation in stability) With the knee extended, hold the patient's heel with right hand and fully internally rotate foot and tibia while applying valgus pressure to the knee with your left hand. Flex the knee from 0° to 30° to detect palpable or visible reduction.

8. *McMurray test:* (for menisci) Flex the hip and knee to 90°, hold the patient's heel with your right hand and hold the knee steady with your left hand. Externally rotate the tibia and slowly

extend the knee. Repeat with internal rotation. If positive, clunk can be felt with some discomfort to the patient.

13. EXAMINATION OF THE SHOULDER

Introduction, then you may say: "I'm going to examine your shoulder, if you don't mind expose your top half, please."

Inspection

Inspect the shoulder from the front, side and back for deformity, swelling, muscle wasting, and skin lesion.

Palpation

Swelling, tenderness in anterior aspect, bicepital groove, tip of shoulder, subacromial space and sternoclavicular joint.

Movement

Ask the patient to place the palms at the base of neck with elbows pointing laterally. Then put arms down and reach between shoulder blades with dorsum of hands. Ask the patient to flex elbow to 90° and to do external and internal rotation of shoulder joint.

Test

1. Glenohumeral joint movement: Firmly hold tip of scapula. Ask the patient to flex arm (normally it can be flexed to 90°), and ask the patient to abduct the arm (normally it can be flexed to 90°).
2. If cannot abduct the arm, passively abduct it to 40°, the patient should now be able to abduct it (supraspinatus rupture).
3. *Test for painful arc:* (40° to 120°) passively abduct arm. Ask the patient for any pain during this movement, and then ask him/her to bring the arm down.
4. Elicit impingement pain by passively flexing the shoulder to 90°, and then internally rotate it (Hawkin's sign).

5. Test for bicepital tendonitis by asking the patient to do flexion, and supination of elbow against resistance.

14. EXAMINATION OF THE HIP JOINT

Introduction, then you may say: " I'm going to examine your hip, please undress your bottom half to your underwear and stand for me".

Inspection

- Ask the patient to walk and inspect the gait. In fixed flexion deformity, the buttock is prominent. And in abduction deformity, the patient swings the apparent long leg out and round with each step.
- Ask the patient to stand up and inspect from back for scoliosis. From side for pelvic tilt which may conceal hip deformity.
- Trendelenburg's test: Ask the patient to stand on one leg with flexing the lifted knee to 90° and observe. In normal conditions, the pelvis is tilted up on the lifted side. In abnormal conditions, the pelvis is tilted down.
- Ask the patient to lie on the couch in supine position with pelvic brim at right angle to spine and inspect for deformity (abduction, adduction, flexion), swelling or redness, muscle wasting, and sinus formation. Compare.

Palpation

Palpate for local tenderness over front of hip and greater trochanter.

Measurement of Leg Length

In case of apparent shortening. With legs parallel, do the measurement from xyphosternum to medial malleolus. In case of true shortening, place the normal leg in a comparable position of abduction or adduction to abnormal one and measure from anterosuperior iliac spine to medial malleolus.

Movement

1. Stabilise iliac crest with left hand and use right hand to flex hip with knee flexed to 90° and note the range of movement. The normal range is 0° to 120°.
2. *Thomas' test:* Place one hand between the patient lumbar spine and the couch. Flex the unaffected hip to its limit and continue to push to straighten lumbar spine. In normal conditions, the opposite leg will remain flats, whereas in abnormal one, the leg will rise from the couch and the degree of rise is the amount of flexion deformity.
3. Stabilise the opposite iliac crest with left hand, then abduct with right hand (normal is 45°) and adduct (normal is 25°).
4. Roll each leg on the couch and measure the range of rotation of foot as indicator (90°).
5. Flex hip and knee to 90° and rotate internally, the normal is 30°. And rotate it internally, the normal is 45°.

15. EXAMINATION OF THE THYROID

Inspection

Thyroid gland can only be seen if it is enlarged.

- Pizzillo's method: Patient's hands are placed behind the head and the head pushed backward against the clasped hands.
- Thyroid swelling moves upward on deglutition.
- Thyroglossal cyst moves upwards on deglutition and protrusion of the tongue.
- The lower border of the swelling also moves up on deglutition. This is not possible in case of retrosternal goitre.
- Congestion of the face and distress may be seen in case of retrosternal goitre due to obstruction of the great veins at the thoracic inlet (Pemberton's sign).
- Identify the position of the trachea.

Palpation

The thyroid gland should always be palpated with the patient's neck slightly flexed. The gland may be palpated from behind and from the front with the four fingers of each hand placed on each lobe.

- Careful assessment of the margins, particularly the lower, is important.
- *Lahey's method:* Palpation of each lobe is best carried out from the front.
- *Surface:* Smooth or bosselated.
- *Consistency:* Firm, soft, hard, uniform or variable.
- *Swelling:* Position, size, shape, and extent
- *Mobility:* In horizontal and vertical planes. Fixity means malignant tumour or thyroiditis.
- Identify the plane of the swelling.
- The patient is asked to swallow and the lower border is palpated to discard the possibility of retrosternal extension.
- *Pressure effects:* On the trachea, larynx (stridor and dyspnoea), the oesophagus (dysphagia), the recurrent laryngeal nerve (hoarseness), the carotid sheath (pulsation of the artery cannot be felt), and the sympathetic trunk (Horner's syndrome).
- Position of trachea should be noted
- Pulsation or thrill in the thyroid.

Percussion

Over the manubrium sterni to exclude the presence of retrosternal goitre.

Auscultation

In primary toxic goitre a systolic bruit may be heard over the goitre due to increased vascularity.

General Examination

- *Primary toxic manifestation (Graves' disease):* Prominent eyes, exophthalmos, von Graefe's (lid lag) sign, tachycardia, wasting, sweating, nervousness, tremors of the extended hands and the tongue, hot and moist palms and elevated sleeping pulse rate, intolerance of hot weather and thyroid bruit.

- *Secondary thyrotoxicosis:* The AF is quite common. CVS is mainly effected. Ejection systolic murmur is present. Cardiomegaly and signs of cardiac failure: ankle oedema, orthopnoea and dyspnoea. Exophthalmos and tremor absent. CVS in secondary and the CNS in primary thyrotoxicosis are mainly affected.
- *CNS:* Look for tremors and exaggerated deep tendon reflexes.
- *Metastasis:* Lymph nodes, bones and lungs.
- Signs of myxoedema: Dry, coarse skin, loss of hair, hypothermia, swelling of the eyelids.

16. Annual Check-up in a Diabetic Patient

1. Measure body weight.
2. Examine the eyes:
   a. Xanthelasma and arcus.
   b. Visual acuity (maculopathy).
   c. Test eye movements (Mononeuritis multiplex, III, IV, VI CN).
   d. Ophthalmoscopy (cataract, rubeosis iridis, retinopathy, vitreous haemorrhage).
3. *Mouth:* Candidiasis.
4. *Neck:* Listen for carotid bruit (atherosclerosis).
5. *Upper limb:*
   a. Blood pressure (sitting and standing for postural hypotension, and hypertension).
   b. Radial pulse (for resting tachycardia).
   c. Inspect hand for wasting of thenar (carpal tunnel syndrome), hypothenar and interossei muscles (ulnar nerve palsy). Index finger for infection of prick site, ask the patient to do prayer sign (joint contracture).
6. *Chest:* Auscultate for signs of TB, pneumonia, or CCF.
7. *Examine lower limb:*
   a. *Inspection:*
   - Foot for ulcer, gangrene, callus, infection at prick site. In between toes and look for small muscle wasting, pes cavus, claw toes.

- Ankle: For deformity (charcot joint, OHCS, 5th ed. p668)
- *Leg:* For muscle wasting.
- *Knee:* For deformity (charcot joint).
- *Thigh:* For injection sites (infection, lipo-atrophy, lipo-hypertrophy), muscle wasting (especially quadriceps for diabetic amyotrophy).
   b. *Foot pulses:*
- *Dorsalis pedis:* On dorsum of foot just lateral to extensor hallucis tendon
- *Posterior tibial:* One to two centimetre below and behind medial malleolus
   c. *Tendon reflexes:*
- *Ankle jerk (S1):* Lower limb flexed at knee and extended at ankle by hand of examiner and ankle put at dorsum of opposite foot (can be abscent in elderly).
- *Knee jerk (L3, L4):* Lower limb flexed at knee to 60° and carried by hand.
- *Plantar reflex (S1, S2):* Stroke with blunt object along lateral border of foot from heel to little toe (can be extended in diabetic amyotrophy).
   d. *Sensory exam:*
- *Joint position:* Ask the patient to close the eyes. Show him up and down positions first. Then start from interphalangeal (IP) joint of hallux holding proximal and moving distal phalanx. If sensation is impaired, move to metatarso-phalangeal (MP) joint, ankle and knee.
- *Vibration:* Ask the patient to close the eyes, apply tuning fork to sternum, to establish baseline sensation. Test base of big toe, medial malleolus, tibial shaft and tuberus of anterior iliac crest.
- *Touch:* Ask the patient to close the eyes, use cotton. Ask the patient to respond verbally. Examine segments in turn and compare.

- *Pain:* Ask the patient to close eyes and to respond verbally. Use disposable pin, establish baseline sensation at the sternum. Test segments in turn and compare. Ask the patient to report if quality of sensations changes (hypo or hyper-aesthesia).

- *Temperature:* Ask the patient to close eyes. Use two containers of warm and cool water; or use a cold subject (e.g., tuning fork). And ask the patient about quality of sensation (test segments in turn and compare).

- *Deep pain:* Ask the patient to close the eyes. Apply firm pressure to nail or squeeze the calf belly. And ask the patient to report pain.

e. *Power (motor system):* Test from proximal to distal.
- Flex, extend, abduct, and adduct hip joint.
- Flex, and extend knee joint.
- Dorsiflex (L5), plantarflex (S1), invert, and evert foot.
- Flex, and extend toes.

f. *Sensory loss in DM:*
- *Early:* Vibration, deep pain, and tempera ture.
- *Later:* Joint position sensation.

g. *Investigations:*
- *Glycosylated Hb (HbA$_{1c}$):* Relates to blood glucose level over 6 to 8 weeks (normal: 2.3 to 6.5%).
- *Glycosylated plasma proteins (fructosamine):* relates to blood glucose level over 1 to 3 weeks.
- Urine for glucose, ketones, and albumin (macro and micro-albuminuria).
- Blood for plasma creatinine, and lipids.

17. PRIMARY AND SECONDARY SURVEY

Firstly, you have to stabilise the neck if there is any risk of neck injury.

Primary Survey

1. Hello, how are you? Would you please open your mouth and put out your tongue? (Check airway if it is clear. If not, remove any obstructions, such as blood, teeth, and foreign bodies.

2. Inspect respiratory rate and bilateral chest movement. Then auscultate to check for air entry on both sides. If there is no respiration, intubate and ventilate. If respiration is compromised, put O$_2$ mask. If there is tension pneumothorax, insert a wide bore cannula in the second intercostal space at midcalvicular line.

3. Check pulse. If pulse is absent, then consider the patient is arrested and treat accordingly. If in shock, start shock treatment.

4. Determine level of consciousness according to AVPU, **not GCS.**
   AVPU: Alert, response to vocal stimulus, response to pain, unresponsiveness.

5. Exposure to check for further injuries, and covering the patient to avoid hypothermia.
   N.B: Ask the patient if he/she feels any pain (assess verbal response), ask him/her to raise hand and to squeeze fingers (motor) and look for eye opening.
   The X-rays before secondary survey—chest, cervical spine and pelvis.

Secondary Survey

1. *Head:* Signs of injury as bruising, laceration, bony deformity, depressed skull fracture.
   a. *Eyes:* Any foreign bodies, redness, perforation, size of pupil. Papillary reflexes, corneal reflexes, bruises around the eye (suggestive of anterior cranial fossa fracture).
   b. *Nose:* Blood, discharge, (bright red discharge suggestive of rhinorrhoea).
   c. *Ear:* Blood, discharge (let blood discharge on sheet, and look for double ring: mixed blood and CSF). Bruises over mastoid (consider middle cranial fossa fracture).

d. *Mouth:* Check stability of maxilla and mandible. Check for airway, any unstable false teeth or foreign body.

2. *Neck:* Check for subcutaneous emphysema, cervical spinous processes, venous dilatation, tracheal deviation.

3. *Chest:* Inspect respiratory movement, check for any penetrating or sucking injury. Paradoxical movement of flail chest. Palpate for tenderness, crepitus or rib fracture. Percuss and auscultate checking for haeamo/pneumo-thorax.

4. *Heart:* Auscultate for heart sounds.

5. Abdomen: Inspect for injury or echymosis, laceration, distension. Palpate for tenderness, and guarding. Auscultate for bowel sounds. Do digital rectal examination, check sphincter tone, and prostate.

6. *Diagnostic peritoneal lavage:* (if in doubt) Below umbilicus, put drip of 1L N/S and aspirate.

7. *Pelvis:* Compressed and distracted manually to check for stability or pain, examine penis for blood drops (if present, do not catheterise).

8. *Extremities:* Inspect for bruises, laceration, or deformity. Palpate for tenderness and stability. Check pulses, sensory exam, reflexes, motor exam and muscle tone.

18. EXAMINATION OF THE EYE

Inspection
In all, looking for asymmetry, deformities, discoloration, redness, discharge, lesions.
- Diagnostic facies.
- *Orbit, rim:* palpate for lumps.
- *Brow:* lost sweating (Horner's).
- *Eyelids:* xanthelasma, ectropian, entropian.
- *Eyelids:* pus on lids (blepharitis).
- Ptosis.
- Exophthalmos.

- *Iris:* colour, defects.
- *Cornea:* transparent vs. opaque, corneal arcus, band keratopthy, Kayser-Fleischer rings, lesion, scars.
- Ask the patient to look up and pull down both lower eyelids to inspect the conjunctiva and sclera.
- *Conjunctiva:* clear/infected. If conjunctivitis, wash hands immediately: viral form contagious.
- *Sclera:* jaundice, pallor, injection.
- Spread each eye open with The doctor's thumb, index finger. Ask the patient to look to each side and downward to expose entire bulbar surface.
- Eyeball tenderness.

Visual Acuity
If eye pain, injury, visual loss, check visual acuity before rest of the exam or inserting medications into eyes.
- Let the patient use glasses, contacts if available.
- Put patient 20 feet from Snellen eye chart, or hold Rosenbaum pocket card 14 inches away.
- The patient covers an eye at a time with a card, reading the smallest letters possible.
- Record smallest line read, e.g., 20/40.

Visual Fields
- Stand 2 feet in front of patient, who looks in The doctor's eyes at eye-level.
- The doctor's hands to side half way between doctor and the patient, wiggle fingers, ask which they see move.
- Repeat 2-3 to test both temporal fields.
- If suspect abnormality, test 4 quadrants of each eye while card covers other.

Ophthalmoscopic (fundi)
- Darken room, adjust scope so light is no brighter than necessary.
- Adjust aperture to a plain white circle.

- Set diopter dial to zero, unless have a preferred setting.
- The doctor uses left hand and left eye to examine the patient's left eye.
- The doctor's free hand onto the the patient's shoulder or forehead for control.
- Tell the patient to stare at wall.
- Look through scope, shine light into the patient's eye from 2 feet away at a 45° angle.
- See the retina as a "red reflex.". Reflex: clear vs. opaque (cataract). Follow red colour to move within a few inches from the patient's eye.
- Adjust diopter dial to bring the retina into focus. Find a blood vessel and follow it to the optic disk, use this as a point of reference.

- *Inspect Optic Disk*
  - Colour of disc: pink vs. pale.
  - Margins clear.
  - State of cup.

- *Inspect vessels:*
All 4 quadrants, veins are darker than arteries:
  - Bleeding, exudate.
  - Pigmentation, occlusion.
- Inspect macula, by moving the scope nasally:
  - Foveal light reflex.
  - Bleeding, exudate.
  - Oedema, drusen.

Pupils

- Shape, relative size.
- *Light reaction: dim lights if needed:*
  - The patient looks in distance, shine light in from side to gauge pupil's light reaction. Record size, irregularity.
  - Assess both direct (same eye) and consensual (other eye) responses.
- Assess afferent pupillary defect by moving light in arc from pupil to pupil, and if left eye light makes right eye dilate, not constrict (Marcus Gunne).

Optionally

As do arc test, have the pateint place a flat hand extending vertically from his face, between his eyes, to act as a blinder so light can only go into one eye at a time.
- *Accommodation:* The pateint alternates between looking into distance, and a hat pin 30 cm from nose.

Corneal Reflections

- Shine a light from directly in front of the the patient.
- Corneal reflections should be centered over pupils.
- Assess asymmetry (extraocular muscle pathology).

Eye Movements

- "Follow finger with eyes without moving head": test the 6 cardinal points in an H pattern.

Assess

  - Failure of movement.
  - Nystagmus [pause to check it during upward, lateral gaze]).
- Convergence by moving finger towards bridge of the patient's nose.
- Gaze palsies (supranuclear lesions).
- Fatiguability (myasthenia).

Corneal Reflex

- Corneal reflex: The patient looks up and away.
- Touch cotton wool to other side.
- Look for blink in both eyes, ask if can sense it.
- Repeat other side. [Tests V sensory, VII motor].

PROCEDURES

The content of this exam reflects the standard laid down by the GMC for granting limited registration. Registered doctors must be proficient in certain procedures they would be expected to perform as the SHOs in the UK. You will be asked the to perform at least three procedures in this exam.

BLOOD PRESSURE MEASUREMENT

1. Introduce yourself to the patient and explain to him that you will be recording his blood pressure and the need for it.
2. Have paper and pen at hand for immediate recording of the pressure.
3. Seat the subject in a quiet, calm environment with his or her bared arm resting on a standard table or other support so that the midpoint of the upper arm is at the level of the heart.
4. Estimate by inspection or measure with a tape the circumference of the bare upper arm at the midpoint between the acromium and olecranon process (between the shoulder and elbow) and select an appropriately sized cuff. The bladder inside the cuff should encircle 80 per cent of the arm in adults and 100 per cent of the arm in children less than 13 years old. If in doubt, use a larger cuff. If the available cuff is too small, this should be noted.
5. Palpate the brachial artery and place the cuff, so that the midline of the bladder is over the arterial pulsation, then wrap and secure the cuff snugly around the subject's bare upper arm. Avoid rolling up the sleeve in such a manner that it forms a tight tourniquet around the upper arm. Loose application of the cuff results in overestimation of the pressure. The lower edge of the cuff should be 1 inch (2-.5 cm) above the antecubital fossa (bend of the elbow), where the head of the stethoscope is to be placed.
6. Place the manometer so the center of the mercury column or aneroid dial is at eye level

and easily visible to the observer and the tubing from the cuff is unobstructed.

7. Inflate the cuff rapidly to 70 mmHg, and increase by increments of 10 mmHg while palpating the radial pulse. Note the level of pressure at which the pulse disappears and subsequently reappears during deflation. This procedure, the *palpatory method*, provides a necessary preliminary approximation of the systolic blood pressure to ensure an adequate level of inflation when the actual, auscultatory measurement is made. The palpatory method is particularly useful to avoid underinflation of the cuff in patients with an auscultatory gap and overinflation in those with very low blood pressure.
8. Place the earpieces of the stethoscope into the ear canals, angled forward to fit snugly. Switch the stethoscope head to the low-frequency position (bell). The setting can be confirmed by listening as the stethoscope head is tapped gently.
9. Place the head of the stethoscope over the brachial artery pulsation just above and medial to the antecubital fossa but below the lower edge of the cuff, and hold it firmly in place, making sure that the head makes contact with the skin around its entire circumference. Wedging the head of the stethoscope under the edge of the cuff may free up one hand but results in considerable extraneous noise.
10. Inflate the bladder rapidly and steadily to a pressure 20 to 30 mmHg above the level previously determined by palpation, then partially unscrew (open) the valve and deflate the bladder at 2 mm/s while listening for the appearance of the Korotkoff's sounds.
11. As the pressure in the bladder falls, note the level of the pressure on the manometer at the first appearance of repetitive sounds (Phase I) and at the muffling of these sounds (Phase IV) and when they disappear (Phase V). During the period the Korotkoff's sounds are audible, the rate of deflation should be no more than

2 mm per pulse beat, thereby compensating for both rapid and slow heart rates.

12. After the last Korotkoff's sound is heard, the cuff should be deflated slowly for at least another 10 mmHg, to ensure that no further sounds are audible, then rapidly and completely deflated, and the subject should be allowed to rest for at least 30 seconds.

13. The systolic (Phase I) and diastolic (Phase V) pressures should be immediately recorded, rounded off (upwards) to the nearest 2 mmHg. In children, and when sounds are heard nearly to a level of 0 mmHg, the Phase IV pressure should also be recorded. All values should be recorded together with the name of the subject, and the date and time of the measurement, the arm on which the measurement was made, the subject's position, and the cuff size (when a nonstandard size is used).

14. The measurement should be repeated after at least 30 seconds, and the two readings averaged. In clinical situations, additional measurements can be made in the same or opposite arm, in the same or an alternative position.

BIMANUAL PER VAGINAL EXAMINATION

1. First greet your examiner and introduce yourself.
2. Say that you are asked to do a bimanual vaginal examination. If this is a real patient, introduce yourself to the patient, explain the procedure and obtain her consent. Ask her if she has emptied her bladder. If not, tell her that it is always better to empty the bladder before a per vaginal examination but due to time constraints you cannot allow her to do so.
3. Ask for a chaperone, even if you're a female, and tell her that you will ensure her privacy.
4. Ask the patient to lie on her back, close to the edge of the table, bend her knees, feet together and let her legs drop.
5. Wear your gloves, know your size, ask for jelly.
6. Then let the patient know that you're going to do now the examination.
7. First, inspection; see if there is any swelling, redness or irritation on the vulva, try to part the labia and feel for any bartholins cysts on the side (While doing your examination, better run your commentaries, state what's pertinent), also ask the patient to cough or bear down, to see if there is any prolapse or incontinence.
8. Then introduce your index finger, followed by your middle finger into the vagina, feel for the vaginal walls, note any irregularities, swelling/mass—check laterals, posterior wall and then go to the anterior.
9. Check the fornices and the cervix, including its position, ideally, you also do cervical excitation (any cervical tenderness?), then feel for the uterus.
10. Do the bimanual examination, right hand on top of the lower abdomen, like doing a ballottement, to feel for the uterus, any lumps? size? then also check for the ovaries, any note of cyst? then check the adnexae.
11. Withdraw your examining finger, note for any blood, or any other discharge.
12. Offer tissue to the patient to clean herself.
13. Thank the patient and tell her that you finished and ask her to get dressed and you will go back to her to inform her about your findings
14. You will be asked regarding your impression, usually, normal vaginal examination, but they may come up with some pathology like ovarian cyst, myoma or fistula.

PER RECTAL EXAMINATION

1. Introduce yourself to the patient and take his consent for the examination explaining him the need to do so.
2. Tell him, "I am going to examine the anus,

rectum, and the prostate. I will be inserting my finger into the rectum. You should feel some pressure. If you feel any other discomfort, please let me know ".

2. Place him in the left-lateral (Sims') position. Patient lying on exam table or bed on left side with superior knee flexed into chest.

3. Examiner should be sitting on rolling stool.

4. Glove both hands for the examination.

5. Generously lubricate the index finger of the gloved dominant hand with lubricant.

6. Give the patient instructions on bearing down to reduce discomfort of insertion. "To make the insertion of my finger into the rectum more comfortable, please bear down as though you were going to have a bowel movement but you won't. You will only feel pressure."

7. Ask the patient to lift his gown above the waist.

8. Separate the buttocks with two hands and visually inspect the area for lesions, rashes, and masses.

9. Visually inspect the anus for fissures, haemorrhoids, skin tags.

10. Use thumb and index finger of non-dominant hand to separate buttocks for digital insertion.

11. Place index finger of gloved dominant hand at the anal opening.

12. Ask the patient to bear down. "Please bear down. You should feel some pressure. As I am palpating the prostate, you may feel the urge to urinate. That is a normal reaction. If you feel any other discomfort, please let me know."

13. Apply gentle posterior pressure and slowly insert finger palmar surface down.

14. Insert fingers in downward angle towards umbilicus. Allow a few seconds for the external and internal sphincter to relax.

15. Evaluate the tone of the sphincter muscles as inserting finger.

16. Rotate finger 360° to evaluate anal sphincter muscle ring. Evaluate all four walls of the

rectum: posterior, left lateral, anterior, and right lateral.

17. Examine for any masses, nodules, inflammation, genital warts, or irregularities. Stool is usually present, but is soft and mobile. Tumours or polyps are firmer and fixed.

18. Gently palpate levator ani muscles attached at the posterior and lateral walls of the rectum for muscle tone, if possible.

19. Examine the prostate—
    i. Position finger palmar surface down. Palpate posteriorly to locate prostate.
    ii. Prostate should be 2 to 4 cm long and triangular in shape.
    iii. The two lateral lobes are separated by a deeper central grove.
    iv. Palpate in a circular motion to increase ability to identify the lobes and groove.
    v. Palpate and note the width and length of gland, and presence of groove. Consistency should be firm and rubbery.

20. Examiner should forewarn the patient before removing finger.

21. Slowly remove. finger to avoid any sphincter muscle spasms

22. Any faeces on finger of gloved hand should be tested for occult blood.

23. Remove glove away from and out of sight of the patient.

24. Offer the patient box of tissues to remove lubricant from anus and buttocks.

25. Give the patient reassuring statement.

26. Allow the patient privacy to dress.

27. Discuss findings.

TAKING A CERVICAL SMEAR

1. Greet the patient, introduce yourself, and explain the procedure and purpose of it. Tell her that is not painful, but may be a bit uncomfortable, make sure that she is not menstruating now, and she did not use spermicide or lubricant jelly in the previous 24 hours.

2. Then: Wear gloves; prepare the slide (write the name of the patient, date and time of taking specimen with pencil not pen, where writings disappear with fixation). And prepare the fixator (50/50 mixture of alcohol and ether).

3. Hold Cusco's bivalve speculum with the right hand and separate the labia with the left hand (do not lubricate with jell). Tell the patient that you are introducing the speculum and ask her to relax. Gently insert the speculum on its lateral side and when you are in turn it up for 90°. Handle anteriorly when the patient is in supine position and fix it. Try to identify the cervix and use the notched end of spatula and rotate it 360° to scrape off cells from cervical os. Spread the sample on the slide and fix it immediately with the prepared fixator (50/50 mixture of alcohol and ether), either put a drop or put the slide in a container with the fixator. You should not allow the sample to dry.

4. Tell the patient that you finished and you are going to take speculum out. Take it out in the same way. Give a towel to the patient to wipe herself.

VENEPUNCTURE

1. Explain the procedure and allow the patient time for questions and, if desired, withdrawal of consent.

2. If taking blood for drug or hormone levels, or fasting samples, ascertain the time and dose of last medication, or time last food or drink was taken. This information is essential for assessment of drug efficacy and accurate diagnose.

3. Ask the patient whether or not he or she has had blood taken previously. He or she may be aware of particular problems encountered and of the best site available.

4. Spend time selecting the most appropriate vein in order to achieve successful vene-puncture at the first attemthe patient This

promotes the patient's confidence and is more comfortable.

5. Wash your hands.

6. Attach needle to syringe. If more than one sample is required, create a vacuum in the other syringes.

7. Apply tourniquet to upper arm and rotate limb to face you.

8. Palpate and examine arm to distinguish between veins, tendons and arteries.

9. The vein should be firm and bouncy. Clenching and unclenching the patient's fist can help, but may lead to a minor alteration in test results.

10. Put on gloves and clean area with alcohol swab, allowing to dry passively for 30 seconds.

11. Stretch the skin over the vein with thumb of one hand. Insert the needle, bevel side up, into the vessel at a 30 to 45 degree angle. Do this smoothly: unnecessary swiftness can lead to puncture of the vessel wall; being too slow increases the discomfort

12. Stabilise needle and syringe with your thumb, index finger and middle finger of one hand, and withdraw the syringe's plunger with the other.

13. If blood flows, click the plunger into locked position.

14. If further samples are required, unlock the syringe while stabilising the needle with the other hand, then connect the next syringe.

15. Release the tourniquet and cover the needle with cotton wool, but do not apply pressure until you have withdrawn the needle, as this causes unnecessary pain and venous damage.

16. Apply firm pressure for 30 to 60 seconds to prevent bruising. Check the site.

17. If clotted, apply elastoplasts or gauze and tape.

18. After completing the procedure, dispose of the needle and any contaminated waste in the appropriate container.

19. Tell the patient that the procedure is complete and that you will let him know when the test results arrive.

Note

- If the tourniquet has been on for more than two minutes prior to inserting the needle, release and allow blood to return to the hand before reapplying.
- If a venous valve is entered during the procedure, the patient will feel sudden, acute pain. Discontinue the procedure immediately.
- If after two attempts you are unsuccessful, seek assistance from a colleague.
- Observe the patient throughout the procedure for signs of dizziness, fainting or paraesthesia.
- Be aware that the brachial artery is also sited near the sites most commonly used for venepuncture.

PERIPHERAL VENOUS CANNULATION

Cannula sizes (See Table 22.1).

Table 22.1: Cannula sizes—size, colour and use

Size	Colour	Use
22G	Blue	Small veins, IV drugs
20G	Pink	Slow fluid adm, IV drugs
18G	Green	IV fluids, blood transfusion
15G	Grey	Rapid IV fluids
14G	Brown	Rapid transfusion

Procedure

1. Introduce yourself to the patient, explain the procedure and the need for doing it.
2. Wash your hands and wear surgical gloves.
3. Apply the tourniquet above the elbow on the preferred arm and tighten it.
4. Ask the patient to open and close the fist a few times.
5. Gently tap over the vein to encourage dilatation.
6. Clean the insertion area with an alcohol swab and allow it to dry.
7. Apply traction to the skin with the thumb of the non-dominant hand to fix the vein in place.
8. Hold the cannula with the two wings together with the bevel of the needle pointing upwards.
9. Puncture the skin, holding the cannula at about 15 degrees to the skin and firmly advance the needle through the subcutaneous tissue into the vein. You should get a flush back of blood into the distal end of the cannula as you enter the vein.
10. Hold the cannula steady and advance the plastic cannula over the metal stilette into the vein.
11. Remove the tourniquet.
12. Apply gentle pressure over the vein just proximal to the entry site to prevent blood flow.
13. Remove the needle from within the plastic catheter. Place the cap over the distal end of the cannula.
14. Secure the cannula in place with dressing and tapes.

CATHETERISATION

Female Catheterisation

1. Explain the procedure to the patient and the need for it.
2. Position the patient in a supine position, heels together, knees apart.
3. Aseptic hand wash and prepare sterile field.
4. Arrange sterile equipment on tray.
5. Thirty seconds hand wash and double glove.
6. Cleanse outer labia with tissue disinfectant, wiping towards anal area.
7. Hold labia apart with gauze squares and clean the inner labia and around urethral meatus.
8. Remove outer pair of gloves.
9. Drape the patient with fenestrated drape.
10. Place the catheter in kidney dish, on drape, between patient's legs. The catheter may be lubricated with sterile lubricant.
11. Insert the catheter into the urethra until urine starts to flow, then advance it a further 5 cms.

12. Inflate the balloon with the appropriate amount of sterile water. Gently withdraw the catheter until resistance is felt.
13. Connect sterile drainage system.
14. Instruct the patient not to touch the catheter as there is the danger of acquiring infection.
15. Inform her that the procedure is over and regarding when the catheter will be removed.

Male Catheterisation

1. Explain the procedure to the patient.
2. Place the patient in a supine position.
3. Aseptic hand wash and prepare sterile field.
4. Arrange sterile equipment on tray.
5. Thirty seconds hand wash and double glove.
6. Cleanse penis with tissue disinfectant, from urethral meatus down shaft. Retract foreskin when cleansing.
7. Instill xylocaine gel into the urethra. Apply gentle pressure to clamp the urethra so gel will pass down the urethra to facilitate lubrication.
8. Remove outer pair of gloves.
9. Drape the patient with fenestrated drape.
10. Place the catheter in kidney dish, on drape, between the patient's legs.
11. Holding penis with gauze, extend it to reduce angle of urethra at bulbar urethra. Insert the catheter until urine starts to flow. Further advance the catheter to bifurcation.
12. Inflate the balloon with the appropriate amount of sterile water. Gently withdraw the catheter until resistance is felt.
13. Connect sterile drainage system.
14. Reposition foreskin if uncircumcised.
15. Explain to the patient regarding the care of the catheter and when it is likely to be removed.

OPHTHALMOSCOPY/ FUNDOSCOPY

To undertake successful ophthalmoscopy, it is essential that both you and your patient are comfortable. The patient will be more co-operative when relaxed. Also, you will be more successful if you do not have to stoop uncomfortably. The patients height adjustment is however, limited by the fixed chair height in this clinic.

1. Instruct the patient to look at a distant target, the white spot light on the vision chart is the best and advise them to keep still and concentrate on this spot and to 'pretend' they can still see it even if you obscure it with your head. The patient also needs to be given permission to blink as required.
2. Your left eye and left hand should be used to examine the patient's left eye. The field of view of the fundus is increased, the closer you are to the patient's eye, so for low myopes and low hyperopes it is best to remove their glasses.
3. Using a large diameter aperture and looking around the side of the ophthalmoscope, examine the external features of the eye. This includes lashes, lid margins, palpebral conjunctiva and the sclera. Also, observe the colour of the iris and the size and regularity of the pupil.
4. Dial up a +10DS lens in the lens wheel and observe the eye from 10 cm. Study the red reflex in particular as this provides an excellent way to detect any opacity of the media. Any dark patches or irregularity of the normal uniform red reflex denotes opacity of the cornea, anterior chamber or the vitreous. Look out for a Mittendorff's dot, which is a small congenital lens opacity often present in normal healthy eyes.
5. The position of an opacity can be inferred from its parallax with respect to the pupil. Whilst examining the red-reflex, ask the patient to look up or down slightly. If, when the patient looks up, the opacity appears to move in the same direction within the red-reflex, then it must lie anterior to the pupil

plane (i.e., the cornea or the anterior chamber). One that remains stationary must, i.e., in the plane of the pupil, and one that moves in the opposite direction to that of the patient's gaze must lie posterior to the pupil plane (i.e. the posterior lens or vitreous). You may find it easier to move yourself slightly from side to side rather than ask your patient to move their eye to achieve the same effect.

6. During ophthalmoscopy it is advisable to keep both eyes open and suppress the image from the other eye. It may take some practice to accomplish this.

7. Slowly move closer to the patient and at the same time gradually reduce the power of the lens in the wheel and focus on the crystalline lens, the vitreous and finally the fundus. The power of lens necessary to focus on the fundus will depend on any patient and observer uncompensated refractive error and the patient or observer accommodation. Once a blood vessel on the fundus has been located then move along it and locate the point at which it branches, and move your field of view in the direction in which the apex of the branch is pointing.

8. By moving along a blood vessel in this manner the optic disc will be located. You will need to consider its colour, its margins and the cup if there is one. Also, note the presence of any pigment, choroidal or scleral crescents around the disc. Differentiate between a colour cup and a contour cup.

9. Retinal blood vessels should be examined in each quadrant after locating the disc. The veins are relatively large and dark red, whilst the arteries are relatively thin and pale.

10. Return to the disc and move nasally to view along the patient's visual axis. In this position you will obscure the fixation target, cause the pupil to constrict, dazzle the patient and notice some troublesome corneal reflections. These factors make the macula a difficult area to

visualize. It may be useful to use a smaller aperture beam. The normal macula is the area between the superior and inferior temporal blood vessel arcades and it's centre is the fovea.

11. Finally ask the patient to look in the eight cardinal directions to allow you to view the peripheral fundus—'look up' to see the superior periphery and so on. In a young patient with a large pupil you will be able to get as far as the equator of the eye. You will need to adjust the lens in the wheel slightly as the periphery is closer to you than the optic disc requiring more focusing power (plus lens).

GIVING AN INTRAMUSCULAR INJECTION

Materials Needed

Syringe with the drug to be administered (without air), needle (Gauss 22, long and medium thickness; on syringe), liquid disinfectant, cotton wool, adhesive tape.

Technique

1. Wash your hands.
2. Reassure the patient and explain the procedure.
3. Uncover the area to be injected (lateral upper quadrant major gluteal muscle, lateral side of upper leg, deltoid muscle).
4. Disinfect the skin.
5. Tell the patient to relax the muscle.
6. Insert the needle swiftly at an angle of 90 degree (watch depth!).
7. Aspirate briefly; if blood appears, withdraw the needle. Replace it with a new one, if possible, and start again from point 4.
8. Inject slowly (less painful).
9. Withdraw the needle swiftly.
10. Press sterile cotton wool onto the opening. Fix with adhesive tape.

11. Check the patient's reaction and give additional reassurance, if necessary.

12. Clean up; dispose of waste safely; wash your hands.

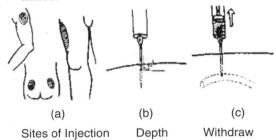

(a)	(b)	(c)
Sites of Injection	Depth	Withdraw

Fig. 22.1: (a) Sites of injection (b) Depth (c) Withdraw

CARDIOPULMONARY RESUSCITATION

Sequence of Actions

• Ensure safety of rescuer and victim.
• Check for consciousness. Gently shake the victim's shoulder and shout, "Are you all right?"

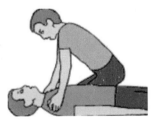

Fig. 22.2

An unconscious casualty will not respond. If they do respond by answering or moving, leave them in the position in which you find them, check their condition and call for help.

If they do not respond by answering or moving:

• Shout for help. Help will be needed either to assist in performing CPR or to call for medical help.
• Position the victim. If the victim is found in a crumpled up position and/or face down, the rescuer must roll the victim over, this is done while calling for help.

A—Airway

• Open the airway. An unconscious casualty's airway may become narrowed or blocked. The main reason for this is that muscular control in the throat is lost which allows the tongue to fall back and block the airway. Use the head-tilt manoeuvre to open airway.
• Place your hand on the casualty's forehead and gently tilt the head well back. Remove any obvious obstructions from the casualties mouth using one finger to hook it out. Then place two fingers under the point of the casualty's chin and lift the jaw.

IF you suspect that the casualty may have an injury to the head or neck, handle the head very carefully to avoid injuring the casualty further. Tilt the head back very slightly—just far enough to open the casualty's airway.

B—Breathing

• Establish breathlessness. After opening the airway establish breathlessness. Kneel beside the casualty, and put your face close to his mouth. Keeping the airway open, look, listen, and feel for breathing (more than an occasional gasp).
• Look for a rise and fall in the victim's chest.
• Listen for sounds of breathing.
• Feel for breath on your cheek.
• Look, listen and feel for up to 10 seconds, before deciding that breathing is absent.

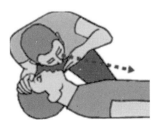

Fig. 22.3

Sometimes, opening and maintaining an open airway is all that is necessary to restore breathing.

If they are *breathing (other than the occasional breath):*
- Turn into recovery position.
- Check for continued breathing.

If they are not breathing:
- Provide artificial ventilation.
- Turn victim onto their back if not already in position.

- Make sure, that the airway is still open with two fingers under the victim's chin and the other hand on the forehead. Remove any visible obstructions from the mouth, including dislodged dentures, but leave well-fitting dentures in place.
- Close the victim's nose by pinching it with the index finger and thumb with the hand that is on the forehead. Take a full breath and place your lips around the victim's mouth making a good seal.
- Give two full breaths by mouth-to-mouth, mouth-to-nose, or mouth-to-stoma ventilation until you see the chest rise. Tke about two seconds for full inflation.
- Remove your lips and allow for lung deflation, which takes about four seconds. Repeat this once and then assess for signs of circulation.

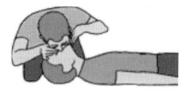

Fig. 22.4

C—Circulation
- Look, listen and feel for breathing, coughing movement, normal colour or any signs of circulation. If there are no signs of life, commence chest compressions immediately.

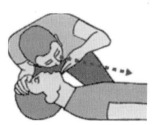

Fig. 22.5

IF circulation is present, continue rescue breathing and about every ten breaths check the pulse.
- Check the victim's pulse.
- Maintain an open airway position by holding the forehead of the victim.
- Place your fingertips on the victim's windpipe and then slide them towards you until you reach the groove of the neck. Press gently on this area (carotid artery).

Check the victim's carotid pulse. Take *no more than ten seconds* to do this.

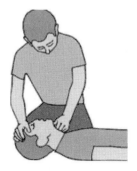

Fig. 22.6

If there are no signs of a pulse, commence chest compressions immediately.

Giving Chest Compressions
- Place the victim in a horizontal position on a hard, flat surface.
- Locate the bottom of the rib cage with the index and middle fingers of your hand closest to the patient's feet.
- Keeping your fingers together, slide your

fingers along the rib to the point where the lowermost rib meets at the sternum (breast-bone).

- Place your middle finger at this point and your index finger on the lower breastbone.

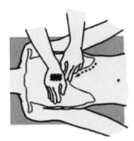

Fig. 22.7

- Place the heel of the other hand on the sternum next to the index finger in the notch in the rib cage.
- Place the hand used to locate the notch at the rib cage on top and parallel to the hand that is on the sternum.
- Keep the fingers off the chest, by interlocking them.

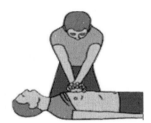

Fig. 22.8

- Lean well over the casualty, keep the arms, elbows in a straight and locked position.
- Position your shoulders directly over the hands, so that pressure is exerted straight downward.
- Exert enough downward pressure to depress the sternum of an adult approximately 4 to 5 cm (1 to ½ to 2 inches).
- Each compression should squeeze the heart

between the sternum and spine to pump blood through the body.

- Totally release pressure in order to allow the heart to refill completely with blood.
- Keep the heel of your hand in contact with the victim's chest at all times.
- Make compressions down and up in a smooth manner.
- Perform 15 cardiac compressions at a rate of 100 per minute, counting "one, two, three fifteen".
- Use the head-tilt/chin-lift manoeuvre and give two full breaths (artificial ventilation).
- Continue the cycle of 15 compressions and two ventilations.
- Continue resuscitation until the victim shows signs of life, qualified help arrives to assist or you become exhausted.

If the victim starts breathing on own his but remains unconscious, turn him into the recovery position. Check his condition and be ready to turn him onto his back and re-start rescue breathing if he stops breathing.

DISPOSING SHARP INSTRUMENTS

Safety Tips When Using Hypodermic Needles and Syringes

- Use each needle and syringe only once.
- Do *not* disassemble the needle and syringe after use.
- Do *not* recap, bend or break needles prior to disposal.
- Decontaminate the needle and syringe prior to disposal.
- Dispose of the needle and syringe in a puncture-proof container.
- Make hypodermic needles unusable by burning them.

Note: Where disposable needles are not available and recapping is practiced, use the "one-handed" recap method:

- First, place the cap on a hard, flat surface; then remove hand.
- Next, with one hand, hold the syringe and use the needle to "scoop-up" the cap.
- Finally, when the cap covers the needle completely, hold the needle at the base near the hub and use the other hand to secure the cap on the needle.

MISCELLANEOUS

A patient with intestinal obstruction, X-ray of abdomen displayed. Call the registrar and explain the situation.

Hello, Dr (Registrar), I am Dr (you), Senior House Officer in the A and E. I have a patient who is a 72-year-old female, she is presented with a history of abdominal pain of 24 hours duration.

The pain is central, was first colicky in nature then became more diffuse aching, she vomited twice, and she has constipation since yesterday.

On Examination (O/E): Vital Signs

She is conscious, pulse rate, blood pressure, temperature all are normal (mention figures according to those given in the exam chart).

Talk about signs of dehydration (according to instructions). Fluid input/output values. Abdomen is distended with tenderness all over the abdomen. Check movement with respiration.

Investigation

We took blood for FBC, U and E, blood chemistry. Results showed increased urea level, increased haematocrit, increased globulin.

We did plain AXR, erect which showed multiple fluid level, the supine film showed dilated large bowel (ascending and transverse colon are located at the periphery). The haustra are on two-third of the way from one wall to another and irregularly spaced.

Barium enema and meal are contraindicated.

Management

1. We put N/G tube to decompress the bowel and to prevent aspiration.
2. We gave N/S to correct fluid and electrolyte imbalance.
3. We took blood for grouping and cross match and save.
4. We gave antibiotic cefuroxime.
5. Analgesia, morphine.
6. Why do you call me? Because I suspect intestinal obstruction with strangulation (may be right inguinal hernia), and an urgent surgery may be indicated.

A mother is seeking advice, over the phone, for her child with diarrhoea.

Hello, this is Dr (you), how can I help you? How long has he been like this?

How many times does he open his bowel? Is it watery, loose or semi-formed? Any blood, mucous, pus? (mucous = slippery).

Any tummy pain or lump? Has he been sick? Any fever (temperature)? How is he feeding?

Ask about signs of dehydration: How is his mouth? His tongue, is it dry or moist? Does he cry without tears? Do his eyes seem to be depressed? Does he pass water as usual? How is his breathing?

Then if the dehydration is mild, give him ORS; if not available, teach the mother how to prepare one. 1 L of water (2 pints of water), boil and let to cool, then add 10 TSF of sugar and TSF of salt. And give the child by spoons as much as he accepts. Don't give ORS if breastfeeding continues.

Describing a Chest X-ray
- Patient details [name, age, sex, date, place]
- Film details [contrast type, level, plane]

Then checklist ABCDEFGHI:
- **A**orta
- **B**ubble [gastric]
- **C**ardiac shadow/ CTR
- **D**iaphragm: inflation, angles

- **O**esophagus (foreign body)/effusion
- **F**ields/fractures [rib]
- **G**as (pneumothorax)
- **H**ila and bronchi
- **I**atrogenic (subclavian line, pacemaker)

Alternatively

- *Airway:* trachea, bronchi, hila, fields, effusion
- Bubble [gastric]
- CTR
- *Diaphragm:* inflation, costophrenic angles
- Oesophagus (foreign body)
- Fractures [rib]
- Gas (pneumothorax)
- *Heart:* shadow, aorta

- Iatrogenic (subclavian line, pacemaker)

Cardiothoracic Ratio (CTR)

- *Measurement:* widest part of heart divided by widest part of chest as measured inside the ribs.
- *Normal value:* <50%, except in:
  - Neonates, infants.
  - Skeletal problems: scoliosis, etc.
  - Athletes.

Tips

- Usual CXR is taken in PA direction during inspiration.
- Echocardiogram better for finding effusion, as CXR needs 250 mL accumulation before visible.

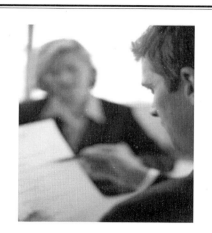

Section *Four*

Enhancing Job Prospects

23 Royal College Exams

> ◆ *Passing the first part of a royal college exam in your desired field will do your job prospects a lot of good. I have provided a breakdown of the five main royal college exams in terms of.... Format of the exam, eligibility, fees, locations, contact addresses, recommended reading and courses available.*

MEMBERSHIP OF THE ROYAL COLLEGE OF OBSTETRICIANS AND GYNAECOLOGISTS— MRCOG PART 1 EXAM

1. What is the exam about?

The examination is on basic sciences and consists of two multiple choice question papers, each lasting two hours. The examination embraces those subjects, which form part of the general education of any specialist and particularly those aspects, which are applicable to obstetrics and gynaecology.

2. Eligibility

Candidates are eligible to enter for the Part 1 examination when they have obtained their medical degree.

Candidates may take the Part 1 examination at any time and must pass the Part 1 examination or obtain exemption before attempting the Part 2 examination.

Candidates *MUST* attempt the Part 2 examination on at least one occasion within *TEN* years of passing the Part 1 examination. Those candidates failing to comply with this regulation will be required to pass the Part 1 examination again.

3. Where to take the exam?

Part 1 examinations are held in March and September. Apart from the UK, the exam is held in various overseas centres—including India (Mumbai, Delhi, Chennai).

4. What is the fee for the exam?

At present the fees for all centres is £ 235.

5. What is the syllabus for the exam?

Paper 1

Anatomy, Embryology, Statistics and Epidemiology, Endocrinology, Microbiology, Immunology, Pharmacology

Paper 2

Physiology, Pathology, Genetics Biochemistry, Biophysics.

6. Whom should I contact?

Royal College of Obstetricians and Gynaecologists

Website: www.rcog.org.uk

7. What books to read?

Recommended Reading

a. *Basic Science in Obstetrics and Gynaecology– a textbook for the MRCOG Part 1*
   M de Swiet, G Chamberlain and P Bennett
   350 pages–2001 edition–*Price:* £ 34

b. *Basic Sciences for Obstetrics and Gynaecology MCQs (2nd edition)*

Tim Chard
122 pages–1998 edition–*Price:* £ 14.95.

c. *MRCOG: Part 1 MCQs—Basic Science for Obstetrics and Gynaecology*
Khaldown W Sharif, Harry Gee and Martin Whittle
226 pages - 2000 edition–*Price:* £ 18.99.

d. *Part 1 MRCOG Examination Multiple Choice Questions and Answers*
Royal College Publication
40 pages–1995 edition–*Price:* £ 10.

e. *MRCOG: Part 1 MCQ Revision Book*
David Ireland–Pastest
192 pages–1995 edition—*Price:* £ 16.50.

f. *The MRCOG: A Guide to the Examination*
Ian R Johnson, Iain T Cameron, Elizabeth J
pages–2003 edition–*Price:* £ 10.

8. What are the courses available?
1. **Pastest MRCOG Course—London**
   Scheduled to begin in January 2004 for the March exam
   Duration: 5 days, *Course Fee :* £ 600.
2. **Vishwa Medicals Course–Mumbai, India**
   Held approximately two months before every exam
   Duration: 3 days, *Course Fee:* INR 10000
3. **India Education Foundation– Delhi, India**
   Held about 3 months before every exam
   Duration: 6 days, *Course Fee:* INR 7000

MEMBERSHIP OF THE ROYAL COLLEGE OF PAEDIATRICS AND CHILD HEALTH—MRCPCH PART 1 EXAM

1. What is the exam about?
The MRCPCH examination for the Diploma of Membership of the Royal College of Paediatrics and Child Health. It consists of two parts, MRCPCH Part 1and MRCPCH Part 2.

The examination consists of 60 multiple choice questions to be answered in two and a half hours.

Each question consists of an initial stem followed by five statements, each of them being true or false. Candidates are asked to answer T = True, F = false or DK = Don't know. Each correct answer will be awarded a score of (+1), and each DK or incorrect answer will be awarded a score of (0). There is no negative marking for this exam.

2. Eligibility
Candidates will not be permitted to sit Part 1 unless 18 months have elapsed since the date of graduation given on their diploma of medical qualification. There is no limit to the number of attempts to sit the Part 1 examination.

3. Where to take the exam?
The examination can be taken at eight centres in UK and at various centres overseas (not India).

However, registration to take the exam in these centres is limited to doctors working in the same country as the exam centre.

4. What is the fee?
For 2003, the fee to sit the MRCPCH Part 1 examination is £245 in the UK and £330 overseas.

5. What is the syllabus?
Number of Questions from each topic

General paediatrics	7
Nephrology	6
Infectious diseases	5
Metabolic	5
Immunology	4
Growth and Development	4
Cardiology	4
Neurology	4
Respiratory	1
Rheumatology	1
Pharmacology	3
Genetics	3
Gastroenterology	3
Endocrinology	2

Psychiatry	2
Neonates	2
Statistics	1
Haematology	1
Basic Sciences	1
Oncology	1

6. Whom should I contact?

Royal College of Paediatrics and Child Health Examination Department, 50 Hallam Street London W1W 6DE
Tel: 020 7307 5600
Fax: 020 7307 5652
Email: http://www.rcpch.ac.uk/

7. What books to read?

Recommended Reading

a. *400 MCQs for the MRCPCH Part 1*

Nagi G. Barkat-2001 edition–*Price:* £ 15.95

b. *Qbase Paediatrics: MCQs for the MRCPCH*

Sidwell, Thompson-2001 edition–*Price:*£ 23.50.

c. *Extended Match Questions for the PLAB* (Medicbyte MRCPCH Best Seller Series) Asrar Rashid, Vijay—2002 edition–£ 22.50.

d. *MRCPCH part 1 MCQ's with individual chapter summaries*

Mark Beattie—2000 edition–*Price:* £ 16.95.

e. *Essential Revision Notes in Paediatrics for the MRCPCH.*

Beattie, Champion—2002 edition–*Price:* £ 39.95.

8. What are the courses available?

a. *Pastest Course*
Highlights all key topics
5 days–£ 640

b. *Onexamination.com online courses*
Over 900 MCQs
2 months subscription for £ 30

c. *Mcqs.com online.courses*
Over 1000 MCQs
One time access fee of £ 26

d. *123doc.com lecture courses*
Various options in courses
3-4 days–£ 385-495

e. *123doc.com online courses*
Monthly access for £ 22.50

MEMBERSHIP OF ROYAL COLLEGE OF PHYSICIANS OF LONDON, EDINBURGH, GLASGOW AND IRELAND—MRCP PART 1 EXAM

1. What is the exam about?

The MRCP examination consists of two parts and is usually taken during the period of general professional training in medicine, which follows registration in the UK. This period should normally last at least two years.

There are now two papers for the Part 1 examination.

Each paper of the MRCP Part 1 Examination will contain 100 "best of five" format multiple choice questions, where the MRCP 1 candidate must choose the best answer from five possible answers. These questions will test a candidate's knowledge of a wide range of common and important disorders in General Medicine, as set out in the published Syllabus. The candidates will have 3 hours to write each paper.

Score

For each answer, candidates receive a mark of +1 if the answer is correct and no mark will be deducted if the answer is incorrect. Marks will not be awarded for answers in excess of the number required (e.g., where two answers are given in response to a 'Best of Five' question, no marks will be awarded for that question) or where the answersheet is spoiled and unreadable by the optical marking scanner.

Pass Rate

At each session, it is the top 35% of the candidates who pass, regardless of their absolute scores. As a result, it is important that candidates planning to take the examination are aware of their relative level in comparison to other candidates.

2. Eligibility

Candidates will not be permitted to sit Part 1 unless 18 months have elapsed since the date of graduation given on their diploma of medical qualification. There is no limit to the number of attempts to sit the Part 1 examination.

3. Where to take the exam?

The exam can be taken at the following centres in the UK: Belfast, Birmingham, Bristol, Cambridge, Cardiff, Edinburgh, Glasgow, Leeds, Leicester, Liverpool, London, Manchester, Newcastle, Oxford, Sheffield, Southampton.

The MRCP exam can be taken in a number of exam-centres overseas. However, registration to take the exam in these centres is limited to Doctors working in the same country as the exam centre. Manipal, India has recently been incorporated as a centre not for the MRCP but the MRCPI (Ireland) exam.

4. What is the fee?

For 2003, the Fee to sit the Part 1 examination is £275.

5. What is the syllabus?

No. of questions from each topic

Clinical Pharmacology/Therapeutics/Toxicology	20
Cardiology	15
Clinical Haematology/Oncology	15
Endocrinology	15
Gastroenterology	15
Infectious Diseases, Sexually Transmitted Diseases	15
Neurology	15
Psychiatry	15
Respiratory Medicine	15
Rheumatology	15
Dermatology	8
Nephrology	8
Ophthalmology	4
Genetics	3
Cell, Molecular and membrane biology	2
Clinical Anatomy	3
Clinical Physiology	4
Clinical Biochemistry and Metabolism	4
Immunology	4
Statistics, epidemiology and evidence-based medicine	5

6. Whom should I contact?

- *Royal College of Physicians of Edinburgh*
  9 Queen Street, Edinburgh EH2 1JQ
  Tel: (44) 131 225 7324
  Fax: (44) 131 225 2053
  Email: http://www.rcpe.ac.uk

- *Royal College of Physicians and Surgeons of Glasgow*
  242 St. Vincent Street, Glasgow G2 5RJ
  Tel: (44) 141 221 6072
  Fax: (44) 141 248 3414
  Email: http://www.rcpsglasg.ac.uk

- *Royal College of Physicians of London*
  11 St Andrew Place, Regent's Park, London NW1 4LE
  Tel: (44) 20 7935 1174
  Fax: (44) 20 7487 2628
  Email: http://www.rcplondon.ac.uk

- *Royal College of Physicians of Ireland*
  Email: members@rcpi.ie

7. What books to read?

Recommended Reading

a. *Get Through MRCP Part 1: 1000 MCQs and Best of Fives (Get through)*
   Una Coales—2002 edition–£ 19.95

b. *Basic Medical Sciences for MRCP: Part 1*
   Philippa Easterbrook—1999 edition–£ 21.99

c. *500 MCQs for the MRCP Part 1*
Ragavendra Baliga—1997 edition—£ 16.99

d. *MRCP Part 1 Pocket Book series by Pastest*
January 2002 edition–each costing £ 11.50

8. What are the courses available?

a. *Pastest courses*–www.pastest.co.uk
All key topics, pre-and-post-course exams, material
5-6 days—fees in excess of £ 700

b. *Onexamination.com online courses*
Over 2000 MCQs and 'Best of Fives'
2-month access for £ 40

c. *Mcqs.com online courses*
Over 1000 MCQs
One-time access fee of £ 26

d. *123doc.com lecture courses*
Various options of courses
2-6 days—fees ranging from £ 250-600

e. *123doc.com online courses*
Various discount packs
Monthly membership of £ 25

MEMBERSHIP OF THE ROYAL COLLEGE OF SURGEONS OF ENGLAND, EDINBURGH, GLASGOW AND IRELAND—MRCS PART 1 EXAM

1. What is the exam about?

All these exams are known as the MRCS exams except for the Ireland exam, which is the AFRCSI exam–Associate fellow of the Royal College of Surgeons of Ireland. All these exams have different formats. The MRCS Part 1 exam is divided into two MCQ papers–core modules and system modules. As for the AFRCSI exam, here too there are two papers—Basic Sciences (Anatomy, Physiology and Pathology) and Clinical Surgery.

Paper 1 is a True/False type whereas Paper 2 is in the form of taking one of two options—either a, c and e are correct or b and d are correct. Seems easy but the questions are pretty confusing.

From January 2004, the individual College MRCS/AFRCS examinations will be replaced by a new intercollegiate MRCS examination. This will be introduced in phases over the next two years. The individual Colleges will continue to administer the examination as they do today and candidates may continue to apply to the College of their choice; however, the examination they sit will be the same irrespective of the College (or other centre) in which it is held. Candidates may thus continue to apply to the College of their choice, but the examination they sit will be the same.

The first part of the intercollegiate examination to be offered will be a common written examination consisting of two MCQ papers and these will be available from January 2004 onwards. The new intercollegiate MCQ papers will differ in format from the old examination in that the first paper will be entirely on the applied basic sciences and the second paper will be devoted to clinical problem solving. The examinations will also be held simultaneously at all centres at home and overseas.

2. Eligibility

Except for the AFRCSI exam candidates are permitted to apply for the exam once they have started their basic surgical training. One can apply for the AFRCSI exam after completing their pre-registration (Internship) year.

3. Where can I take the exam?

The exam can be taken at various centres in the UK and Dublin and at overseas centres too. The exam cannot be taken in India.

4. What is the fee?

For 2003 the fees for the MRCS exam. is £ 175 and for the AFRCSI exam is Euros 300.

5. What is the syllabus?

1. Preoperative Management
2. Intraoperative Care
3. Postoperative Management

4. Surgical Sepsis and its Prevention
5. Surgical Technique and Technology
6. ***Trauma and Critical Surgical illness—*** General Principles of Management. The applied basic sciences relevant to the clinical assessment of critically ill or severely injured patients and to the understanding of disorders of function caused by trauma, haemorrhage, shock and sepsis.
7. ***Neoplasia:*** The applied basic sciences relevant to the understanding of the clinical behaviour, diagnosis and treatment of neoplastic disease.
8. ***Haemopoietic and Lymphoreticular Systems:*** The anatomy, physiology and pathology of the haemopoietic and lymphoreticular systems appropriate to the understanding of clinical signs and special investigations.
9. The Evaluation of Surgery and General Topics
10. ***The Alimentary System:*** The surgical anatomy of the abdomen and its viscera and the applied physiology of the alimentary system, relevant to clinical examination, to the interpretation of special investigations, to the understanding of disorders of function and to the treatment of abdominal disease.
11. ***Vascular System:*** The surgical anatomy and applied physiology of the vascular system relevant to clinical examination, to the interpretation of special investigations and to the understanding of the disorders of function caused by diseases and injuries of the blood vessels.
12. ***Head and Neck:*** The surgical anatomy, applied physiology and pathology of the head and neck relevant to clinical examination, to the interpretation of special investigations and to the understanding of disorders of function and to the treatment of diseases and injuries involving the head and neck.
13. ***Endocrine System:*** The surgical anatomy, applied physiology and pathology of the endocrine glands relevant to clinical examination, to the interpretation of special investigations, to the understanding of disordered function and to the principles of surgical treatment of common endocrine disorders.
14. ***Breast:*** The surgical anatomy, applied physiology and pathology of the breast
15. ***Respiratory System:*** Heart and Great Vessels: The surgical anatomy and pathology of the heart, great vessels, air passages, chest wall, diaphragm and thoracic viscera.
16. ***The Genito-urinary System:*** The surgical anatomy, applied physiology and pathology of the genito-urinary system, relevant to clinical examination, to interpretation of special investigations, to the understanding of disordered function and to the principles of the surgical treatment of genito-urinary disease and injury.
17. ***Central Nervous System:*** The anatomy and physiology relevant to clinical examination of the central nervous system, to the understanding of its functional disorders, particularly those caused by cranial or spinal trauma, and to the interpretation of special investigations.
18. Locomotor Systems
19. Paediatric Surgery

6. Whom should I contact?

- *Royal College of Surgeons of England* Website: www.rcseng.ac.uk
- *Royal College of Surgeons of Edinburgh* Website: www.rcsed.ac.uk
- *Royal College of Surgeons of Glasgow* Website: www.rcpsglasg.ac.uk
- *Royal College of Surgeons of Ireland* Website: www.rcsi.ie

7. What books to read

Recommended Reading

a. *MRCS Core Modules Essential Revision Notes*
   Sam Andrews—2002 edition—£ 34.95

b. *MRCS System Modules: Essential Revision Notes*
   Smith, Hernon—2000 edition—£ 34.95

c. *MCQs and EMQs for the MRCS*
   Ghnaneim, Benjamin—1999 edition—£ 19.99

d. *MRCS Examination: MCQs and EMQs*
   Chatrath —1999 edition—£ 16.95

e. *MRCS Core Modules Practice Papers*
   Chris Chan—2000 edition—£ 17.95

f. *MCQs for the MRCS/AFRCS*
   Mokbel—2000 edition—£ 12.95

8. What are the courses available?

a. *Pastest course*—www.pastest.co.uk
   Pre course Exam material, Course binder with detailed explanations and Mocks
   2/3-day courses with fees of £ 500-600

b. *Mcqs.com*—www.mcqs.com
   Over 1000 MCQs
   One time access fee of £ 26

c. *Fahmida's course*—www.easyexamltd.com
   £ 150 for a 5-day course

d. *SELECT course*—www.rcsed.ac.uk
   Covers all modules, available in printed or CD format
   £ 200 for books and £ 100 for CD

e. *BEST course*—www.intumed.com
   Comprehensive course for MRCS/AFRCSI
   Euros 1500

MEMBERSHIP OF THE ROYAL COLLEGE OF OPHTHALMOLOGISTS— MRCOPH PART 1 EXAM

1. What is the exam about?

a. *Two multiple-choice question papers each of 60 questions*

Duration: 2 hours each paper

In Paper 1, some of the questions will relate to anatomy of the head and neck, CNS and visual systems, including embryology, and to general and ocular physiology, biochemistry and cell biology.

In Paper 2, some of the questions will relate to general and ocular pharmacology, immunology, general pathology, microbiology, molecular biology, genetics and epidemiology and statistics.

b. *One written paper (12 short questions including problem solving, completion of diagrams etc).*

Duration: 3 hours

2. Eligibility

A medically qualified candidate will be eligible to sit the examination provided that he/she

a. holds a medical qualification approved by the General Medical Council for the purpose of registration, and

b. has completed one year in House Officer posts in medical and surgical specialities.

3. Where to take the exam?

The exam can be taken at various centres in UK and overseas including India—Chennai

4. What is the fee?

For giving the exam in the UK—£ 370
For giving the exam overseas—£ 630

5. What is the syllabus?

a. Anatomy and embryology of the head and neck to include CNS.

b. Specialised anatomy and embryology of the visual system.

c. Ocular and visual physiology.

d. General principles of physiology, genetics, basic statistics, biochemistry, molecular biology, pharmacology, immunology, microbiology and pathology.

6. Whom to contact?

Royal College of Ophthalmologists
www.rcophth.ac.uk

7. What books to read?

Recommended Reading

a. ***The Eye:*** *Basic Sciences and Practice.* Forrester JV, Dick AD, McMenamin P, Lee WR, WB Saunders Ltd, London.

b. ***Adler's Physiology of the Eye.*** Ed Hart WM. Mosby.

c. ***Clinical Anatomy of the Eye***. Snell RS, Lemp MA. Blackwell Scientific Publications.

d. ***Pathology for the Primary FRCS.*** Gardiner DL, Tweedle EF. Arnold Publishers.

e. ***Havener's Ocular Pharmacology.*** Mauger TF, Craig EL. Mosby.

f. ***MCQs in Ophthalmology.*** Vivian A, Manners R. Butterworth-Heinemann.

g. ***MCQs in Basic Science Ophthalmology.*** Ferris J. Foreword by Easty D. BMJ Publishing Group, London.

24 *Clinical Attachments*

◆ *They are not as difficult to acquire as the jobs themselves, but nonetheless, it takes some effort to get a clinical attachment. You will find in the following pages, information on how and where to apply for these.*

CLINICAL ATTACHMENT

A clinical attachment is the association of a novice clinician (junior doctor) with an experienced clinician (consultant) to introduce the novice to a clinical discipline or environment.

The principal purposes of clinical attachments are to provide overseas doctors with experience of NHS health care and an opportunity to gain a reference from a clinician based in the United Kingdom. Overseas doctors gain confidence through clinical attachments and are more likely to pass the Professional Linguistic Assessments Board (PLAB) exam and secure their first post.

The attachment should provide first hand experience of health care in the United Kingdom. The supervisor should be able to assess whether the attached doctor is ready for limited registration to work as a Senior House Officer and provide appropriate constructive feedback throughout the attachment.

For Overseas Doctors, Clinical Attachments

- Provide learning in the NHS and the United Kingdom's medical, legal, and cultural traditions.
- Refresh clinical knowledge and skills
- Are the only ways in which qualified overseas doctors (especially refugees) can get a reference from a British consultant, which is very helpful for getting a job.

For NHS providers, Clinical Attachments

- Are an investment in a medical professional who is likely to join the workforce
- Are an opportunity to attract new doctors into trusts and areas outside the traditional teaching hospital circuit
- Invest in future staff that is likely to stay on permanently (especially refugees and people with permanent residence rights).

FINDING A CLINICAL ATTACHMENT

There is no central organisation that arranges clinical attachments for doctors. Although in 1970s, the GMC did organise clinical attachments for foreign doctors coming into the NHS, it no longer does.

You can arrange a clinical attachment on your own by writing to a hospital consultant or to a hospital medical staffing officer.

Overseas doctors are concentrated in large urban centres in the United Kingdom (probably at least 60% in London, followed by Birmingham, Manchester, and Glasgow), and they are likely to be familiar with the names of the bigger teaching hospitals. According to anecdotal evidence, however, district general hospitals have much to offer. They are less crowded with students and provide a broad exposure to health care, which is better preparation for the PLAB examination. Overseas doctors may be understandably reluctant to move to an unknown area, but district general hospitals with a track record of providing clinical attachments sometimes also provide temporary accommodation.

You can find a list of consultant's names in Dr Foster's Guide to Healthcare services in the UK.

Tel: 0906 190021

Website: www.drfoster.co.uk

Each year the Royal Medical Colleges publish handbooks with names and addresses of their members and fellows. Copies of these handbooks may be found in public libraries.

Writing to Consultant

You have to write to a hospital consultant requesting to spend several weeks on a clinical attachment is his/her department. The consultant may offer you an attachment and ask you to sort out administrative details with the medical staffing office.

Write to a few consultants at a time, wait a few weeks before writing again. If you are unable to take up an offer, write back, thank the consultant and explain why you will not be taking up his offer.

Writing to Hospital

You can write to a hospital's medical staffing officer and ask her to find you a clinical attachment in a hospital. If the hospital offers clinical attachments, she will contact the consultant in the speciality of your interest. If a consultant agrees to supervise you, the medical staffing officer will then tell you how to sort out administrative details.

ETHICAL AND LEGAL CONSIDERATIONS

Medical Indemnity Matters

The supervising doctor is liable for the actions of the attached doctor, as the attached doctor has no indemnity. It is a matter of judgement about what the doctor can be permitted to observe and do. Talking to patients and routine physical examination should be encouraged; performing invasive procedures and intimate physical examinations are best avoided. As with medical students, the patient must give free and informed consent to their involvement in training of any personnel and must be aware that the doctor is not registered to practice in the United Kingdom. With the advent of structured clinical attachments with guidelines for supervision, the medical defense unions may be able to review their position, particularly where the attached doctors have passed the PLAB exam, which indicates eligibility for limited registration in a supervised medical job as an SHO.

Who Pays?

Some trusts in the past have charged all overseas doctors for clinical attachments. But many clinicians have offered excellent clinical attachments for years for no remuneration. If supervisors or their trusts expect to be paid, the risk is that this cost will be transferred to the overseas doctors or the voluntary sector.

PLAB 2 COURSE PROVIDERS

The following course providers arrange for clinical attachments in the UK:

1. PLABWISE—Manchester
2. MEDICBYTE—London
3. NHS RECRUITS—London

25 *Curriculum Vitae*

> ◆ *This is your "sales" document—information about you that allows the selection panel to decide whether you have the skills,* personal attributes, experience, and qualifications for the post being advertised. Let's make sure it is good enough for the recruiters…

A Curriculum Vitae (CV) is a summary of an individual's professional life and work. CV's are also called Career Summaries, Biodata *or* Resume.

Many overseas doctors come from very different cultures and medical systems, where qualifications and "years in post" can be strong factors in appointment. It is a common mistake to think that merely listing experience and qualifications is enough. These days it is not. But with stiff competition the final decision can rest on more generic skills, such as evidence of team working and teaching, which will need to come under an "additional skills" subheading.

Application Forms

Currently, an increasing number of posts have an application form either in addition to or instead of a **CV**. An application form allows the selection panel to have information about candidates in a standardized format, which makes comparisons between candidates easier and also finding relevant information easier. The disadvantage to the candidate is that there is less room for creativity and a greater requirement to be succinct. Application forms also tend to ask more essay-type questions such as "give an example of how you deal with a difficult patient" or "explain a case where you feel you learnt a lot."

This format is considerably more searching than a **CV**, where you are merely listing jobs, procedures, and papers. The answers people give are often much more revealing than they realize.

Get it Edited

Once you have completed your **CV** and/or job application get several people to read through it. Firstly, ask someone who has excellent spelling and grammar to check for mistakes. Secondly, try to find a doctor in your own speciality to read through the documents and point out anything that looks odd or things you could do to improve it.

Some CV "don'ts"

- Do not use the same **CV** for every job application (if you do this, you are not "targeting" appropriately).
- Do not include copious details about schooling on the front page.
- Do not repeat the same information under several job headings.
- Do not write huge paragraphs that is, more than five lines of unbroken text; bullets are better.
- Do not use a chatty style, a **CV** is a professional presentation.
- Do not make grammar and spelling mistakes
- Do not adopt poor chronology. You should start with current jobs and work logically backwards.

- Do not use inappropriate terminology.
- Do not use an inconsistent layout for example, fonts, headings.

STRUCTURE OF A CV

Curricula vitae are as different as the individuals they describe. Nevertheless, they follow common formats. The CV should display personal details, qualifications, career plans, education, work history, other relevant information and hobbies clearly.

1. Personal Details

State your address, telephone number and Email address; Give your full names, Date of birth, Nationality and Sex.

2. Qualifications

State your qualifications (BSc, MBBS, MD, etc); Memberships of professional bodies (MRCP, MRCS, etc.)are included in this section. Passes in Part 1 of various professional examinations should be listed separately and clearly identified as such. Do not claim full qualifications after passing Part 1. In case you are expecting a qualification in the near future, mention it.

3. Career Plans

Briefly state your future plans and how the job will help you achieve them. Your reason for applying for the job should be on the front page in the career plan. Your Career Plan should be short and clear.

There is no need for long paragraphs and personal statements. When the recruiter is short-listing, he wants to know why the candidate wants the job, not what he/she wanted as a teenager.

4. Education

Give the dates, names of addresses of the institutions you attended, courses taken and examinations passed. Outstanding non-academic achievements too should be described briefly with dates.

5. Work History

Give dates, job titles, names of employers, their addresses and your duties and responsibilities. Briefly state your achievements in each position. Employers are interested in what you have done and can do, and not empty years of experience. Also, list your main skills and abilities concisely, e.g., supervising and teaching medical students and Junior House Officers.

6. Research and Publications

If you have done any research and published papers, cite them. If you have contributed chapters to books or written whole books, include them here. List your publications giving names of author(s), title of paper or book, the journal (name, date, volume and pages) or publisher of the book.

Citing a Published Book
Wasim Shaikh PLAB SIMPLIFIED; Jaypee Brothers Medical Publishers (P) Ltd., India - 2003

7. Interests and Hobbies

The purpose of this section is to show that you have life outside medicine. Name and briefly describe your hobbies and leisure activities.

8. Additional Information

This is the where you may state other information you wish the recruiter to know, but could not fit into other sections.
- General and professional courses you have attended, or are attending
- Special professional, linguistic, technical skills, etc.

9. Referees

These are people who know you socially, from university or college or from work who are able and willing to commend you to a new employer. Ask them if they would be willing to act as referees.

List the names, addresses, telephone and fax numbers of two or three people who have agreed to support you with regards to your character and skills.

PROFESSIONAL HELP

1. www.plabwise.co.uk
2. www.medicbyte.com
3. www.fischtest.co.uk

PRINTING CV'S

This aspect is something which not many would have thought about...

A reminder again, that each of your CV's should be tailored to the paticular post, and photocopying the same CV and sending it to various recruiters would be detrimental.

Let's consider that during your quest for getting a job, you send about 25 new applications per week. Each application requires an average of around 3 CV's and each CV is—say 4 pages.

This means you will be printing $25 \times 3 \times 4 = 300$ pages/week.

A print out in any cyber in the UK will cost you around 20 p, so you will be spending £ 60 a week or £ 240 a month!!! Hunting for a job for 4 months you will be spending around £ 1000 on print-outs. Apart from this you should consider your monthly expenses on computer and internet access to search for jobs—around £ 30.

Now consider this: You buy a second-hand laptop for £ 400, a laser printer for £ 200 and 10 bundles of 500 pages each for £ 50; a total of £ 650 is what you will be spending for four months—this way you would have a laptop to yourself, and you can always plug it into a telephone cable wherever you stay. You would be saving at least £ 100 a month on computer and internet access. (Internet access through land phone is £15 pounds a month for unlimited access—check www.bt.com)

Therefore, if you really want to cut down on your expenses for printing out CV's, think of the above option!

26 *Useful Courses*

> ◆ *Apart from helping you in obtaining a job, these courses will also enhance your clinical knowledge and skills. Find here, information on their contents, fees and application process.*

1. BASIC SURGICAL SKILLS COURSE

The Royal College of Surgeons of Edinburgh runs eight basic Surgical Skills Courses per year in the College. Courses are also run at several centres overseas including India (Mumbai).

The course has now become mandatory for those taking the MRCS exam. The course runs over 3 days and costs £ 495, which includes all course material, lunches and refreshments.

Day 1

Theatre gowning; basic instrument skills; knot tying and tissue handling; skin incision and suturing; dissection techniques; intestinal anastomosis.

Day 2

Vascular anastomosis; tendon repair, debridement; principles of fracture management; plastering techniques.

Day 3

Introduction to minimal access surgery. Before the course each participant receives a detailed course manual and video to introduce the main topics covered.

For further details see www.rcsed.ac.uk
To register in India Contact:
Professor Gautam Sen FRCSEd,
Secretary ICRCSEd,

51 Jupiter Apts,
Cuffe Parade,
Mumbai 600 005
Tel: 91 22 2282 4479/
Fax: 91 22 22188864/
Email: drgsen@vsnl.com

2. EARLY TRAUMA AND CRITICAL CARE COURSE

This **two-day** course is designed to cover the aspects of emergency care that basic Surgical Trainees need to know.

It focuses on problems that trainees are likely to meet and the skills that they will actually need to manage them. This course is held only in the UK.

The course is divided into two days. The first day covers early trauma management and resuscitation. The second day consists of the management of the day-to-day critical care problems that the trainee faces.

The format of the course is a series of lectures covering early trauma care and critical care. Skill stations appropriate to the lecture follow these. A manual covering the lectures and skill stations is supplied.

The course is a strongly recommended component of Basic Surgical Training and fulfils College requirements in the area of trauma and critical care.

The course costs £ 485 that includes course fees, course dinner, lunches and refreshments.

For further details and to apply for the course go to www.rcsed.ac.uk.

3. MASTERING CLINICAL AUDIT COURSE—ONLINE

This is a new online course, which is run by the University of Edinburgh Office of Lifelong Learning.

The aim of the course is to provide participants with the understanding and skills to promote and conduct effective multi-professional clinical audit

The emphasis of the course is on the skills to do audit. The emphasis is on 'how to do audit' rather than 'why audit?'

Participants can do different modules of the course over a period of 28 days. Modules can be repeated if necessary.

Each module comprises:

1. Slide presentation with audio and corresponding textual commentary.
2. Intermittent multiple-choice questions with feedback of correct responses and previous participants responses.
3. 'My Audit'. Opportunity for participants by answering simple questions to build their own audit.

The course costs £ 95 and at the end of the course you will receive an embossed certificate from the University of Edinburgh.

For more details visit
www.clinicalaudit.mvm.ed.ac.uk

4. CLINICAL GOVERNANCE—HEALTH INFORMATICS—ONLINE

The University of Bath in association with the University of Edinburgh conducts this course.

The aim of this course is to provide healthcare professionals with quality training in order to achieve the nationally and internationally described competencies in health informatics.

This module provides a brief introduction to the philosophy and scope of activities encompassed by Clinical Governance. The module commences with a definition of the term and then expands on the following aspects of practice:

- Risk Management
- Needs Assessment
- Clinical Audit
- Evidence Based Practice
- Professional Development

Assessment will take place at the end of each module, usually in the form of a multiple-choice questionnaire. Students will receive feedback on their performance.

The cost of the course is £ 60.

For further details log on to
www.healthcare-informatics.info

5. MEDICAL INTERVIEW TEACHING ASSOCIATION

The course offers Practice of communication and teaching communication skills with access to patients, students, patient-simulators (actors) and videos.

The cost is £495 inclusive of meals and refreshments during the course times and supper on the first day.

Contact person:
Lesley Millard, MITA Hon. Sec.,
1, Summerlands Cottage, Botley Road,
Curdridge,
Southampton, SO32 2DS, UK
Phone: 07815 765355
Email: ajm56@tutor.open.ac.uk
Website: www.mita.soton.ac.uk/mita

6. FUNDAMENTAL CRITICAL CARE SUPPORT COURSE

"A two-day comprehensive course addressing fundamental management principles for the first 24 hours of critical care."

Topics include:

- Mechanical Ventilation I & II

- Basic Trauma and Burn Management
- Hemodynamic Monitoring
- Neurologic Support
- Diagnosis and Management of Shock
- Management of Life-threatening Electrolyte and Metabolic Disturbances
- Myocardial Ischaemia and Infarction
- Life-threatening Infections

The course is held worldwide and has been conducted twice in India in Jaipur.

The fees for the course in India are INR 3500 and the course lasts 2 days.

To register contact:
Indian Society of Critical Care Medicine, Jaipur branch
Course Director: Narendra Rungta MD
Course Coordinator: Shri R. S. Mittal
Phone: 91 1412 525684/ Fax: 91 1412 524082
Email: drnrungta@yahoo.com
Website: www.sccm.org

7. HOUSE OFFICER INDUCTION COURSE

All non-UK doctors (from within or outside the EEA), refugee or not, should be encouraged to go on an International Doctors' Induction Course. These are short courses (2-5 days) run throughout England by the Postgraduate Medical Deaneries. They are completely free (accommodation and travel are paid) and open to all doctors who have passed PLAB Part 2 and are eligible for the GMC registration.

The aim of the induction is to introduce non-UK doctors to the culture of the NHS, and the courses are suitable for doctors looking for posts, about to begin their first post, or already in post. In addition to providing guidance about living in the UK and working in the NHS, it gives delegates an opportunity to reinforce their clinical and communication skills.

Individual hospital trusts may also offer their own induction course for overseas doctors, and possibly a period of work shadowing.

Information about such courses can be obtained from the *Postgraduate Centre Manager* at the hospital concerned.

Information about this course can be obtained from
NHS Professionals 0845 120 3146 or email lyndsay.towers@wymas.nhsprofessionals.nhs.uk.

8. PG DIPLOMA IN ACCIDENT AND EMERGENCY—ONLINE

1. Online study along with printed study material for 6 months.
2. Practical training with logbook for one month at Emergency Department in a hospital located near to you and approved by Medvarsity.

Eligibility: MBBS Doctors registered with Medical Council of India.

Duration: 6 months (including practical training)

The course deals with important emergencies in the following areas:
1. Organization of Emergency Medicine Dept., Disaster preparedness and management.
2. Management of Cardiac, Respiratory, Neurologic emergencies.
3. Dealing with Surgical, Obstetrical, ENT and Paediatrics emergencies.
4. Management of shock burns.
5. Management of environmental emergencies.
6. Anaesthesia and mechanical ventilation.

The course costs INR 17000 or INR 20000 paid in installments.

For further information log on to
www.medvarsity.com

9. IMMEDIATE TRAUMA LIFE SUPPORT COURSE

Organised on the lines of the internationally acclaimed advanced trauma life support (ATLS) course this 3 day course, though not very useful in improving your chances of getting a job, will be a sound addition to your Trauma Management skills. By far the stress will be on hands on training of the delegates on models and animal torsos. Each delegate will perform all major emergency procedures listed below:

Endotracheal, Intubation, Cricothyroidotomy, Tracheostomy, Central Venous Cannulation, Venous cut down, Pericardiocentesis, Diagnostic peritoneal lavage, Intercostal drainage, Cardio-pulmonary resuscitation

The course is conducted at the Ernakulam Medical Centre in Kochi, Kerala and the fees for the course is INR 2500, which includes the course dinner, lunches and refreshments.

To register contact:
Dr.C.G. Raghu MS FRCS, Course Director,
Ernakulam Medical Centre, N.H Bypass,
Cochin-682 028
Phone: 91-484-2807101 to 109/
Fax: 91-484-2805011
Email: ernmed@vsnl.com/
Website: www.emccochin.com

10. NATIONAL TRAUMA MANAGEMENT COURSE

National Trauma Management Course is an authentic course on acute trauma management, being organized in India.

This two-day course consists of core content lectures, case presentations, discussions, development of life saving skills, practical laboratory experience and a final performance proficiency evaluation. There will also be a voluntary post course test.

The Course costs INR 2000.
Contact:
Dr.Harsh Shah
Email: contact@indiatrauma.org

11. EUROPEAN COMPUTER DRIVING LICENSE

At the core of the modernisation of the NHS is the use of information systems and new techno-

logy to help patients receive the best possible care and make informed decisions on their own treatment. New information systems, access to e-mail and online services, and 24 hour access to electronic patient records (EPR) means the need for a workforce that is skilled in the use of lT.

The NHS Information Authority (NHSIA) has been commissioned to implement a basic IT skills reference standard for all staff employed by the NHS in England—the European Computer Driving License (ECDL).

For an individual to gain accreditation for the ECDL, they have to complete seven modules. Each module has been designed to be free standing so training can be delivered in any order. Participants will be awarded the ECDL qualification when they have passed a test at the end of each module. The test includes one theoretical test and six practical tests that must be taken at an accredited test centre.

Modules of the ECDL
* Basic concepts of IT
* Using the computer and managing files
* Word processing
* Spreadsheets
* Data base
* Presentation
* Information and communication.

The International version of the ECDL is known as the International Computer Driving License (ICDL), and can be taken in various countries including India.

The total cost of the seven modules is 105 euros.

For more information, contact
Mr.Gunaseelan/Mr.Murthy
FourthR India
Email: fourthr@fourthrindia.com
Tel: 044-28229533 / 28267745/
28200108 / 28200110

27 Audit, Research and Presentations

> ◆ These days a lot of emphasis is given on the above when considering the eligibility of a candidate for a particular job. You need to get at least one of them under your belt before you apply.

CLINICAL AUDIT

Basically, an audit means to account for, to balance, check, examine, to verify something against expectations, what should have been done.

Clinical audit is the review of clinical performance, the refining of clinical practice as a result and the measurement of performance against agreed standards—a cyclical process of improving the quality of clinical care.

The Audit Cycle

What should be happening? What is happening? ↑ ↓

What changes are needed?

↑ ↓

← ← ← ←

NICE States That:

"Clinical Audits monitor the use of particular interventions, or the care received by patients, against agreed standards. Any departures from 'best practices' can then be examined in order to understand and act upon the causes."

Clinical audit aims to lead to an improvement in the quality of service providing:

- Improved care of patients
- Enhanced professionalism of staff
- Efficient use of resources
- Aid to continuing education
- Aid to administration.

STEPS IN CLINICAL AUDIT

Step 1

Identifying problems, choosing a topic
Choose a subject that you consider to be important or significant.

Ways of spotting audit topics	Examples
Important clinical events	Admissions for asthma
"Significant events"	Patient died of MI—no record of smoking history or BP
Patients' complaints	Too long to get an appointment
Observation	No system for ensuring bag drugs up-to-date
NICE subjects	Post-MI patients on aspirin

Tips

- Choose something that interests you.
- Check with others that would be involved with making changes—do they agree with your proposal? This is important—you won't get changes made if you don't carry people with you from the start.
- There's no point in auditing something that you think is already being done well–you will find plenty of problems that need to be sorted out first!

Step 2

Setting Priorities

You may come up with a number of possible subjects to audit.

To help yourself prioritise, ask yourself:
- Is the problem common?
- Does it have serious consequences?
- Can I do something about it?

Step 3

Setting the Criterion

"An audit criterion is a specific statement of what should be happening."

Example: "All eligible women aged 25 to 65 should have had a cervical smear in the last 5 years."

Tips

- Make sure that there is evidence for your criterion—do a literature search.
- Ensure that the criterion is measurable "asthmatics should have had yearly PFs" is difficult to measure (how many years will you go back?); "asthmatics should have had a PF recorded in the past year" is more practical.
- For the quickest results, make sure that what you are doing is fairly easy to measure, e.g., is Read-coded, though don't let other data-gathering methods put you off if you you're really interested in the subject

Step 4

Setting Standards

"An audit standard is a minimum level of acceptable performance for that criterion."

Example: "At least 80 per cent of eligible women aged 25 to 65 should have had a cervical smear in the last 5 years."

The standard should reflect the clinical and medico-legal importance of the criterion.

- In the example above, 80 per cent of women should have had a cervical smear.
- But of those who've had an abnormal smear, 100 per cent should have had action taken.

Tips

- Some criteria are so important that they need 100 per cent standard.
- However, 100 per cent standards are unusual—patients or circumstances usually conspire against perfection and the standard needs to reflect that.

Step 5

Comparing Results with Standards

Example:

Criteria	Standards	Results
All eligible women aged 25-65 should have had a cervical smear in the last 5 years	Minimum 80%	55%

Step 6

Introducing Change

Medical audit shows what changes are needed—it isn't a method for changing care; actually making the changes is the most difficult part of audit!

Actions to Remedy Identified Deficiencies

- Emphasise what has been achieved.
- What are we proud of?
- What are we not so proud of?
- How can we correct any deficiencies?

Changes Must be Practical!

How are you actually going to make the changes?
- Simply saying "We've got to do better" won't result in change.
- You need to think through in detail—what needs to be done, which's going to do it, when, and how.

Step 7

Reauditing

You need to choose a suitable time period when you would like to reaudit. This is to make sure that the changes you have introduced have had an effect.

RESEARCH

Research means 'to search for information'. It is very different from an audit. In an audit, you know what is the best way to do something, whereas in a research you are trying to find out what is the best way to do something.

For most clinicians, research involves looking for answers from clinical problems. Published authors are well regarded by their colleagues. They make presentations at scientific meetings, publish articles in journals and chapters in learned books.

Doing research gives you the opportunity to learn the science of medical enquiry and the opportunity to differentiate your CV.

Details of research are beyond the remit of this book.

PUBLICATIONS

As mentioned in the CV section, publications do a world of good in enhancing your CV's.

Your publications may be:
- A book you have authored
- Contributions to chapters in a book
- Articles in journals
- Articles in magazines.

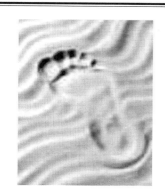

Section *Five*

Heading for the United Kingdom— the Nuts and Bolts

28 About the UK

> ◆ I will include in this chapter, information on those aspects about the UK which could make that little difference in making the transition from here to there, as smooth as possible.

MAP OF UNITED KINGDOM

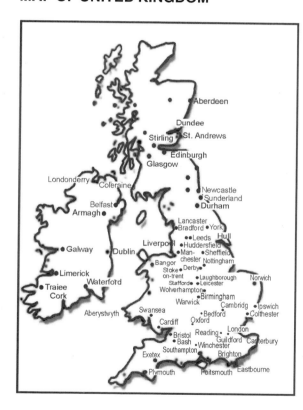

Fig. 28.1: Map of United Kingdom

England dominates both the political entity that is the United Kingdom and the geographical entity that is the island of Great Britain. Although the Scots and the Welsh made an enormous contribution to the British Empire, it was, and in some ways remains, an English empire.

GEOGRAPHY

Enveloping over 50000 square miles, England is the largest of the three political divisions within the island of Great Britain. England is no more than 32 kilometres from France across the narrowest part of the English Channel. England can be divided into a number of geographical areas—London is in the southeast of the country, on the River Thames.

CLIMATE

Climatologists classify England's climate as temperate maritime—mild and damp. Despite the country being in the north, temperatures in England are moderated by light winds that blow in from seas warmed by the Gulf Stream. In winter this stops the inland temperature from falling below 0 degree celsius and in summer, it keeps the temperature below 30 degree celsius. The typical high in London from June to August is 21 degree celsius and the average low is 12 degree celsius. It tends to be colder in the north but not as cold as in Scotland.

Rainfall is greatest in the hilly areas and in the west of the country. Some areas receive up to 4500 mm of rain every year. You can, however, expect some cloudy weather and rain anywhere in England, at anytime. An umbrella or a raincoat is suggested. Once you have seen the blue skies suddenly cloud over and a gloomy day-long downpour begin, you will understand why London, Manchester and other English cities have so many chartered flights to Ibiza, Tenerife and other hot spots!

GOVERNMENT AND POLITICS

At present, the United Kingdom does not have a written constitution, but operates under a mixture of parliamentary statutes, common law and convention. The Parliament is made up of three separate elements—the Queen, the House of Lords, and the House of Commons. In practice, the supreme body is the House of Commons, which is the only one to be elected directly every five years.

POPULATION AND PEOPLE

Britain has a population of around 60 million, or around 625 inhabitants per square mile, making it one of the most crowded islands on the planet. Most of the populace is concentrated in and around London.

EDUCATION

Schooling is compulsory for those aged between 5 and 16, and an increasing number of young people stay on at school until they are 18. For those aged up to 18, education is free.

SOCIETY AND CONDUCT

It is intricate to generalise about the British and their culture, but there is no doubt that they are creative, energetic and aggressive people who have had an impact on the world that is entirely out of proportion to their numbers.

The British are reasonably tolerant and it is not particularly easy to cause offense (without meaning to). All said, it is as well to be aware that most locals would no sooner speak to a stranger in the street than fly to the moon. If you are obviously a tourist battling with directions, there is no problem—but try starting a general conversation at the bus stop and people will stare at you as if you are nuts!

CLOTHING

England is relaxed about how you dress in the street or in churches, for that matter. Some classy restaurants and many clubs operate strict dress codes. In restaurants, it usually means a jacket and a tie for men. In clubs, it can vary from night to night.

AIRPORT CUSTOMS

On entering the UK, if you have nothing to declare go through the Green channel; if you may have something to declare, then go through the red channel. If you are arriving from another European Union (EU) country, go through the Blue channel. For goods purchased at airports outside the EU, you are allowed to import 200 cigarettes or 250 g of tobacco, 2L of wine + 1L of spirits over 22%, 50 g of perfume, 250 cc of toilet water, and other duty-free goods to the value of £ 136 (INR 10000)

TIME

The British Summer Time (BST) muddies the water so that even Britain itself is ahead of Greenwich Mean Time (GMT) by one hour from late March to late October. For the rest of the year, the British time coincides with the GMT. To give you a further idea, India is 5 ½ hours ahead of GMT.

CURRENCY

The British currency is the pounds sterling, which is divided into 100 pence (p). Coins of 1 p and 2 p are copper, 5 p, 10 p, 20 p and 50 p coins are silver; and the bulky £ 1 coin is gold-coloured. The £ 2 coin is gold coloured on the edge with a silver centre. Notes come in £ 5, £ 10, £ 20 and

£ 50 denominations. The £ 50 notes can be difficult to change—avoid them.

Remember to check the exchange rates when heading for the UK.

OTHER CURRENCY MATTERS

Cash

Nothing can beat cash for convenience—or risk. However, it is a good idea to carry some cash in sterling £. You can land sterling—less at any English airport; they usually have good value exchange counters open for incoming flights.

Travellers Cheques

They offer protection from theft. Ideally your cheque should be in £ and preferably issued from American Express or Thomas Cook, which are widely recognised, well represented, and do not charge anything for cashing their own cheques. Bring most cheques in large denominations. Traveller's cheques are rarely accepted outside banks or used for everyday transactions in England so you need to cash them in advance.

Keep a record of the numbers of your cheques and which cheques you have cashed, even if they are lost or stolen, you will be able to tell the issuing agency where exactly the cheques are gone. Keep this list separate from the cheques themselves.

As soon as you realise that the cheques are missing, you should contact the issuing office or the nearest branch of the issuing agency.

American Express: Tel—029 2066 6111
Thomas Cook: Tel—01733 318 950

These will arrange replacement cheques for you within 24 hours.

ATM Cards

Debit cards are widely linked internationally. Credit cards may not be hooked up to ATM networks unless you specifically ask them to do so. You have to ask your local bank regarding which UK bank ATM's will accept your card, and whether you will be charged a fee to use them.

Credit Cards

Visa, MasterCard, AMEX and Diners Club cards are widely accepted in England, although small businesses such as B & B prefer cash. Businesses sometimes make a charge for accepting payment by credit card so this is not always the cheapest way to go.

If a card is lost or stolen, you must inform the police and the issuing company as soon as possible.

Visa: Tel: 0800 895082
Master Card: Tel: 01702 362988

International Transfers

If you instruct your bank back home to send you a draft, make sure you specify the bank and the branch to which you want your money directed. Money sent by telegraphic transfer should reach you within a week, by mail—allow two weeks. The charge for converting it to local currency would be around £ 20. You can also transfer money using AmEx or Thomas Cook or MoneyGram.

Money Changers

Changing your money is never a problem in the major cities, with banks, bureau de change and travel agencies all competing for your business. Just make sure you get the best deal possible.

TIPPING AND BARGAINING

Many restaurants now add a 'discretionary' service charge to your bill, but in places they do not, you are expected to leave a 10 per cent tip unless the service was unsatisfactory. Taxi drivers also expect a tip of 10 per cent, especially in London.

Bargaining is virtually unheard of, even at markets, although it is fine to ask if there are discounts for students, young people or youth hostel members. Some 'negotiation' is acceptable if you are buying an expensive item such as a car or a motorcycle.

POST

Although the queues in the post offices can be long, the Royal Mail delivers a competent service. Most post offices are open from 9 am to 5 pm. A first-class mail reaches anywhere in the UK the next day and costs 28 p whereas a second-class mail takes 2 days and costs 20 p. These are charges for standard documents less than 60 g.

TELEPHONE

To call England from abroad, dial your country's international access code (00 for India), followed by 44 (UK's country code), then the area code (dropping the initial 0), followed by the phone number.

British Telecom's famous red boxes survive only in conservation areas. Most common these days are the glass cubicles with phones that accept coins, prepaid phone cards and/or credit cards.

British Telecom (BT) offers phone cards for £ 2, £ 5, £ 10 and £ 20 that are extensively available from all sorts of retailers. A digital display on the telephone indicates how much credit is left on the card.

To install a land telephone at the place you stay, just call up the British Telecom and they will arrange for a connection in a weeks time for as little as £ 15.

When making an international call, for most countries it is cheaper to make a call between 8 pm and 8 am Monday to Friday and at weekends.

There is a wide range of local and international phone cards. International Student Travel Card Holders can avail of overseas calls at discounted rates (cost for a call to India—70 p per minute).

For more information visit their website www.isic.org.

There is also the U-turn card—buy 3 for ten £ and you can get an international talk time of about 28 minutes on each card—easy on the pocket!

MOBILE PHONES

England uses GSM 900/1800, which is compatible with the rest of Europe and Australia, but not with the North American GSM 1900 or that of India. So, if you do have any mobile in India that is not tri-band, do not get it to the UK.

If you want the convenience of a mobile in England, the simplest solution would be to buy one of the pay as you talk phones sold in the plethora of high-street shops. For just under £ 70, you get a phone with a descent amount of talk time and your own telephone number. All four major mobile companies in England—Orange, Vodaphone, One 2 One and BT Cellnet—have variations on this scheme.

OWNING A CAR IN THE UK

Once you get an appropriate job, you will find that a car is imperative in the UK. It is a lot economical than the various modes of public transport available.

Two magazines *The Loot* and *Autotrader* form a vital source of information for those in quest of a car. They offer a huge data-base of second-hand cars, and you could get a fitting vehicle not more than 5 years old for around £ 1000. You should, however, make sure that you get a car that is in good condition. For someone coming from overseas, identifying the condition of a foreign car would certainly be a big ask. In these situations, you can approach a number of auto consultants who charge about £ 50 to £ 100 for a comprehensive check-up of a car, but at least they make sure you get a good deal.

All cars require a MOT (Ministry of Transport)

safety certificate valid for one year and issued by a licensed garage, full third party insurance (around £ 300), a registration form signed by the buyer and seller and a proof of VED (Vehicle Excise Duty) which costs about £ 82. You are strongly advised to buy a car, which has all these documents.

ELECTRICITY

The standard voltage throughout England and Britain is 240V AC, 50 Hz. Plugs have three-square pins and adapters are widely available.

LAUNDRY

Almost every high street boasts of a launderette where you have a number of washing machines. You just dump the clothes in with a little of soap powder. On an average, the cost for a single load is about £ 2 to £ 3.

TOILETS

Those at train stations, bus terminals and motorway service stations are good quality. At some, you will have to pay a charge of 20 p, but you can be confident that they will be clean.

NEWSPAPERS AND MAGAZINES

Breakfasts are never dull in the UK, with a number of dailies to choose from—*The Sun, The Mirror, The Daily Star* and so on. Leaving behind newspapers in tubes and trains in the mornings is considered as public service. In the evenings, it is just garbage!

England boasts of magazines catering to almost any interest—*Time Out* being one of the most popular, especially for tourists.

INTERNET ACCESS

You will find not as many cyber café's in the UK as they are in India. The usual surfing charge is £ 1 to £ 2 per hour. However, as mentioned before, if you take an internet connection from the British Telecom in the place you stay, you can surf unlimited for £ 15 a month.

WOMEN TRAVELLERS

Apart from the occasional wolf-whistle on the London underground aside, women will find England reasonably enlightened. Some restaurants persist in assigning the table by the toilet to lone female diners, but places like this are becoming fewer by the year.

Solo travellers should have a few troubles, if common sense is observed. Hitching is always unwise.

EMERGENCIES

The National Emergency Services number in the UK is 999. It is good for police, fire and medical emergencies.

29 *Before Travelling*

◆ *You don't just pass your Part 1 and take the next available flight to Heathrow. There are a number of things that have to be considered before traversing that distance...*

1. BANK ACCOUNTS

Although there are not many problems in attaining a visa to travel to the UK as it is in getting one for the US, a few documents are essential in satisfying the visa officials. Details about these can be found in the chapter on 'Visa formalities'. One of the most imperative of these documents is a proof that you have sufficient funds to support yourself during your stay in the UK. Evidence in support of this could be your salary certificate, income tax returns, and letter from a sponsor in the UK or your bank statement.

Therefore, it is important for you to show ample funds in your account for a good period—say six months. Deposits in the months preceding your travel, could make the visa officials apprehensive. It is, therefore, best to have an account with funds of over £ 2000 for at least six months.

It is a very thorny and cumbersome process to open an account in the UK without any introducer. Therefore, you should also be selective in choosing the bank you have your account in your home country. Having an account in Banks such as HSBC and Citibank would enable you to transfer your account to their branches in the United Kingdom. The ICICI Banking Corporation would have started their branches in the UK by the time you are reading this book.

Recommended: *6 months before travel or earlier.*

2. HEPATITIS VACCINATION

This is not an obligation prior to entering the UK, but before being given a job, you will have to undergo a Hepatitis B and C test to prove that you are free of these viral illnesses. It is desirable to take the three doses required for the vaccination of Hepatitis B if you have not already taken them. Also, get a Hepatitis B and Hepatitis C antibody test done, just to make sure that all the effort and travel that you are going to put in will not be in vain.

Recommended: *6 months before travel or earlier.*

3. INTERNATIONAL STUDENT/YOUTH TRAVEL CARD

Provided by the International Student Travel Federation, this card is crucial before traveling to the UK, or for a traveller to any country for that matter. Endorsed by the UNESCO, this card provides cheap or free admission to museums and sights, inexpensive meals in some restaurants and discounts on many forms of transport. More importantly, you can get a heavy discount on your air ticket if you travel by the Emirates Airlines, which have collaborated with the Student Travel Federation.

To avail of the International Student Travel Card (ISTC), all you need is a College identity card which states that you are a full time student (even postgraduate), a passport copy, two photographs and a duly filled and signed application form which you can download from the ISTC website.

If you are not a full time student but are aged under 26, you are entitled for the International Youth Travel Card (IYTC) provided by the same federation. The number of discounts offered is, however, less than the ISTC. You will need to provide the documents listed above except for the identity card. Your passport copy will be the proof of your age.

There is also an International Teacher Travel Card that is available for those Teachers who are engaged in full-time employment at any registered institution.

The ISIC and the IYTC also provide you with the benefit of making International Calls at discounted rates by their service known as the ISIC connect. Calls made through the ISIC from the UK to India would cost 70 pence a minute.

For further details, you can refer to their website www.isic.com

Recommended: *5 months before travelling.*
Cost: £ 5 or INR 200
Contact: www.isicweb.net—search for an office close to you or contact STIC travels in your city.

4. MEMBERSHIP OF YOUTH HOSTELLING ASSOCIATION

If you are travelling on a budget, which most of the plabbers do, Membership of the International Youth Hostelling Association (IYHA) or Hostelling International (HI) could prove beneficial. There are over 200 hostels in England and members are eligible for all sorts of discounts.

On applying, along with the membership card, you will also receive a booklet, which will provide you with details of all youth hostels in Europe and the discounts and facilities offered. This card will serve as a useful escort to you when travelling for interviews, exams and courses. On an average, you will be able to get a respectable and secure room for £ 10 per day including breakfast.

For travellers from India, this card will also prove useful in obtaining discounts at youth hostels, which are located in all the major cities of India. Details about their locations will be provided in the accompanying booklet.

Recommended: *5 months before travelling*
Price: £ 12 or Rs.300 per year.
Contact: www.yha.org.uk

5. APPLY FOR PLAB PART 2
Recommended: *5 months before exam date*

6. APPLY FOR PLAB PART 2 COURSE/ SPONSORSHIP SCHEME
Recommended: *4 months before*

7. BOOKING YOUR TICKET
Once you have received a letter from the GMC confirming your test date, do not waste anytime before you book your ticket. Booking does not mean purchasing the ticket. You are entitled to block a seat on the day you wish to travel without having to pay anything.

There are various options available in booking your tickets. The airline you travel by depends on which city you are intending to travel to, the common choices being London and Manchester. Candidates who have travelled earlier had the false notion that a return ticket is required on a PLAB visa. This is not true—if you have the required documents to prove to them that you have the funds to support yourself while in the UK and to purchase a return ticket, no one can stop you from buying a one-way ticket. Candidates purchasing a return ticket would invariably find themselves losing a significant amount of money because most of them would not return within the stipulated time of four months.

Emirates Airlines
The Skytrax airline of the year for the last few

years. It is also the cheapest option thanks to its partnership with the International Student Travel Federation. You can book your flight from Mumbai/ Delhi/ Chennai/ Kochi/ Hyderabad to London or Manchester via Dubai. The one-way fare would be in the order of INR 21000 including taxes. The halt in Dubai would be for about 1 to 2 hours, but, having stayed in Dubai for 17 years, I would suggest you to allow yourself a day or two in this extraordinary tourist destination. The Emirates Airlines allows you the chance to see the sights of Dubai for 2 days for just INR 2500 including star accommodation with breakfast, visa and airport pick-up and drop. You can add another INR 2500 for luxury travel and for an assortment of scrumptious food in the Food capital of the World.

Air India
This is for the patriotic ones who say, 'When you fly to or from India, fly Air India.' The only advantage that this airline offers is a direct flight from Mumbai/Delhi/Bangalore to London and so will be favourable for single travellers who have never travelled alone. However, the standard of service provided is far less than the Emirates Airlines or Lufthansa, and a one-way fare to London would be around INR 29000 all-inclusive.

Lufthansa
This highly reputed German airline has recently started direct flights from Bangalore/Chennai/ Mumbai/Delhi to Frankfurt with convenient connections to all major cities in the UK. The one-way fare would be the same as the Air India.

Other options would be those of the British Airways, Gulf Air, Sri Lankan Airlines, KLM, Swiss Airlines and Royal Jordanian Airlines. These, however, are either too costly or travel around the world before they reach the UK.

Recommended: *4 months before travelling*

8. DRIVING LICENSE
This forms a very important content of your wallet. Once you get a job, you will find that having a car would be very convenient and also cheaper than the expensive tubes, trains, buses and other forms of public transport in the UK. Your normal Driving License obtained in your country is valid for 12 months from the date you last entered the United Kingdom; you can then apply for a driving license at British post offices. The International Driving Permit, though not an absolute essential, is recommended. It can be obtained at your local Transport Authority office for INR 500 to 1000.

Recommended: *3 months before travelling*

9. TRAVEL INSURANCE
You have to make sure you take out a comprehensive travel insurance policy that covers you for medical expenses and luggage theft or loss and for cancellation or delays in your travel arrangements. There are all sorts of policies, but the international student travel policy handled by STA travel, Thomas Cook and other student travel organisations are usually of good value. Paying for your ticket with a credit card often provides limited travel accident insurance, and you may be able to reclaim the payment if the operator does not deliver.

Recommended: *2 months before travelling*

10. SHOPPING
As mentioned before, the British are not very strict in adopting any finicky dress sense. However, the following are a few guidelines on what kind of attire to carry along:
- Most importantly, carry as little as possible, a little more than the bare minimum requirements. Airlines would not permit a checked luggage of more than 25 kgs and hand luggage of more than seven kgs.
- 1 Executive suit, preferably a branded one—like Louis Phillippe or Van Heussen for men; and Allen Solly for women would take care of the PLAB Part 2 exam and any short-listing interviews that you may have to attend. This

would cost you more than INR 4000, but believe me; it is worth buying one of them.

- For your Clinical Attachments, you will need a few formal wears. About five pairs would be useful. Buy them such that you can wear them in different combinations.
- Apart from these, a couple pair of jeans, few T-shirts and shorts would be sufficient.
- Thermal wear is an absolute must, and it is worth spending a hefty amount on them. Choose the ones that are also rainproof. One thick jacket and one jersey would do. Thermal undergarments will also prove useful in winters!
- A pair of goggles would do you many good if you are travelling during the summer time that is June to October.
- One pair of formal shoes and one pair of sneakers or sandals.
- A good branded but mild cologne for your interviews and exams, even otherwise!
- If you have space in your suitcase, you could add supersaver shampoos, soaps, shaving foam, and other cosmetics. If not, you can buy them for a little higher price in the UK. You might take all this stuff and think that you would not be spending on them in the UK, but in the meantime your luggage would cross the 25 kg mark and you could end up paying the airline 2000 bucks.
- A couple of things, which though would seem very costly, are recommended. Firstly, a laptop computer and secondly a laser printer. Nevertheless, because of the problems in customs, it would be better to buy them in the UK and you would not be paying more there.
- Allow yourself to buy a strong suitcase, preferably a samsonite or Echolac—they really protect your stuff!
- Stationery including pens, staplers and pins, punchers, clip files, envelopes, bond papers for printing purposes.

Recommended: *1 month before travelling*

11. VISA APPLICATION

Recommended: *1 month before travelling.*

12. BOOKING YOUR ACCOMMODATION

If you have opted for a sponsorship scheme or you have a relative in the UK who has agreed to accommodate you, then you do not have to be bothered. If not, then it would be wise to advance book a room in a youth/independent hostel at least for 2 to 3 days. It can be a pain to carry your 30 kg luggage and look around for accommodation. Within those three days at the hostel, you can look for alternate cheaper accommodation in flat shares or rental flats.

Recommended: *1 month before travelling*

13. YOUNG PERSONS RAILCARD

It is simple. Absolutely anyone between 16 and 25 (or mature full-time students) can get away with a third off most rail fares anywhere in Britain. All you have to do is buy a Young Persons Railcard.

It costs only £18 a year and it usually pays for itself in one or two trips. Even on short journeys, the savings really mount up.

There are plenty of ways to use your Railcard, for both long and short trips, and you can use it at anytime on weekends, Bank Holidays, and during the week. The only restriction is that if you travel at or before 10 am Monday to Friday (except during July and August), a minimum fare will apply.

You will have to catch a relative or a friend in the UK to get a railcard made for you. If you do not have any, get it on the first day you arrive in the UK from any ticket booking office.

The International Student Identity Card and International Youth Travel Cards are accepted as proof of student or youth status.

Recommended: *1 month before/ the day you reach UK*

30 *Visa Concerns*

◆ *After all that effort you have put in clearing the Part 1 and applying and preparing for the Part 2—after all the dreams that you have had about travelling to and living in the UK—you will not want this to come in your way, would you?*

The Visa you will need to write the PLAB Part 2 exam is branded as the PLAB VISA which is a form of Visit Visa valid for 6 months from the time you step foot in the UK. Unlike the US, it is not very hard procuring a visa to the UK; very few are denied of it. However, having taken so much of sweat to clear the Part 1 and to make other preparations, it is important that you do not lose out on such a silly matter. You can avert this by keeping all the essential documents geared up and by being as honest as possible.

As stated by the Home Office, the requirements to be met by a person seeking leave to enter the United Kingdom as a visitor are that she:

i. is genuinely seeking entry as a visitor for a limited period as stated by him, not exceeding 6 months; and

ii. intends to leave the United Kingdom at the end of the period of the visit as stated by him; and

iii. does not intend to take employment in the United Kingdom; and

iv. does not intend to produce goods or provide services within the United Kingdom, including the selling of goods or services direct to members of the public; and

v. does not intend to study at a maintained school; and

vi. will maintain and accommodate himself and any dependants adequately out of resources available to him without recourse to public funds or taking employment; or will, with any dependants, be maintained and accommodated adequately by relatives or friends; and

vii. can meet the cost of the return or onward journey.

DOCUMENTS REQUIRED

Absolute

1. Visa application forms (enclosed)
2. Passport with a validity of at least one year
3. General Medical Council test place confirmation letter
4. Medical degree certificate/ Postgraduate qualification certificate
5. IELTS result certificate
6. PLAB Part 1 pass certificate
7. Bank statements preferably of the last six months
8. Sponsorship letter from either a person in the UK or a course provider. This should be accompanied by the sponsor's passport copy, copy of bank statement and a declaration that he will be taking care of your accommodation and other expenses in the UK.

Handy

- Pay slips of last 6 months/ Income tax returns
- Documents of any immovable assets, i.e., property, etc.
- Any special awards

The above documents should be accompanied by a covering letter to the consulate stating that you are requesting them to issue you a visit visa for the PLAB exam. You will also have to state that your intention is to acquire post-graduate training during the stipulated time.

APPLICATION

The British High Commission has commenced new improved visa application facilities and procedures throughout India. Visa application centres are located in: New Delhi, Jalandhar, Chandigarh, Mumbai, Ahmedabad, Pune, Chennai, Hyderabad, Bangalore and Kolkata.

Trained staff will accept the applications at each centre, explain the latest visa rules and offer advice where necessary. The Application Centres are manoeuvred by Visa Facilitation Services (VFS). The VFS are responsible only for accepting applications and providing advice and guidance where necessary.

For the purposes of PLAB visa, the VFS provide same day service. You can present all the documents at the collection centre and collect the visa in the afternoon. An interview may be required.

ADDRESSES OF VISA FACILITATION CENTRES IN INDIA

New Delhi
B 2/3 Africa Avenue,
Safdarjung Enclave (Opposite St Thomas's Church)
New Delhi
Tel: (011) 51651510
E-mail: vfsuk.north@visa-services.com
Opening hours: 0800-1200, 1300-1600

Jalandhar
Balbir Tower (3rd Floor),
Namdeo Chowk, GT Road
Jalandhar
Tel: (0181) 5095600
E-mail: vfsuk.north@visa-services.com
Opening hours: 0800-1200, 1300-1500

Chandigarh
SCO 61-63, Madhya Marg, Sector 9 D
(Above Bank of Punjab)
Chandigarh, Tel: (0181) 5095600
E-mail: vfsuk.north@visa-services.com
Opening hours: 0800-1200, 1300-1500

Mumbai
Stadium House, (Above Kaysons)
Veer Nariman Road, Churchgate
Opening hours: 0800-1200, 1300-1600
Email: vfsuk.south@visa-services.com

Ahmedabad
Gujarat Chamber Building
Ashram Road
Opening hours: 0800-1200, 1300-1500
Email: vfsuk.north@visa-services.com

Pune
158, Sohrab Hall (1st floor)
Sassoon Road
Behind Pune Station
Opening hours: 0800-1200, 1300-1500
Email: vfsuk.south@visa-services.com

Chennai
"Jaishanker's Bungalow"
3, College Lane; Off Haddows Road,
Behind SBI Circle Office
Nungambakkam,
Chennai 600006
Timings: 0800-1200, 1300-1600
Email: vfsuk.south@visa-services.com

Hyderabad
208, Prajay Corporate House
Chikoti Garden
Begumpet, Opp. Shoppers' Stop
Hyderabad 500016
Timings: 0800-1200, 1300-1500
Email: vfsuk.south@visa-services.com

Bangalore
304, Prestige Centre Point,
7 Edward Road,
Cunningham Road LVL,
Bangalore 560052
Timings: 0800-1200, 1300-1500
Email: vfsuk.south@visa-services.com

Kolkata
Om Towers, 14th floor
32 J.L. Nehru Road
Opp. Park Street Metro Station
Opening hours: 0900-1700 Mon-Friday

For auxiliary information on visas you can contact

New Delhi
Visa DePartment,
British Deputy High Commission
Shantipath, Chanakyapuri,
New Delhi 110 021
Tel: 011-24100017-22 (Six Lines)

Kolkata
Visa DePartment,
British Deputy High Commission
1 Ho Chi Minh Sarani,
Kolkata 700 071
Tel: 033-288-5172-76 (Five Lines)
Fax: 033-288-3996/3435

Mumbai
Visa DePartment,
British Deputy High Commission
Makers Chambers IV,
2nd Floor
222 Jamna Lal Bajaj Road,
PO Box 11714
Nariman Point, Mumbai 400 021
Tel: 022-22830517/22832330/22833602,
Fax: 022-22027940

Chennai
Visa DePartment,
British Deputy High Commission
20 Anderson Road,
Chennai 600 006
Tel: 044 52192308/52192310,
Fax: 044 52192320

Websites: www.ukinindia.org
www.ukvisas.gov.

EXTENSION OF VISA

In case you do not dig up a job within six months of your arrival in the UK, it is possible to extend your visa for a further six months by contacting the Immigration authorities in the UK. Any further extensions are not permitted, though according to some, they are given in 'exceptional circumstances'. Contact the General Medical Council for further details.

31 Survival in the United Kingdom

◆ *Wouldn't you feel better if before taking your flight, you already have an accommodation booked; and if you had information on how you could cut down on your expenses, in probably the costliest country in the world?*

ACCOMMODATION

This will be almost certainly your single greatest expense.

You have the following options:
1. Youth Hostels
2. Independent hostels
3. Bed and Breakfast
4. Renting a Flat
5. Flat share
6. Accommodation provided by Course organisers.

YOUTH HOSTELS

Membership of the Youth Hostelling Association (YHA) gives you access to a network of hostels throughout England, and you do not have to be young or single to use them.

The local YHA for England can be contacted at Tel: 0870 870 8808;

email: customerservices@yha.org.uk

Expect to pay anywhere from £ 7 in the country to £ 23 in London for adults, and £ 6 to £ 20 for youths.

Facilities

All hostels provide facilities for self-catering, and some provide cheap meals. Advance booking is advisable, especially at weekends, bank holidays and at any time over the summer months. Most hostels accept phone bookings and payment with Visa or Master Card. Some will accept same day booking, although they will usually only hold a bed until six.

Advantages of hostels are primarily price and the chance to meet other travellers. The disadvantages are that some of them are still run dictatorially, you are usually locked out between 10 to 5. In addition, many of them are closed during winter.

INDEPENDENT HOSTELS

Independent hostels offer the opportunity to escape curfews and lockouts for a price of around £ 9 to £ 18 per night. Like the YHA, these are places to meet other travellers and they tend to be in town centres rather than out in the sticks.

BED AND BREAKFAST

B and B's are a great English institution and pretty cheap compared to the hotels. At the bottom end, £ 14 to £ 20 per person, you get a bedroom in a private house, a shared bathroom and an enormous cooked breakfast. Small B & B's may only have one room to let and you can really feel like a guest of the family.

Guesthouses, which are often just large converted houses with half a dozen rooms, are an extension of the B and B concept. They range from £ 12 to £ 50 a night, depending on the quality of food and accommodation. In general, they are less personal than B and B's, and more like small budget hotels.

RENTING A FLAT

There has been an upsurge in the number of houses available for short-term rent. A double bedroom flat accommodating four can cost as little as £ 80 to £ 100 per week. Outside London, they could come down to £ 60 per week. This means that you can expect to pay £ 60 per month (around INR 4500) for a decent place.

The best tool for hunting down such flats is the weekly magazine *The Loot* or you can check out their website at www.loot.com. Also, check out www.fishforhomes.co.uk

FLATSHARE

This essentially means that someone who has rented a flat finds it too huge or too expensive and would like someone to join him/her. You could be sharing a single bedroom or may have a separate bedroom for yourself. Ideal for single women as this would be a safe and secure place to share, particularly if she is of a conservative nature. Flat shares cost between £ 60 to £ 100.

Adverts for flat shares can be found in *The Loot* magazine or their website stated above.

ACCOMMODATION PROVIDED BY COURSE ORGANISERS

Apart from providing the accommodation for the duration of the course and that for the sponsorship schemes, some course organisers also offer additional accommodation if required. These are unquestionably on the pricey side, but convenient in the sense that they can be booked in advance while applying for the course and you get an opportunity to stay with fellow plabbers and struggle together!

Plabwise

Provides accommodation during the course for £ 35 a week and otherwise for £ 50 a week.

Plab Doctors

Provides accommodation with food for £ 60 a week.

Plabtutor

Provides accommodation for £ 50-60 per week.

Fahmida's

Provides accommodation for £ 50 a week

The rule is that if you are not fussy about a budget, you can book your accommodation in one of the youth or independent hostels; or ask your course organisers to arrange an extended stay. However, if you are stiff on your budget, and have not opted for a sponsorship stay, you can book a youth hostel for 3 days, and during those three days search for a rental flat or a flat share.

FOOD

England is the nation that brought us fatty sausages, mushy peas and margarine sandwiches, a cuisine so undesirable that there is no English equivalent for the French phrase *Bon appetit.*

It is an image that has proved hard to shake off but, fortunately, things are improving fast, especially in the South. In the main towns and cities, a decent range of cuisine is available. Particularly if you like Pizza, pasta and curry, you should be able to get a reasonable meal pretty well anywhere.

Vegetarianism has taken off in a big way— most restaurants will have at least a token vegetarian dish, although menus at better places often offer several choices. All said, as anywhere, vegans would find the going tough.

Takeaways

Every high street has its complement of takeaway restaurants, from McDonald's and Pizza Hut to the ubiquitous local curry house and fish and chop shops.

Cafes

Usually referred to as caffs or greasy spoons, they

are warm, friendly, very English places that serve cheap breakfast and English Tea. They also provide plain but filling lunches.

Restaurants

There are many superior and outstanding restaurants in England. Seafood, various meats, roasts and many other dishes are often very well prepared. London has scores of restaurants that could hold their own in major cities worldwide.

Self-Catering

This is by far, the cheapest way to eat. Even if you lack great culinary skills, you can buy good quality pre-cooked meals from the supermarkets —Marks and Spencer are the most highly regarded. You could be spending around £ 30 a month on food if you cook on your own.

Drinks

Takeaway alcoholic drinks are sold from neighbourhood off-licenses rather than pubs. Some stay open until 9 or 10 pm. Pubs are allowed to stay open any twelve hours and most maintain the 11 to 11 scheme.

TRAVELLING

Getting around in England is simple but expensive. For a visitor from India who is used to explore an entire city in a bus drive costing 4 rupees, spending £ 4 for a trip on the tube from Heathrow to East Ham could be outrageous.

Buses are nearly always the cheapest way to get around. Unfortunately, they are also the slowest. With discount passes and tickets bought in advance, trains can be competitive on price; they are quicker and often take you through beautiful countryside relatively unspoiled by the modern age.

AIR

Most cities are linked to each other and London by air. However, unless you are travelling from the outer reaches of Britain, in particular northern Scotland, flights would be marginally quicker than trains if you consider the time taken to go to the airport.

BUS

Road transport in the UK is almost entirely privately owned and run. The National Express runs the largest network and completely dominates the market. You can refer to their website: *www.gobycoach.com*

In Britain, long distance express buses are usually referred to as coaches, and in most towns and cities, the bus and coach stations are separate.

Table 31.1: Approximate bus fares from London to various cities

Destination	Duration hrs	Single	Return
Manchester	4	15	25
Birmingham	2 ½	10	15
Liverpool	4 ½	15	25
Cardiff	3 ½	14	24
Edinburgh	8	22	33

Discount Card

The National Express sells discount coach cards that give you 20 to 30 per cent off on standard adult fares. They cost £ 9 and can be purchased from all the National Express agents. The ISIC cards are acknowledged as proof of student status and passports for date of birth.

TRAIN

Despite the damage that has occurred by privatisation, Britain still has a useful rail service. Fast trains that travel at speeds of up to 140 mph serve the main routes—for example, you can take a trip from London to York in just over 2 hours.

You can refer to *www.thetrainline.com* for information on train timings, fares and online purchase.

Finding the best ticket for your journey is not easy. The thing to do is to tell the ticket seller exactly what you want to do and let them find the best option for you. Alternatively, you can find your best bet by surfing the above mentioned website.

Table 31.2: Approximate rail fares from London

Destination	Duration hrs	Single	Cheap return
Manchester	2 ½	11	18
Birmingham	1 ½	10	15
Liverpool	2 ½	13	20
Cardiff	2	14	23
Edinburgh	4	18	30
Glasgow	5	30	53

Discount Cards

The Young Persons Railcard is the most popular. It costs just £ 18 and gives you a discount of 33 per cent on most rail fares and ferries. Details are given in the chapter—*Before Travelling.*

TRAVELLING TO IRELAND

There is a great array of ferry services between Britain and Ireland using modern car ferries. There are often special deals worth investigating and off-season fares are low. The journey from Liverpool to Dublin via Catamarans takes about 4 hours and costs £ 50.

The Ryan Air offers special fares to and from Ireland and if you are lucky, you could get a one-way flight for under £ 50. Check out their website www.ryanair.com for further details.

THE TUBE

The London Underground or Tube, as it is universally known, first opened in 1863, and sometimes it feels as if not a whole lot has changed since then. It is slow, unreliable and breakdowns are common.

The TfL and the Underground operate information centres that sell tickets and provide free maps. The TfL divides London into six concentric zones.

The basic fares are as follows:

Zone 1	£ 1.50
Zone 1 and 2	£ 1.90
Three zones	£ 2.20
Four zones	£ 2.70
All six zones	£ 3.60

Daily and Weekly Travel Cards are available, and the Weekly Travel Card requires identification and a passport sized photograph. It costs £ 4 for a single-day travel card for zones 1 and 2; and £ 19 for a weekly travel card for the same zones.

Appendix

1. PULSE AND ITS ABNORMALITIES

Rate
- <60: bradycardia
- >100: tachycardia.

Rhythm
- Regular
- Regularly irregular
- Irregularly irregular.

Character
- *Bounding pulse:*
  - CO_2 poisoning.
- *Collapsing pulse, and 'water hammer pulse':*
  - Aortic regurgitation
  - Heart block
  - PDA.
- *Plateau pulse:*
  - Aortic stenosis.
- *Pulses alternans [alternate strong, weak beats]:*
  - LVF
  - Pulses paradoxus [volume decreases on inspiration more than normal: by >10 mm Hg]
  - Constrictive pericarditis
  - Tamponade
  - Severe asthma.
- *Small volume:*
  - Aortic stenosis
  - Shock
  - Pericardial effusion.

Delays
- Radioradial delay
- *Radiofemoral delay:* test in patients with HTN or ejection systolic murmur:
  - Coarctation of aorta.

Surface Anatomy of Pulses
- *Radial:*
  - Palmar side of wrist, between flexor carpi radialis tendon and radius.
- *Brachial:*
  - Cubital fossa, medial to biceps tendon.
- *Carotid:*
  - Just lateral to upper border of thyroid cartilage.
- *Superficial temporal:*
  - Anterior to ear as crosses temporal bone's zygomatic process.
- *Abdominal aorta:*
  - In midline, at umbilicus pressing into abdomen.
  - Use caution if large AAA, to avoid rupture.
- *Femoral:*
  - Below inguinal ligament, midway between ASIS and pubic symphysis [not pubic tubercle].
  - May be reduced or absent in arteriosclerotic dz.
- *Popliteal:*
  - Flex knee before palpating.
  - In midline, on popliteal side of lower end of femur.
  - Most difficult one to palpate.

- *Alternative method:* The doctor's one hand on the patient's knee, other hand under knee. Push flexed knee downwards [into extension] until can feel popliteal.
- *Posterior tibial:*
  - Posterior, inferior to medial malleolus, between flexor digitorum longus and flexor hallucis longus.
- *Dorsalis pedis:*
  - Lateral to extensor hallucis longus, over tarsal bones.
  - Palpate with three fingers along artery.
  - May be reduced or absent in peripheral vascular dz.

2. ABNORMAL APEX BEAT

Absent Apex Beat Causes
- *DOPES:*
- **D**eath
- **O**besity
- **P**ericarditis
- **E**mphysema, other COPD
- **S**inus inversus

Apex Deviation Causes
With trachea shift also:
- Mediastinal shift.

Without trachea shift:
- Cardiomegaly
- Scoliosis
- Pectus excavatum
- Sinus inversus.

Abnormal Apex Beat Types
- *Double impulse:* Systole has 2 impulses.
  - *DDx:* Hypertrophic cardiomyopathy.
- *Dyskinetic:* Uncoordinated, easily palpable.
  - *DDx:* MI.
- *Hyperdynamic:* Forceful, sustained apex beat.
  - DDx: AS, HTN.

- *Hyperkinetic:* Coordinated, palpated beat is distributed over greater area.
  - *DDx:* LV dilation.
- *Tapping Apex:* S1 sound is palpable.
  - *DDx:* mitral stenosis.

3. HEART SOUNDS

First Heart Sound
- *Loud DDx:* Mitral stenosis.
- *Soft DDx:* MR.

Second Heart Sound
- *Aortic component loud DDx:* Aortic HTN.
- *Pulmonary component loud DDx:* Pulmonary HTN.
- *Soft DDx:* AR, calcification of aortic valve.

Splitting
- *Increased normal splitting [wider split when inspire] DDx:*
  - Delayed RV emptying (pulmonary stenosis, RBBB).
- Fixed wide splitting DDx: ASD.

Third Heart Sound
- *Sound:* In early-mid diastole, low-pitched, "gallop sounding".
- *DDx:*
  - Normal in children
  - Constrictive pericarditis
  - Mitral regurgitation
  - Tricuspid regurgitation
  - LVF, RVF.

Fourth Heart Sound
- *Sound:* Higher pitch, late diastole, "gallop sounding"
- *DDx:* HTN, MI, AS, Heart block

Opening Snap
- *Sound:* High-pitched click after S2.
- *Where:* Lower L sternal edge.
- *DDx:* Mitral stenosis.

Systolic Click

- *Sound:* high-pitched click, soon after S1. Click followed by AS or PS murmur.
- *Where:* aortic, pulmonary auscultation sites.
- *DDx:* AS.

Murmurs: Grading

Graded on scale of 1 to 6.
1. Only cardiologist can hear.
2. Trained doctor can hear.
3. Student can hear. No thrill.
4. Thrill barely palpable.
5. Thrill easily palpable.
6. Can hear murmur by being in the room without a stethoscope.

4. JVP

Kussmaul's Sign

- Place the patient sitting up at 90°.
- JVP becomes more distended during inspiration (classically constrictive pericarditis, currently severe RHF). This is opposite of what happens in normal patient
- Usually negative in cardiac tamponade.

Hepatojugular Reflex

- Exert pressure on liver for 15 sec.
- Venous return to right atrium increases.
- JVP will rise transiently in normal person.
- Check if remains elevated (RVF).

5. DERMATOMES

Landmarks

- **T4:** Nipple
- **C6:** Thumb, index finger
- **C7:** Middle finger
- **T10:** Umbilicus
- **L3:** Knee
- **S1:** Sole
- **S5:** Anus.

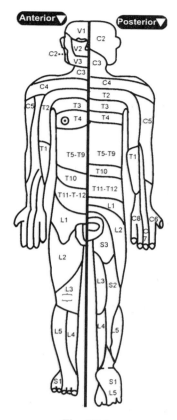

Fig. 32.1

6. NERVE ROOTS

- **C4:** Spontaneous breathing
- **C5:** Shoulder shrug, deltoid
- **C6:** Biceps, wrist extension
- **C7:** Triceps, wrist flexion
- **C8/T1:** Finger flexion
- **T1-12:** Intercostals, abdominal
- **L1/L2:** Hip flexion
- **L2/L3/L4:** Hip adduction, quadriceps
- **L4/L5:** Hip abduction
- **L5:** Great toe dorsiflexion
- **S1/S2:** Foot plantarflexion
- **S2-S4:** Rectal tone.

Quick Screen

- *Shoulder*
  - Abduct (C5)
  - Adduct (C5-C7).
- *Elbow*
  - Flex (C5-C6)
  - Extend (C7).
- *Wrist*
  - Flex (C7-8)
  - Extend (C7).
- *Finger*
  - Flex (C7-8)
  - Extend (C7)
  - Abduct (T1).
- *Hip*
  - Flex (L1/L2)
  - Extend (L5/S1).
- *Knee*
  - Flex (S1)
  - Extend (L3/L4).
- *Ankle*
  - Dorsiflex (L4)
  - Plantar flex (S1/S2).

7. SPEECH ABNORMALITIES

Dysphasias

- *Conductive*
  - Repeat statements and names poorly.
  - Can follow commands.
- *Expressive*
  - Understands, but cannot answer appropriately (including objects can't be named).
  - Other speech aspects normal.
  - *Cause:* Broca's area lesion.
- *Receptive*
  - Cannot understand spoken or written word.
  - *Cause:* Wernicke's area lesion.
- *Nominal*
  - Specifically can't name objects, but everything else OK.

Dysarthria

- Difficulty of articulation only.
- Can't say "British Constitution".
- *Causes*
  - Alcohol intoxication (commonest)
  - Cerebellar
  - Bulbar or pseudobulbar palsy
  - Extrapyramidal disease.

Dysphonia

- Husky voice, decreased volume.
- *Causes:*
  - Laryngeal nerve palsy
  - Recurrent laryngeal
  - Hysterical.

8. APGAR SCORE

- Score 0-2 in each category.
- Take scores at 1min post-birth and 5 min post-birth.
- Don't waste time doing scoring, if baby is in difficulty.
- Perfect score is 10.

Colour

- 0: All blue
- 1: Trunk pink, limbs blue
- 2: All pink.

Heart Rate

- 0: 0 beats/min
- 1: <100 beats/min
- 2: >100 beats/min.

Reflex Irritability

- 0: None
- 1: Grimace
- 2: Grimace and cough.

Muscle Tone

- 0: Limp, no tone
- 1: Some limb flexion
- 2: Active movement.

Respiratory effort
- 0: None
- 1: Slow, irregular
- 2: Strong cry, regular.

9. VITAL SIGNS-NORMAL VALUES
Normal values by age
Age: Neonate

Respiratory rate	: 30-60
HR awake	: 100-180
HR sleeping	: 80-160
Systolic BP	: 70-100
Diastolic BP	: 50-65

Age: 6 Months

Respiratory rate	: 25-50
HR awake	: 120-160
HR sleeping	: 80-180
Systolic BP	: 87-105
Diastolic BP	: 53-66

Age: 2 Years

Respiratory rate	: 18-35
HR awake	: 80-150
HR sleeping	: 70-120
Systolic BP	: 90-106
Diastolic BP	: 55-67

Age: 5 Years

Respiratory rate	: 17-27
HR awake	: 80-110
HR sleeping	: 60-90
Systolic BP	: 94-109
Diastolic BP	: 56-69

Age: 10 Years

Respiratory rate	: 15-23
HR awake	: 70-110
HR sleeping	: 60-90
Systolic BP	: 102-117
Diastolic BP	: 62-75

Age: >10 Years

Respiratory rate	: 55-100
HR awake	: 50-90
HR sleeping	: 105-128
Systolic BP	: 66-80
Diastolic BP	: 10-23

10. DUTIES OF A DOCTOR
- Make the care of your patient your first concern;
- Treat every patient politely and considerately;
- Respect patients' dignity and privacy;
- Listen to patients and respect their views;
- give patients information in a way they can understand;
- Respect the rights of patients to be fully involved in decisions about their care;
- Keep your professional knowledge and skills up-to-date;
- Recognise the limits of your professional competence;
- Be honest and trustworthy;
- Respect and protect confidential information;
- Make sure that your personal beliefs do not prejudice your patients' care;
- Act quickly to protect patients from risk if you have good reason to believe that you or a colleague may not be fit to practise;
- Avoid abusing your position as a doctor; and
- Work with colleagues in the ways that best serve patients' interests.

In all these matters you must never discriminate unfairly against your patients or colleagues. And you must always be prepared to justify your actions to them.

11. REFERENCE BIOCHEMICAL VALUES

Biochemical Test	*Reference Range*
BLOOD	
Albumin	35-50 g/L
Amylase	28-238 iu/L
Bilirubin, direct	< 7 umol/L

Contd...

Contd...

Biochemical Test	Reference Range
Bilirubin, total	4-22 umol/L
Calcium	2.1-2.6 mmol/L
Carbon dioxide (HCO_3)	23-29 mmol/L
Chloride	100-108 mmol/L
Cholesterol, total	4.1-7.4 mmol/L
Creatinine phosphokinase	25-200 iu/L (Male)
	25-275 iuL(Female)
Creatinine	60-120 umol/L (Male)
	48-97 umol/L (Female)
Lactic dehydrogenase	211-423 iu/L
Gamma glutamyl transferase	11-50 iu/L (Male)
	7-32 iu/L (Female)
Glucose	3.9-5.8 mmol/L (fasting)
	6.7-9.4 mmol/L (1 hour)
	3.9-6.7 mmol/L (2 hours)
Iron	9.5-29.9 umol/L (Male)
	8.8-27.0 umol/L (Female)
Iron binding capacity, total	50-72 umol/L
Phosphatase, prostatic	< 4.0 iu/L
Phosphatase, alkaline	31-93 iu/L
Phosphate, inorganic	0.81-1.45 mmol/L
Potassium	3.5-5.2 mmol/L
Protein, total	60-84 g/L
Sodium	135-145 mmol/L
Transferase, alanine amino	8-37 iu/L
Transferase, aspartic amino	8-40 iu/L
Triglycerides	0.4-2.1 mmol/L
Urea	3.0-7.3 mmol/L
Uric acid	0.2-0.415 mmol/L (Male)
	0.14-0.34 mmol/L (Female)

URINE

Calcium	2.5-7.5 mmol/24 hour
Creatinine	9.0-18.0 mmol/24 hour
Creatinine clearance	85-125 ml/min (Male)
	75-115 ml/min (Female)

Contd...

Contd...

Biochemical Test	Reference Range
Phosphate, inorganic	15-50 mmol/24 hour
Potassium	25-150 mmol/24 hour
Protein, total	0.01-0.1 g/24 hour
Sodium	40-220 mmol/24 hour
Urea	330-580 mmol/24 hour
Uric acid	1.5-4.5 mmol/24 hour

CSF

Chloride	1210-130 mmol/L
Glucose	2.8-4.4 mmol/L
Protein, total	0.15-0.45 g/L

Haematology Test	Reference Range
Haematocrit	0.38-0.59 L/L (Male)
	0.31-0.43 L/L (Female)
Mean cell volume	80-97 fL
Mean cell haemoglobin	26-33 pg
Mean cell Hb concentration	31.0-34.5 g/dL
Reticulocyte count	0.2-2.0%

ESR (Westergen 1 hr)	Men	Women
17-50 yr	1-7 mm	3-9 mm
> 50 yr	2-10 mm	5-15mm
Thrombocyte count	120-500 × 10^9/L	
Total WBC count	4-11 × 10^9/L	

WBC differential count	× 10^9/L	%
Neutrophils	2.00-7.50	40-75
Lymphocytes	1.50-4.00	20-45
Monocytes	0.20-0.80	2-10
Eosinophils	0.04-0.40	1-6
Basophils	0.01-0.10	0-2

Prothrombin time	11-14 seconds
Activated partial thromboplastin time	25-43 seconds
Thrombin time	9.5-12.0 seconds
Glycosylated haemoglobin	4.0-8.0%
HbA_2	1.5-3.5%
HbF	< 1.0%

12. ADDRESSES

ACCIDENT & EMERGENCY MEDICINE (Faculty of)
Royal College of Surgeons of England
35-43 Lincoln's Inn Fields
London
WC2A 3PN
Tel: +44 (0)20 7405 3474
Fax: +44 (0)20 7831 9438
Website: www.rsceng.ac.uk

BRITISH COUNCIL
Medlock Street
Manchester
M15 4AA
Tel: +44 (0161) 957 7000
Fax: +44 (0161) 957 7111

BRITISH COUNCIL
(Education Information Centre)
10 Spring Gardens
London
SW1A 2BN
Tel: +44 (0)20 7930 8466
Fax: +44 (0)20 7839 6347
Website: www.britcoun.org

BRITISH DENTAL ASSOCIATION
64 Wimpole Street,
London,
W1M 8AL.
Tel: +44 (0)20 7935 0875
Fax: +44 (0)20 7487 5232
Website: www.bda-dentistry.org.uk

BRITISH MEDICAL ASSOCIATION
North East Office
First Floor, Holland Park C
Holland Drive
Fenham Barracks
Newcastle upon Tyne, NE2 4LD.
Tel: +44 (0)191 261 7131
Fax: +44 (0)191 261 6203

BRITISH MEDICAL ASSOCIATION
Tavistock Square
London
WC1H 9JP
Tel: +44 (0)20 7387 4499
Fax: +44 (0)20 7383 6400
Website: www.bma.org.uk

BRITISH MEDICAL JOURNAL
Tavistock Square
London
WC1H 9JP
Website: www.bmj.com

COMMONWEALTH SCHOLARSHIP COMMISSION
John Foster House
36 Gordon Square
London
WC1H 0PF
Tel: +44 (0)20 7387 8572
Fax: +44 (0)20 7387 2655

Website: www.acu.ac.uk

DENTAL SURGERY (Faculty)
Royal College of Surgeons (England)
35-43 Lincoln's Inn Fields
London
WC2A 3PN
Tel: +44 (0)20 7405 3474
Fax: +44 (0)20 7831 9438
Website: www.rcseng.ac.uk

DEPARTMENT OF HEALTH NHS EXECUTIVE HQ
Quarry House
Quarry Hill
Leeds
LS2 7UE
Tel: +44 (0)113 2545 0000

ENGLISH LANGUAGE CENTRE
University of Newcastle
Newcastle upon Tyne
NE1 7RU
Tel: +44 (0)191 222 7535
Fax: +44 (0)191 222 5239
Website: www.ncl.ac.uk/langcen/

FAMILY PLANNING AND REPRODUCTIVE CARE
(Faculty of)
Royal College of Obstetricians and Gynaecologists
27 Sussex Place
Regents Park
London
NW1 4RG
Tel: +44 (0)20 7262 5425
Fax: +44 (0)20 7723 0575
Website: see RCOG entry

GENERAL DENTAL COUNCIL
37 Wimpole Street
London
W1M 8DQ
Tel: +44 (0)20 7486 2171
Fax: +44 (0)20 7224 3294

GENERAL MEDICAL COUNCIL
178-202 Great Portland Street
London
W1N 6JE
Tel: +44 (0)20 7580 7642
Fax: +44 (0)20 7915 3641
Website: www.gmc-uk.org

IMMIGRATION AND NATIONALITY
DEPARTMENT
Home Office
Lunar House
40 Wellesey Road
Croydon
CR9 2BY
Tel: +44 (0)181 686 0688
Website:
www.homeoffice.gov.uk/ind

INTERCOLLEGIATE SPECIALTY BOARD
Central Administrative Office
11 Hill Square
Edinburgh
EH8 9DR
Tel: +44 (0)131 662 9222

JOINT COMMITTEE ON
POSTGRADUATE TRAINING IN
GENERAL PRACTICE
14 Princes Gate
Hyde Park
London
SW7 1PU
Tel: +44 (0)20 7581 3232
Fax: +44 (0)20 7225 3047

MEDICAL DEFENCE UNION
3 Devonshire Place
London
W1N 2EA
Tel: +44 (0)20 7486 6181
Fax: +44 (0)20 7935 5503
Website: www.the-mdu.com

NATIONAL ADVICE CENTRE FOR
POSTGRADUATE
MEDICAL EDUCATION
British Council
Medlock Street
Manchester
M15 4AA
Tel: +44 (0161) 957 7218
Fax: +44 (0161) 957 7029
Website: www.britcoun.org

MEDICAL PROTECTION SOCIETY
33 Cavendish Square
London
W1M 0PS
Tel: +44 (0)20 7637 0541
Fax: +44 (0)20 7399 1301
Website: www.mps.org.uk

MEDICAL WOMEN'S FEDERATION
Tavistock House North
Tavistock Square
London
WC1H 9HX
Tel: +44 (0)20 7387 7765
Fax: +44 (0)20 7387 7765

OCCUPATIONAL MEDICINE (Faculty)
Royal College of Physicians (London)
6 St Andrew's Place
London
NW1 4LB
Tel: +44 (0)20 7487 3414
Fax: +44 (0)20 7487 5218

OVERSEAS DOCTORS' ASSOCIATION
28-32 Princess Street
Manchester
M1 4LB
Tel: +44 (0)161 236 5594
Fax: +44 (0)161 228 3659

OVERSEAS DOCTORS' ASSOCIATION
Local Secretary
Mr H Fawzi,
North Tynesiode General Hospital,
Rake Lane,
North Shields,
NE29 9NH.
Tel: +44 (0)191 957 6660

OVERSEAS LABOUR SERVICE
W5 Moorfoot
Sheffield
S1 4PQ
Tel: +44 (0114) 259 4074
PLAB
178 Great Portland Street
London
W1N 6JE

POSTGRADUATE INSTITUTE FOR MEDICINE AND
DENTISTRY
10 - 12 Framlington Place
Newcastle upon Tyne, NE2 4AB
Tel: +44 (0)191 222-6762
Fax: +44 (0) 191 222-8620
e-mail: a.j.rich@ncl.ac.uk
Website: www.ncl.ac.uk/pimd

PUBLIC HEALTH MEDICINE (Faculty)
4 St Andrew's Place
London
NW2 4LB
Tel: +44 (0)20 7935 0243
Fax: +44 (0)20 7224 6973

ROYAL COLLEGE OF ANAESTHETISTS
48-49 Russell Square
London
WC1B 4JY
Tel: +44 (0)20 7813 1900
Fax: +44 (0)20 7813 1876
Website: www.rcoa.ac.uk

ROYAL COLLEGE OF GENERAL PRACTITIONERS
14 Princes Gate
Hyde Park
London
SW7 1PU
Tel: +44 (0)20 7581 3232
Fax: +44 (0)20 7225 3047
Website: www.rcgp.org.uk

ROYAL COLLEGE OF OBSTETRICIANS &
GYNAECOLOGISTS
27 Sussex Place
London
NW1 4RG
Tel: +44 (0)20 7262 5425
Fax: +44 (0)20 7723 0575
e-mail: Coll.Sec@rcog.org.uk
Website: www.rcog.org.uk

ROYAL COLLEGE OF
OPHTHALMOLOGISTS
17 Cornwall Terrace
London
NW1 4QW
Tel: +44 (0)20 7935 0702
Fax: +44 (0)20 7935 9838
Website: rcophth.ac.uk

ROYAL COLLEGE OF PAEDIATRICS AND
CHILD HEALTH
50 Hallam Street
London
W1N 6DE
Tel: +44 (0)20 7307 5600
Fax: +44 (0)20 7307 5601
Website: rcpch.ac.uk

ROYAL COLLEGE OF PATHOLOGISTS
2 Carlton House Terrace
London
SW1Y 5AF
Tel: +44 (0)20 7930 5861
Fax: +44 (0)20 7321 0523
Website: rcpath.org.uk

ROYAL COLLEGE OF PHYSICIANS
(EDINBURGH)
9 Queen Street
Edinburgh
EH2 1JQ
Tel: +44 (0)131 225 7324
Fax: +44 (0)131 220 3939
Website: www.rcpe.ac.uk

ROYAL COLLEGE OF PHYSICIANS
(LONDON)
11 St Andrew's Place
London
NW1 4LE
Tel: +44 (0)20 7935 1174
Fax: +44 (0)20 7487 5218
Website: www.rcplondon.ac.uk

ROYAL COLLEGE OF PHYSICIANS OF IRELAND
6 Kildare Street
Dublin 2
Ireland
Tel: +353 1 661 6677
Fax: +353 1 676 3989
Website: www.rcpi.ie

ROYAL COLLEGE OF PSYCHIATRISTS
17 Belgrave Square
London
SW1X 8PG
Tel: +44 (0)20 7235 2351
Fax: +44 (0)20 7245 1231
Website: www.rcpsych.ac.uk

ROYAL COLLEGE OF RADIOLOGISTS
38 Portland Place
London
W1N 4JQ
Tel: +44 (0)20 7636 4432
Fax: +44 (0)20 7636 4432
Website: rcr.ac.uk

ROYAL COLLEGE OF SURGEONS (EDINBURGH)
Nicholson Street
Edinburgh
EH8 9DW
Tel: +44 (0)131 556 6206
Fax: +44 (0)131 557 6406
Website: www.rcsed.ac.uk

ROYAL COLLEGE OF SURGEONS (ENGLAND)
35-43 Lincoln's Inn Fields
London
WC2A 3PN
Tel: +44 (0)20 7405 3474
Fax: +44 (0)20 7831 9438
Website: www.rcseng.ac.uk

ROYAL COLLEGE OF SURGEONS IN IRELAND
123 St Stephen's Green
Dublin 2
Ireland
Tel: +353 1 402 2100
Fax: +353 1 402 2454
Website: www.rcsi.ie

ROYAL COLLEGE OF PHYSICIANS AND SURGEON (GLASGOW)
232-242 St Vincent Street
Glasgow
G2 5RJ
Tel: +44 (0)141 221 6072
Fax: +44 (0)141 221 1804
Website: www.rcpsglasg.ac.uk

ROYAL SOCIETY OF MEDICINE
1 Wimpole Street
London
W1M 8AE
Tel: +44 (0)20 7290 2991
Fax: +44 (0)20 7290 2929
Website: www.roysocmed.ac.uk

SCOTTISH COUNCIL FOR POSTGRADUATE MEDICAL EDUCATION
12 Queen Street
Edinburgh
EH2 1JE
Tel: +44 (0131) 225 4365
Fax: +44 (0131) 225 5891
Website: www.scopme.org.uk

SPECIALIST TRAINING AUTHORITY
1 Wimpole Street
London
W1M 8AE
Tel: +44 (0) 20 7935 8586
Fax: +44 (0) 20 7935 9031
Fax: +44 (0)20 7935 8601
Website: www.sta-mrc.org.uk

IELTS Application Form

Please return to:

Centre Stamp

Candidate's photo

1. Preferred Date of Test

   _____/_____/_____
   (day / month / year)

   Second Choice

   _____/_____/_____
   (day / month / year)

2. Family Name _____   3. Dr Mr Mrs Miss Ms
                                                 (circle as appropriate)

4. Other name(s) _____
   (These names must be the same as the names on your national identity document)

5. Address for correspondence _____

   _____

   _____

6. Tel. No _____   7. Fax No _____   8. e-mail _____

9. Date of Birth_____/_____/_____   10. Sex   F / M
   (day / month / year)   *(circle as appropriate)*

11. ID Type: Passport / National ID Card   ID Document Number _____
    (circle as appropriate)   *(This document must be brought to the test)*

For questions 12-15 please enter codes. Codes will be found at the end of the IELTS Handbook.

12. Nationality_____ [ ][ ]   13. First Language_____ [ ][ ][ ]

14. Occupation (Sector)_____(Level)_____ [ ][ ][ ]

15. Why are you taking this test? [ ]

16. Which country are you applying/intending to go to? *(circle as appropriate)*
    Australia/Canada/New Zealand/Republic of Ireland/United Kingdom/United States of America/Other

17. Which IELTS Modules are you taking?   Academic   General Training   *(circle as appropriate)*
    (Please turn over)

18. Which IELTS test are you taking?

Pen and Paper test ☐ or Computerised test (CBIELTS) ☐ *(tick one box)*

Are you taking the Writing on paper   Yes   No   *(circle as appropriate)*

19. Have you taken IELTS before?   Yes   No   *(circle as appropriate)*   If yes how many times? ☐
(You are not allowed to repeat the test within 3 months at any centre)

20. Most recent test details: Centre Name_____   Date _____/_____/_____
(day / month / year)

Centre Number ☐

21. What level of education have you completed? *(circle as appropriate)*
Secondary up to 16 years / Secondary 16-19 years / Degree or equivalent / Post-graduate

22. How many years have you been studying English? *(circle as appropriate)*

Less   1   2   3   4   5   6   7   8   9
than 1   or more

23. Please give details below where you would like your results sent to *(if known)*

Name of Person/Department ——————————————————————————

Name of College/University/Institution_____

Address_____

_____

IELTS entry requirement (Band, *if known*) ☐

Name of Person/Department_____

Name of College/University/Institution_____

Address_____

_____

IELTS entry requirement (Band, *if known*) ☐

24. Do you have any special needs?_____

I certify that the information on this form is complete and accurate to the best of my knowledge.

I understand that I must not attempt to re-take IELTS at any centre within 3 months.

I have received a copy of the IELTS Handbook.

Signature_____   Date   _____/_____/_____
(day / month / year)

APPLICATION FORM

Personal Information:

First Name _____

Last Name _____

Date of Birth _____

Address _____

_____

_____

Phone _____

Nationality

University/College _____

_____

E-mail ID _____

Note: A Demand Draft of Rs.230/- (Rs.200 /- Enrolment fees and Rs.30/- Courier Charges)
in favour of STIC Travels Pvt.Ltd. payable at Delhi at the address given below.

I am applying for (Please tick one):
  [ ]   International Students Identity Card—Rs.200/=
          (Full time /Part time Student & 12 yrs & above)
  [ ]   International Youth Travel Card—Rs.200/= (Youth under 26 yrs)
  [ ]   International Teachers Identity Card—Rs.200/=
          (Full time teacher/lecturer at a recognised educational institution)

SIGNATURE _____

DATE _____

Please attach following with the application form
• One passport size photo
• Photocopy of your student/teacher status
• Photocopy of your age proof(for ISIC, IYTC)

FOR OFFICE USE

Issued By   :
Date of Issue   :
Folio No.   :

Student and Youth Division
STIC Travels Pvt.Ltd.
Room #2, Hotel Janpath,
Janpath, New Delhi-110001
Tel: 23368462, 23368760

APPLICATION FORM FOR PART 1 OF THE PLAB TEST

Once you apply to sit a PLAB examination, the information you provide will be used to update, administer and maintain your record, process complaints, compile statistics, and send you relevant material. We supply data to the Department of Health, professional, educational and training bodies so that they can correct their own information and compile statistics.

PLEASE COMPLETE THIS FORM IN CAPITAL LETTERS

PLEASE NOTE INCOMPLETE FORMS WILL DELAY ALLOCATION TO A TEST DATE
Please read *Advice to Candidates* carefully before completing this form. This can be accessed from the website (www.gmc-uk.org) or by phoning the GMC enquiry line on 020 7915 3630, or email plab@gmc-uk.org.

GMC Reference Number (if known):	☐ ☐ ☐ ☐ ☐ ☐ ☐
Have you made a previous application for PLAB?	Yes ☐ No ☐

Personal Details

Family Name:	Address:
First Name:	
Other Names:	
Title:	
Day Month Year	
Date of Birth:	Telephone:
Sex:	Mobile:
Nationality 1st:	Email:
Nationality 2nd:	
First language:	

Qualifications

Primary Medical Qualification (eg: MB BS, MB ChB)

University or conferring body: Date awarded:

Country of qualification:

Language of instruction:

Other qualifications:

Title: Field of Medicine: Date awarded:

Title: Field of Medicine: Date awarded:

Information about Ethnic Origin

We are committed to eliminating bias and promoting equality of opportunity, irrespective of race or ethnic background. We regularly review the ethnic background of all PLAB test candidates to make sure we are as free from bias as possible.

This information will not be given to examiners but will be used to monitor the PLAB test. It will be treated confidentially and will be published only in a form that does not allow individuals to be identified. You do not have to complete this section but you will be providing us with vital information if you do so.

Please tick the appropriate box below to indicate the ethnic group to which you belong. The list of categories has been drawn up in consultation with the Commission for Racial Equality.

[ ] Bangladeshi   [ ] Indian

[ ] Black African   [ ] Irish

[ ] Black Caribbean   [ ] Pakistani

[ ] Black Other (please specify)   [ ] White

....   [ ] Other (please specify)

[ ] Chinese   ....

IELTS results

Please complete your IELTS results

| Listening | Reading | Writing | Speaking | Overall Band |

Date of IELTS examination _____

I would like to take Part 1 of the test on one of the dates specified below:

1 (Date)_____ (Venue)_____

2 (Date)_____ (Venue)_____

3 (Date)_____ (Venue)_____

NB: Please ensure you put three different dates. If you do not your application may be delayed.

I hereby declare that:
- The information given in this application is true and accurate.
- I understand that if a test admission letter is sent to me, I will be charged a cancellation fee if I decide to postpone or cancel my test place.

Please check that the information above is correct. Your original documents (primary medical qualification and IELTS scores) will be checked when you apply for limited registration. If you have given false information, you may not be granted registration even if you have passed the PLAB test.

_____   _____

Signature of applicant   Date

If you wish to take the examination in the UK:

Send this form, and the fee of £145 (payable to the General Medical Council by cheque or sterling banker's draft, money order or postal order) to: The Registration Directorate, General Medical Council, 178 Great Portland Street, London W1W 5JE

For those wishing to take the examination outside the UK:

Send this form and the fee of £145 (payable to the General Medical Council by cheque or sterling banker's draft or money order) to the appropriate British Council office (see Advice to Candidates).

APPLICATION FORM FOR PART 2 OF THE PLAB TEST

Once you apply to sit a PLAB examination, the information you provide will be used to update, administer and maintain your record, process complaints, compile statistics, and send you relevant material. We supply data to the Department of Health, professional, educational and training bodies so that they can correct their own information and compile statistics.

PLEASE COMPLETE THIS FORM IN CAPITAL LETTERS

PLEASE NOTE INCOMPLETE FORMS WILL DELAY ALLOCATION TO A TEST DATE

When completing this form, please refer to *Advice to Candidates* for Part 2 of the PLAB test and the list of examination dates. This can be accessed from the website (www.gmc-uk.org) or by phoning the GMC enquiry line on 020 7915 3630, or email plab@gmc-uk.org.

GMC Reference Number:
Family Name:
First Name:
Other Names:
Address:
Telephone:
Mobile:
E-mail:

Please indicate below the dates on which you would like to take the examination. Please enter dates for five different examinations. Your application may be delayed if you do not do this.

Please note that where the examination is run over two days we cannot guarantee on which day you will be allocated a place. For example, you may not put your first choice as 9 October 2002 and your second choice as 10 October 2002 as these dates are for the same examination.

	Date	*Place*
1.		
2.		
3.		
4.		
5.		

I hereby declare that:
- The information given in this application is true and accurate.
- I understand that if a test admission letter is sent to me, I will be charged a cancellation fee if I decide to postpone or cancel my test place.

Signed: _____   Date: _____

To give you quick access to your test results we will publish them on the Internet. If you do not wish us to do this, please tick this box.

Please return this form and fee of £430 (payable to the General Medical Council by cheque or sterling banker's draft, money order or postal order) to the Registration Directorate, General Medical Council, 178 Great Portland Street, London, W1W 5JE.